Pilates for Everyone

Pilates FOR EVERYONE

50 POSES FOR EVERY TYPE OF BODY

»» MICKI HAVARD ««

DK

Publisher Mike Sanders
Editor Christopher Stolle
Designer Lindsay Dobbs
Art Director William Thomas
Photographer Kelley Jordan Schuyler
Proofreaders Amy J. Schneider & Chrissy Guthrie
Indexer Celia McCoy

First American Edition, 2021
Published in the United States by DK Publishing
6081 E. 82nd St., Suite 400, Indianapolis, IN 46250

21 22 23 24 25 10 9 8 7 6 5 4 3 2 1
001-322097-JUL2021

ISBN 978-1-6156-4992-1
Library of Congress Catalog Number: 2020950747

Printed and bound in Canada

Contents

FOREWORD

I'm a classically trained Pilates expert and I've dedicated my life to sharing the authenticity of Joseph Pilates's method, originally called Contrology. Joseph's vision for his method was for it to be known across the world because he knew it was beneficial for every body.

This book and Micki Harvard are helping carry on the essence of Joseph's dream—and that makes me happier than words can express. Micki excels at giving modifications and adaptations of the classical work so it's accessible to all bodies while maintaining the principles of the original Pilates method. Micki knows how to help you on your fitness journey without the need of expensive apparatuses.

No matter your age, gender, ability, education, economic status—every body is designed to move. This means every body is a Pilates body. My wish is that you use Micki's guidance in this book to make your body Pilates strong.

CARRIE RUSSO
Pilates instructor
@russopilates

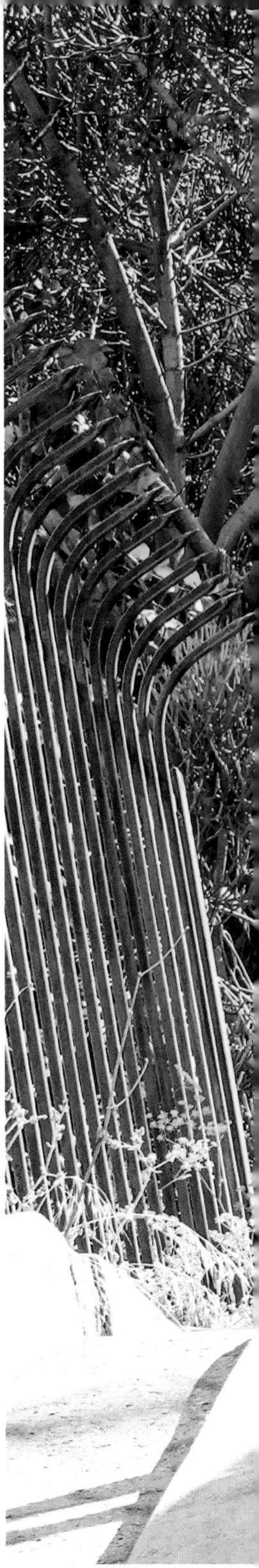

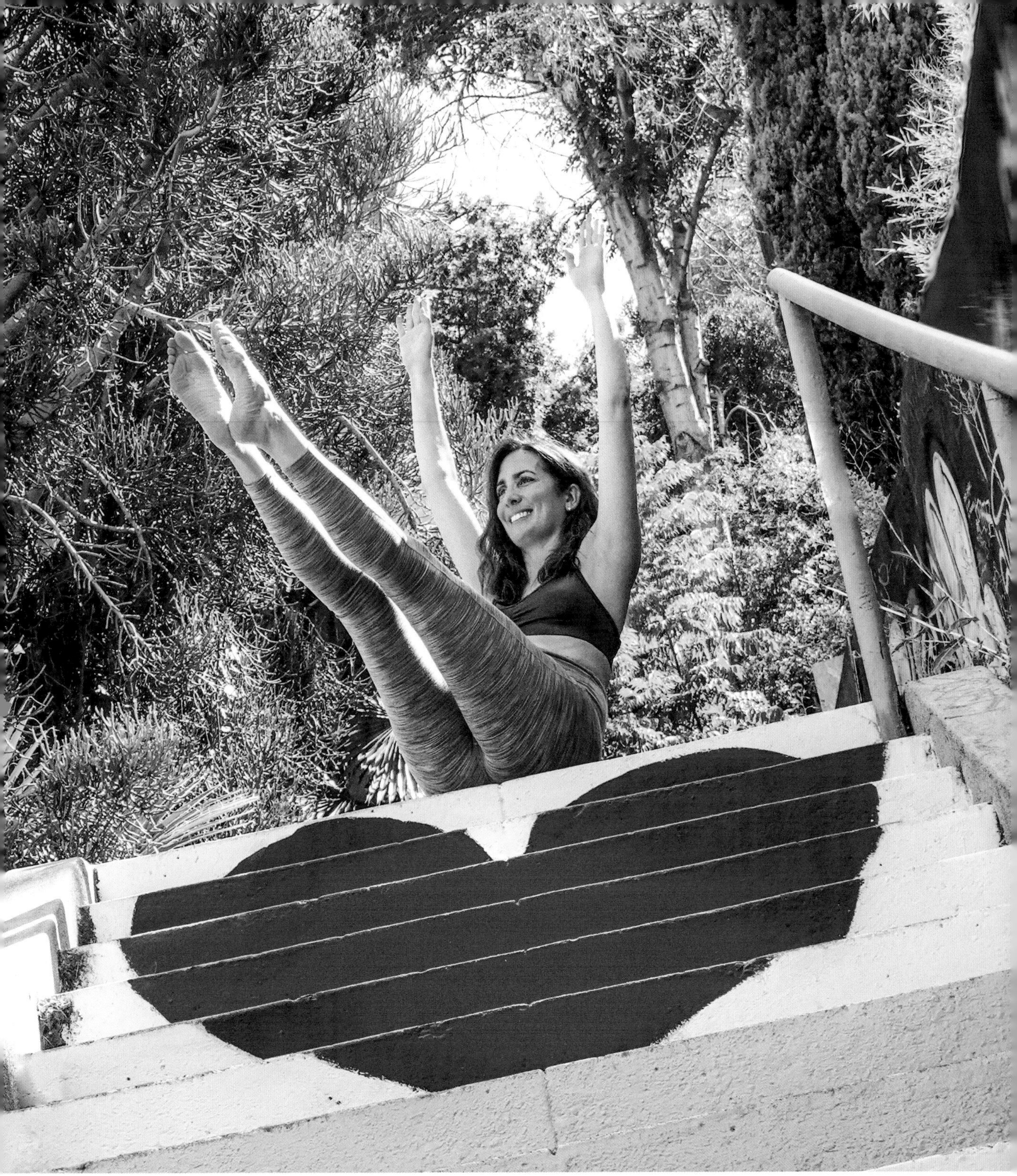

Photo by Shawn Driscoll

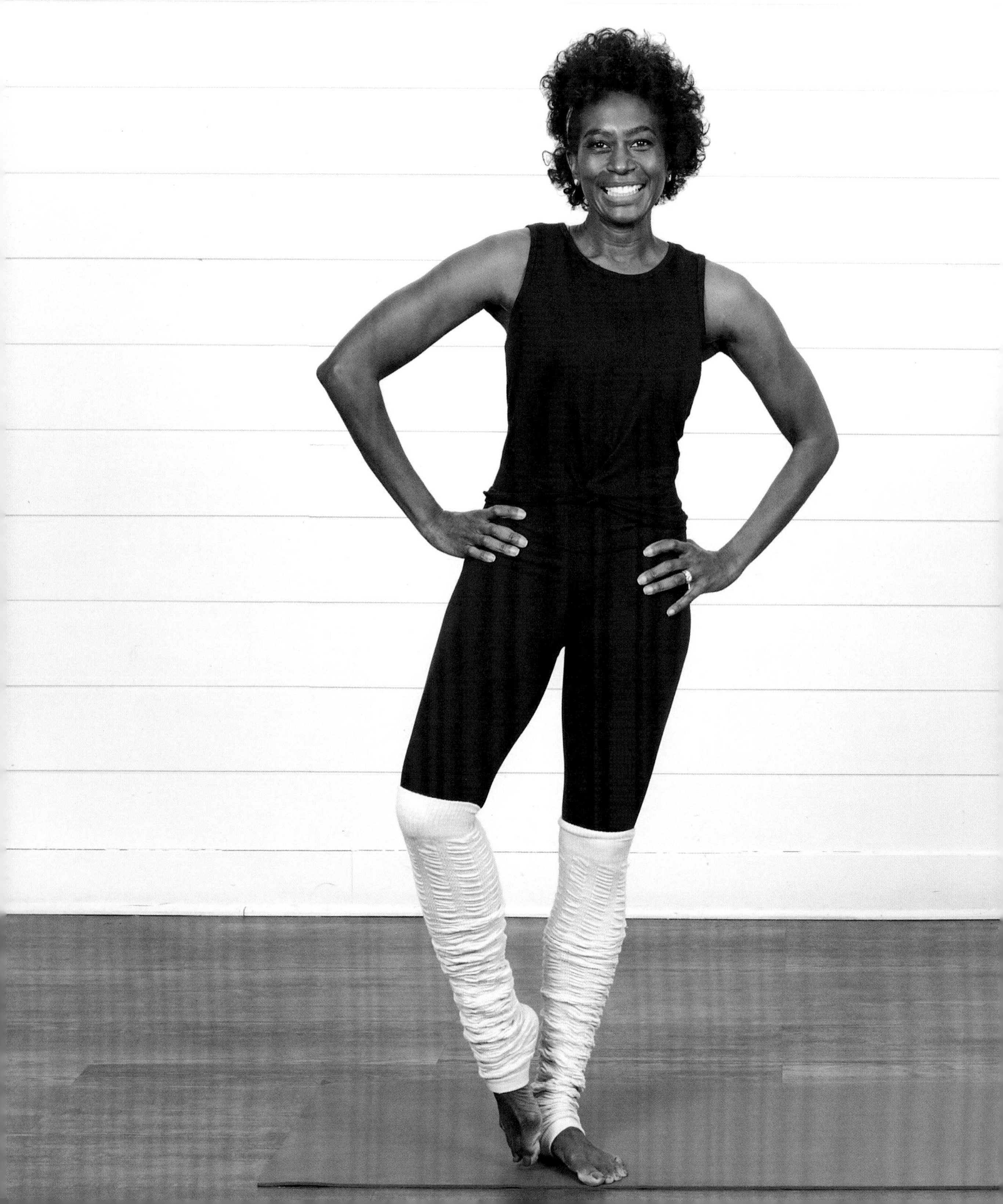

Yes, You Can Do Pilates!

When I started practicing Pilates more than 20 years ago, I was getting in shape for my impending wedding. My goal was to maintain my figure to make sure I'd fit in my wedding dress. I had no idea Pilates would prove to provide so much more. My practice started in my parents' basement with VCR tapes and cable fitness programs. When I branched out of my home practice and went in search of a Pilates studio, I found they were quite homogenous. I didn't find that the classes included a variety of fitness levels, shapes, races, or even ages. There seemed to be an almost "Stepford"-like quality to the instructors and the practitioners. Everyone was twenty-something and slender, and they looked like dancers or models. And even though I fit in physically, something didn't feel right about the environment.

I popped around from studio to studio until I settled in with a small studio owned by an older woman who didn't look like a Pilates magazine cover model. She was fit, a former dancer, and very passionate about inclusivity in her classes. After taking Pilates for just over a year, she suggested I become certified. I knew that when I became an instructor, I wanted to be inclusive and to share Pilates with a wide range of students. I taught in private studios for a few years and then got a job with my local Y to fit with my at-home-mom schedule. That's where I had the opportunity to teach a wide range of fitness levels, shapes, ages, and sizes. I felt at home and connected with my students.

My mission now—as it was then—is to bring Pilates to as many people as possible because I believe Pilates is truly for everybody. I hope this book helps you find your place in Pilates.

MICKI HAVARD
@mickiphit

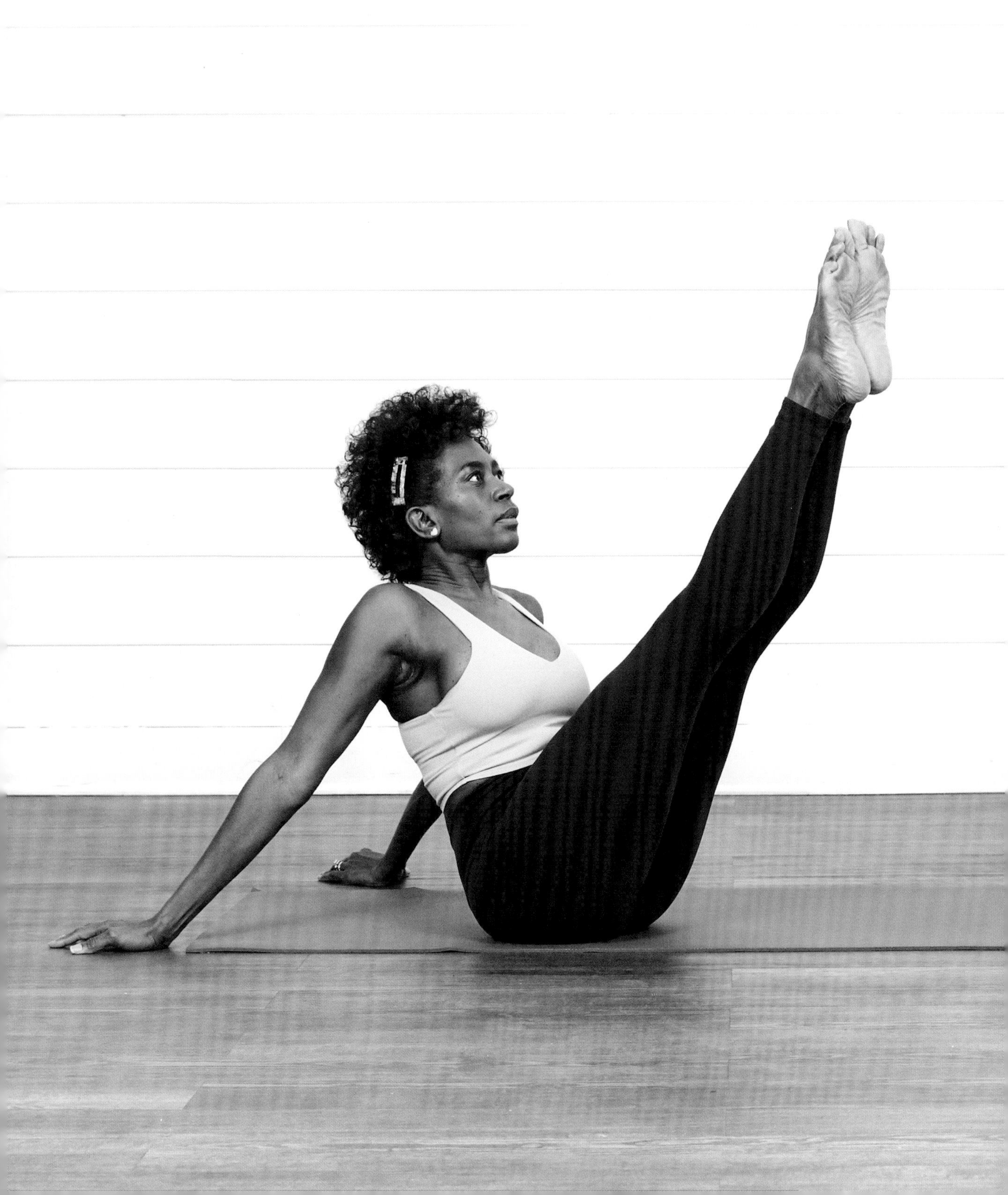

MICKI HAVARD

When I started my Pilates practice more than 20 years ago (in preparation for my wedding), I never thought I'd be still practicing today, not to mention teaching. I started my training in 1998 in a small studio owned by a Black woman. She was the first Black person I had seen practicing or teaching Pilates in the two years of my practice. When I began teaching, I heard the same message from many of my students of color. And unfortunately, this became a recurring theme during my teacher trainings, continuing education, and personal practice.

The first couple years of my teaching, I taught in a couple small studios (including the Black-owned studio where I began my training). I realized how underrepresented WOC (women of color) were in the industry. Once my Black teacher trainer closed her studio, I had a hard time finding a studio where I felt welcomed and where there were students of color in attendance.

In my third year as an instructor, I made the decision to leave the boutique studios and taught exclusively at my local YMCA. Most of my coworkers had a hard time understanding why I'd leave the boutique studios for the Y. I heard things like: "You know you'll be paid pennies" and "You won't have access to quality students."

At the Y, my classes were filled with diverse people. There were many different races, ages, and fitness levels. Most of my students were new to Pilates and many of them had never heard of Pilates. My teaching style was forever changed. In addition to my verbal cues, I was on the mat demonstrating every move and making modifications for most moves to accommodate a large variety of fitness levels. I can honestly say I enjoyed teaching every single class at the Y. I went on to teach at the YMCA for 10 years, and toward the end, I taught a "seniors only" class. That senior Pilates class was easily the most rewarding class I've ever taught. I learned so much more than I taught my students.

After leaving the Y, I began holding Pilates 101 workshops—designed to expose WOC to Pilates and to provide a non-intimidating and welcoming environment. I continue this kind of atmosphere in all the Pilates classes I teach.

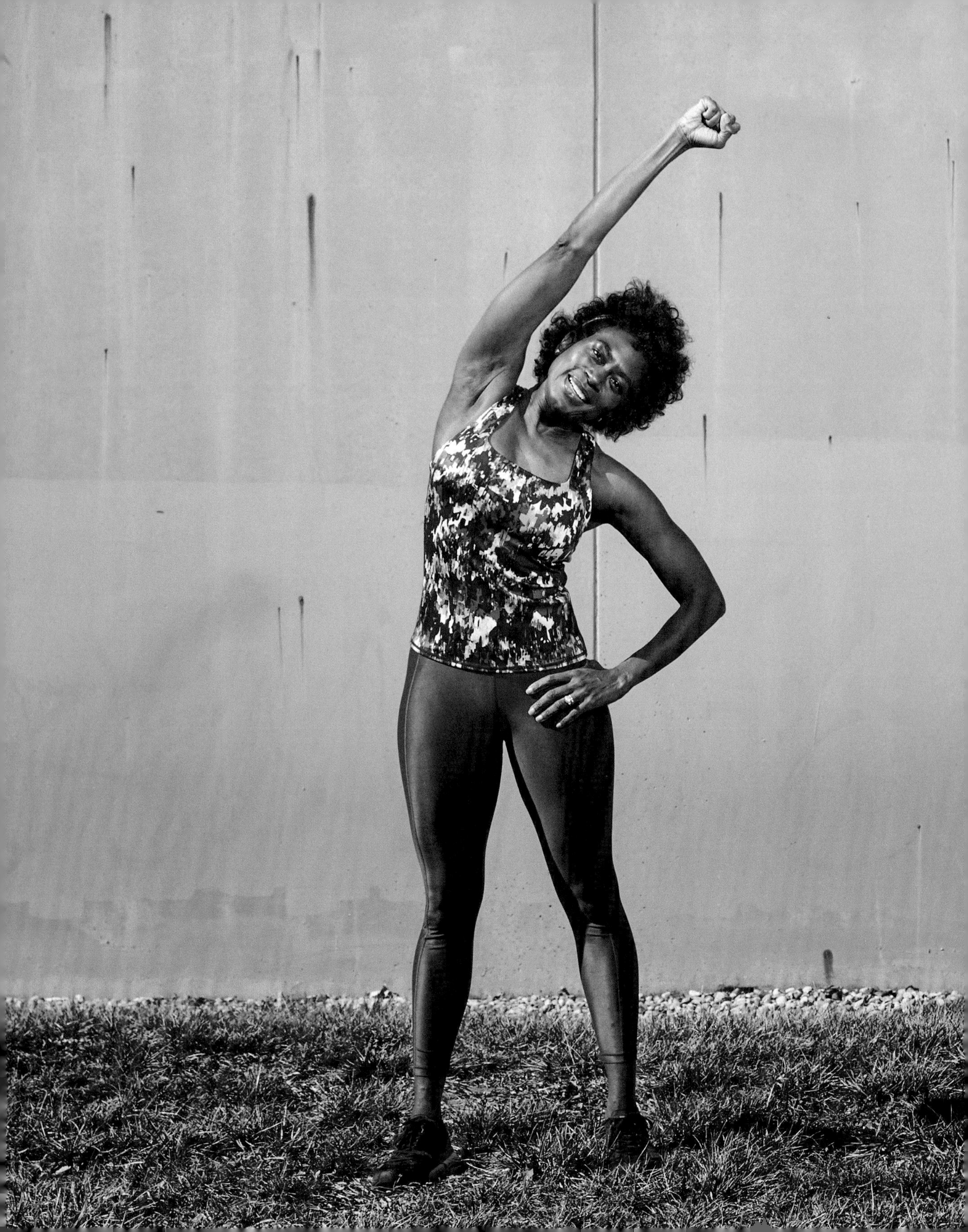

CHAPTER 1
Pilates Facts

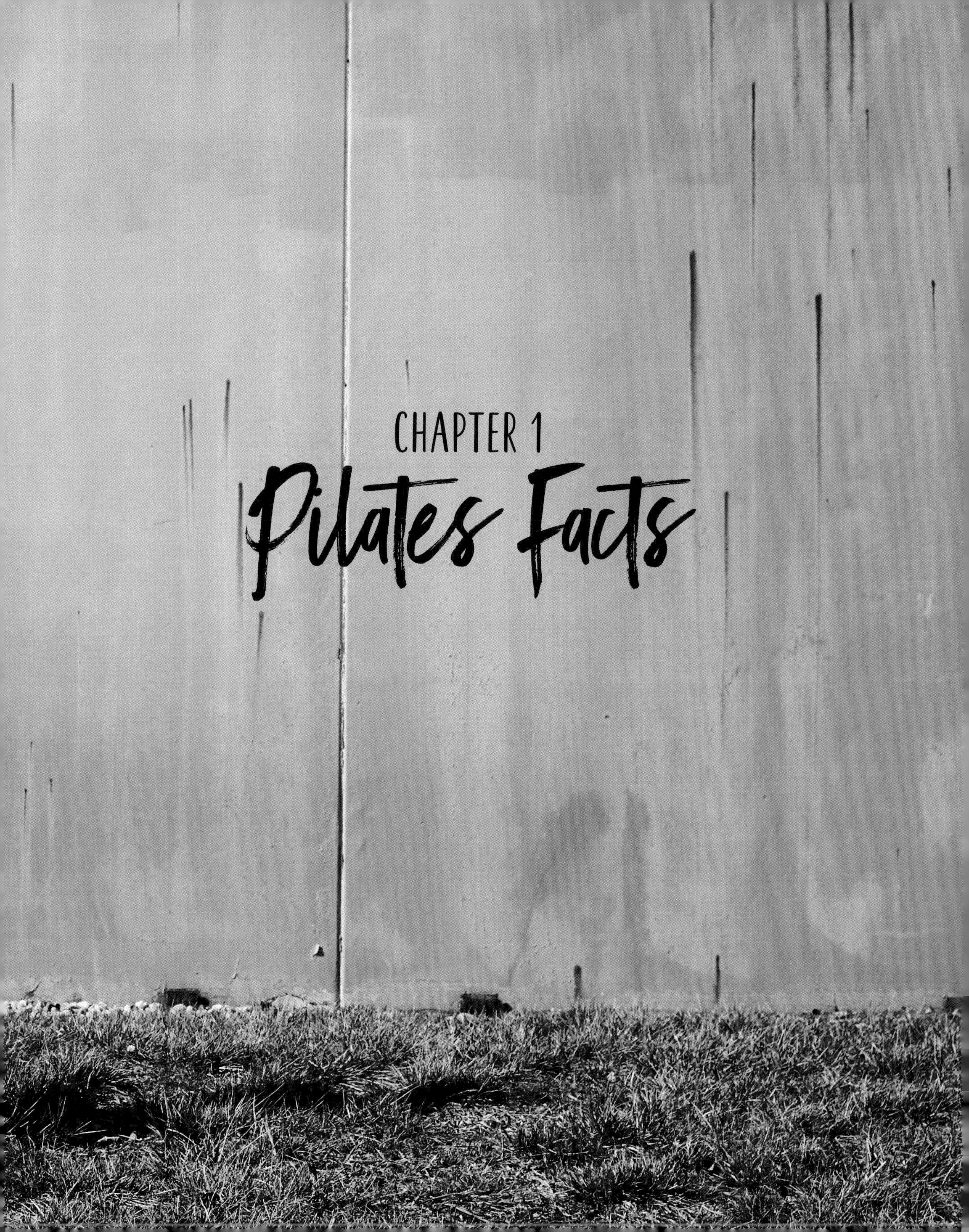

WHAT IS PILATES?

Most of us have heard about Pilates or perhaps even taken a Pilates class. But do you know the history, types, benefits, and goals of Pilates? What follows is a brief introduction to this form of exercise focused on flexibility, strength, and endurance.

HISTORY OF PILATES

Joseph Pilates was born in Mönchengladbach, Germany, in 1883. As a child, he had rheumatic fever, rickets, and asthma. In an effort to restore his health, he began studying anatomy books and a variety of disciplines, including bodybuilding, boxing, and gymnastics. Joseph engaged in a variety of movement arts as a youth, including yoga, skiing, diving, and martial arts.

He continued his work as a physical trainer and athlete in Germany throughout his young adulthood. During this time, Joseph became more aware of the importance of the mind–body connection—a symbiotic relationship with myriad benefits. He developed what we today know as Pilates by focusing on this connection and furthering the correlation between spiritual and physical arts.

Joseph immigrated to England in 1912 and he worked as a martial arts trainer for Scotland Yard. At the start of World War I, he was sent to an English internment camp, where he continued to train others in wrestling, boxing, and self-defense. It was here that he began developing a system of mat exercises he called "Contrology." Joseph continued to develop his system by studying the movements of animals and human anatomy. Some of his exercises were even used to rehabilitate injured war veterans.

After WWI, he returned to Germany. Around 1925, he immigrated to New York City, where he and his wife, Clara, taught Contrology classes. This instruction focused on the core and postural muscles, and the exercises were designed to flow from one move to the next. They met Romana Kryzanowska, a former ballerina who would become Pilates's protégé. They opened a studio in NYC and began building the teacher training program.

When Joseph created the Pilates method nearly 100 years ago, society was becoming more sedentary and people were using their bodies less and less. He designed his methods to counter society's ever-increasing inactive lifestyle and lack of daily movement, which is a problem for so many more today than ever before.

TYPES OF PILATES

Classical Pilates focuses on preserving the original teachings of Joseph and Clara Pilates and the equipment used to practice Pilates, featuring the exact specifications as those built by Joseph Pilates. Classical Pilates is taught within the order of exercises Joseph created for the reformer and the mat. Exercises in this book use Classical Pilates as their foundation.

Contemporary Pilates integrates various traditional Pilates exercises with other forms of exercise, like yoga, fitness training, and physiotherapy. It might also include props, such as resistance bands, foam rollers, and stability balls. Contemporary Pilates includes additional exercises as well as modifications to the original Pilates exercises. Exercises in this book are most closely related to Contemporary Pilates while still maintaining core elements from Classical Pilates.

METHODS OF PILATES

Pilates has two main methods: mat and reformer Pilates. Mat classes use your body weight for exercises, while reformer classes use equipment that works against spring-loaded resistance. Some forms of Pilates also include weights and small equipment that offer resistance and aid in alignment.

Mat Pilates is practiced on the floor and requires little to no equipment. Pilates matwork is the basis for the entire Pilates system of exercises. On the mat, your body weight provides resistance against gravity, making the workout more challenging in many cases. Mat Pilates focuses on developing core strength and it's typically taught in groups, making it more affordable.

Reformer Pilates is taught on a narrow bed with a sliding carriage, straps and pulleys, and springs for increasing or decreasing tension and resistance. Using a reformer, you can target small muscle groups, which help build strength. The reformer acts as a support system for the body by helping assist it into proper form and gives you the option of performing exercises in a variety of different body positions—from your back, side, and stomach as well as while kneeling, standing, or seated.

They're both beneficial to building up your core strength and toning your muscles. Both methods also train you to initiate the movements from your body's powerhouse (your core) and they translate into benefits across your day-to-day activities. The biggest misconception is that reformer Pilates is harder than mat Pilates, but this can be the opposite in an advanced class, which can lead to faster results. What's critical is that regular practice is maintained and that the principles of Pilates (breathing, centering, concentration, control, precision, and flow) are adhered to throughout a class to maximize the results.

All exercises in this book are mat Pilates exercises. While many of these exercises use small props, mat Pilates allows you work out at home without needing specialized equipment. This also makes mat Pilates a more inclusive kind of exercise—a type of fitness for everyone.

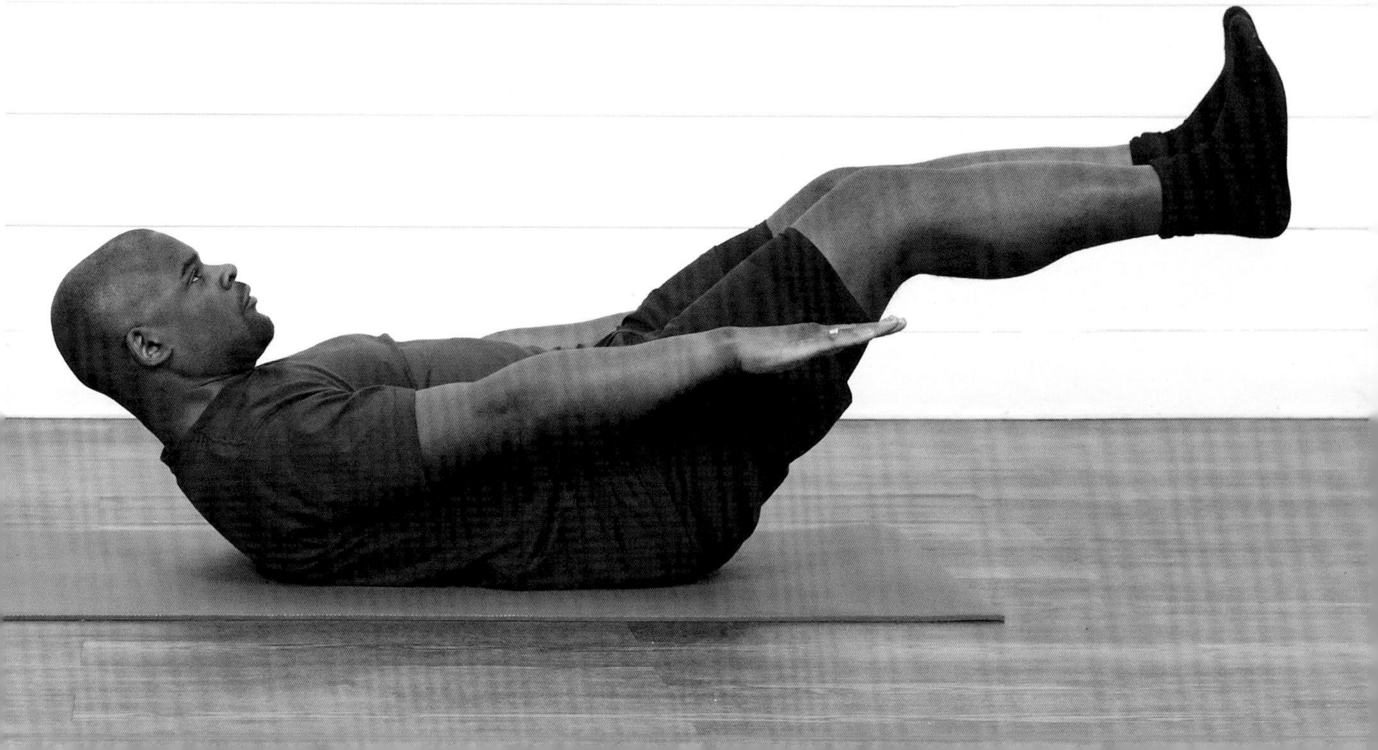

WHAT ARE THE BENEFITS?

Practicing Pilates can improve your core strength (balance), flexibility, spinal and joint mobility (posture and stability), body awareness, and overall physical strength. Let's look at these areas to discover how they can help you reach your fitness goals.

CORE STRENGTH (BALANCE)

Perhaps the biggest advantage of making Pilates a part of your wellness regimen is it can help strengthen your core. Your core is the center of your body, including all the muscles in your midsection (front, back, and sides), and this area can greatly benefit from a regular Pilates routine. Almost every movement you make relies on your core muscles, and when you can develop and enhance these muscles, movements can feel easier. Plus, with a strong core, you'll increase your balance, further making physical activities easier and more efficient.

FLEXIBILITY

Flexibility is the most neglected component of fitness and adding a Pilates practice to your wellness plan is a wonderful way to gain more flexibility. Rather than using static stretches, Pilates focuses on movements while stretching. This means the muscles are warm as you stretch, allowing you to stretch further with less pain and injury. Improving and strengthening your flexibility can also mean better posture and balance, better mobility, and, yes, even a better state of mind—which is a strong aspect of every Pilates exercise.

SPINAL & JOINT MOBILITY (POSTURE & STABILITY)

Pilates encourages students to target the muscles that protect and support their spine. Because Pilates involves stretches and exercises that work to strengthen all the essential parts of your core, when you perform exercises that target your core muscles, you're also going to strengthen your back and gain spinal stability and mobility. This means less back pain, especially in your lower back, which would typically prevent you from fully enjoying all kinds of activities, but with help from Pilates, you'll gain more control over your ability to perform everyday movements.

Pilates can also improve your joint mobility and range of motion by moving your joints through their full range of motion from a stable base. During a balanced Pilates class, you work through all planes of motion and allow the body's joints to mobilize through their natural movement and natural function. The repetitive joint movements in Pilates help stimulate and promote the release of synovial fluid into the joint cavities, which helps protect joints and allows for smooth movement. Because Pilates is a low-impact and low-intensity type of workout, the movements are easy on the joints.

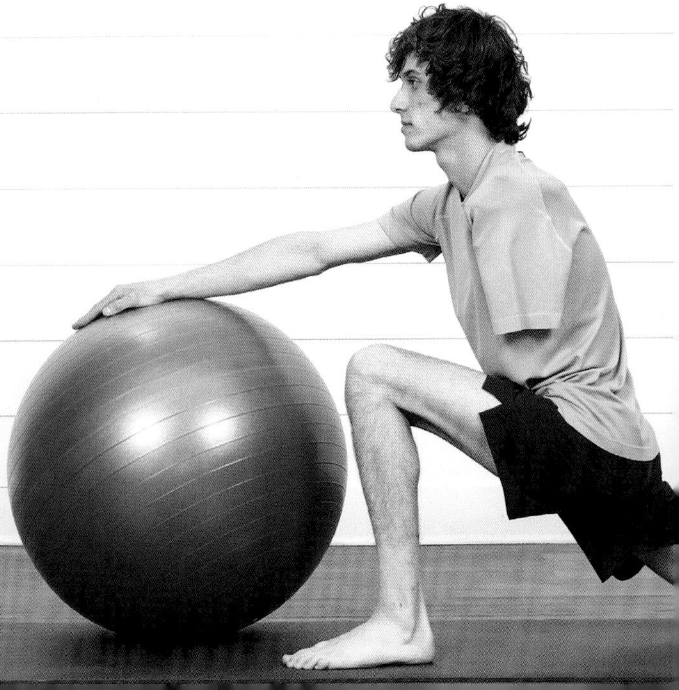

BODY AWARENESS

Pilates can help you connect with your body to learn how to best move and function. This isn't about limitations as much as it's about finding ways to do what you need and want to do. Performing the exercises in this book—whether the main exercises or the modifications (or a combination depending on what feels right to you)—will help you see where you are physically and mentally. Making your practice a regular routine will allow you to take this even further by developing and achieving your exercise goals while continuing to discover your capabilities and full potential.

OVERALL PHYSICAL STRENGTH

Pilates is also a form of strength training. You can perform Pilates on a mat using your body's weight and/or small props or on Pilates equipment that uses spring tension for weight resistance. Practitioners also perform movements that improve their overall strength, working large muscles and often neglected smaller muscles. By practicing the sequences at the back of this book—combining Pilates exercises into routines—you can assure yourself that you'll target many different areas of your body, ensuring you're working on strengthening your body from head to toe.

WHO SHOULD DO PILATES?

You—no matter who you are. Pilates is great for people of all ages, sizes, and fitness levels. The accessibility of mat Pilates makes it the perfect home, studio, or on-the-go workout. Whether you're recovering from an injury, looking to get back into regular exercise to strengthen your body, or a professional athlete trying to stay in shape, the principles of the exercises apply to you. Pilates is low impact in nature, but it can provide high intensity, making it the perfect balance for anyone looking to increase their fitness. All the exercises in this book have been modified to allow anyone and everyone an opportunity to practice Pilates.

MEET THE MODELS

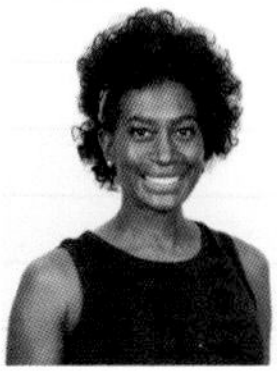

MICKI HAVARD

READ HER STORY ON PAGE 10.

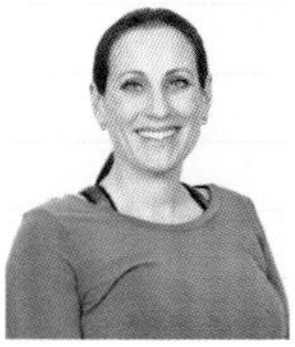

JILLIAN PETERSON

READ HER STORY ON PAGE 42.

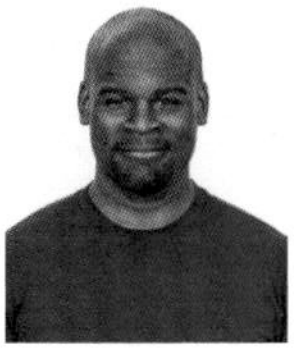

ANDREW PETERSON

READ HIS STORY ON PAGE 90.

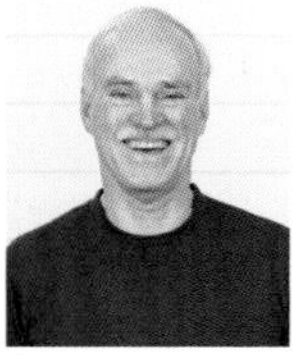

JERRY DENYS

READ HIS STORY ON PAGE 142.

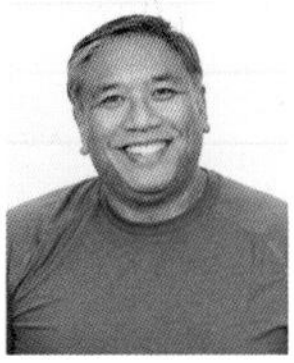

JEROME PASCUA

READ HIS STORY ON PAGE 168.

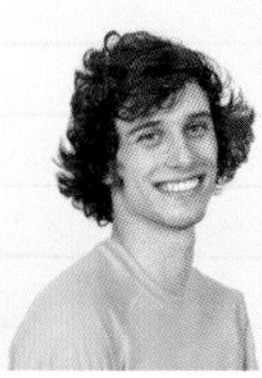

ANDREW BLUM

READ HIS STORY ON PAGE 200.

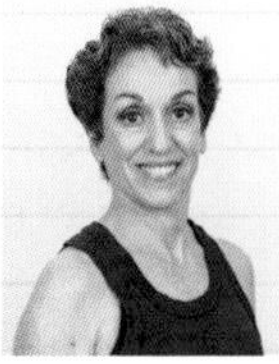

SUSAN HOLEWINSKI

READ HER STORY ON PAGE 240.

WHAT YOU NEED TO PRACTICE PILATES

The great thing about Pilates is all you need is a small space and a willingness to practice. Although you don't need any equipment for your practice, having a mat and wearing fitness clothing can make it more comfortable. Adding Pilates props can enhance your workout by engaging specific muscles, helping with alignment, assisting with modifications, and adapting reformer moves to the mat.

MAT

For Pilates, a thicker mat usually works best. Unlike a yoga mat (which is thinner so you can balance properly), a Pilates mat is ¼ to ½ inch (0.5 to 1.25 centimeters) thick and made with dense compact foam to provide more support for your spine, wrist, hips, etc., as well as help you stay firm on the floor.

MAGIC CIRCLE

The Magic Circle was originally created by Joseph Pilates from the metal ring around a beer barrel and two wooden blocks connected to the sides. Today's version is flexible metal or rubber, is about 13 inches (33 centimeters) in diameter, and has small pads on both sides. It has seemingly endless uses: creating stability, assisting with alignment, providing the body with feedback as to which muscles it's targeting, and increasing flexibility.

RESISTANCE BAND

Resistance bands are affordable, portable, and adaptable. They can provide support during stability moves. Training with resistance bands provides similar muscle activity as weight training and produces less force on the joints. They're helpful when used in stretching and mobility training. Resistance bands are often used during physical therapy rehabilitation sessions to improve mobility, strengthen and lengthen muscles, and increase range of motion.

LOOP BAND

Like resistance bands, loop bands are affordable, portable, and useful for a large number of exercises. They're available in varying levels of resistance and provide options to adjust your workouts according to your fitness level and goals. Loop bands are excellent for warming up, targeting smaller muscle groups, and adapting reformer exercises to mat exercises. They're often used in lower-body exercises that target the gluteal, hip, and leg muscles. Whether you're a beginner or advanced athlete, these bands offer customizable levels of resistance, making them suitable for everyone.

PILATES SMALL BALL

Also known as the Overball, the Pilates small ball is an inflated soft ball that's very common in the Pilates studio. It's a very versatile prop, often used to increase the intensity of a workout. Placing the ball between the ankles, hands, or inner thighs aids in engagement of the surrounding muscles. It creates good alignment and can be used to modify exercises by adding support when placed on your back or side. The Pilates small ball is especially helpful for pregnant people. You can place the ball behind your middle back to avoid lying flat on your back for an extended period of time.

STABILITY BALL

A stability ball is known by many names: balance ball, Swiss ball, fit ball, physio ball, and exercise ball. It's a large inflated vinyl ball that comes in different sizes: 22 inches (55 centimeters), 26 inches (65 centimeters), and 30 inches (75 centimeters). These sizes indicate the diameter of the ball when fully inflated. The ball sizes are designed to ensure body alignment for specific body heights. (See the chart at right.) You can use a stability ball to stretch and warm up your muscles before your workout. It can also improve your mobility, flexibility, balance, and core strength. A stability ball is very useful if you have back problems because it supports your lower back when you stretch and exercise. To that end, the support can help with alignment and act as a weight when executing Pilates exercises.

YOUR HEIGHT	BALL SIZE
5'0" TO 5'5"	SMALL: 22 INCHES (55 CENTIMETERS)
5'6" TO 5'11"	MEDIUM: 26 INCHES (65 CENTIMETERS)
6'0" TO 6'3"	LARGE: 30 INCHES (75 CENTIMETERS)

LIGHT HAND WEIGHTS

Using light hand weights (1 to 3 pounds [450 grams to 1.4 kilograms]) can encourage extra stability work for your shoulders, core, and pelvis. Adding weight to exercises can also increase the amount of energy used (which will increase the number of calories burned), help you build bone mineral density, and tone muscles. Light weights are traditionally used for the Pilates arm series and you can do many reformer exercises on the mat using hand weights.

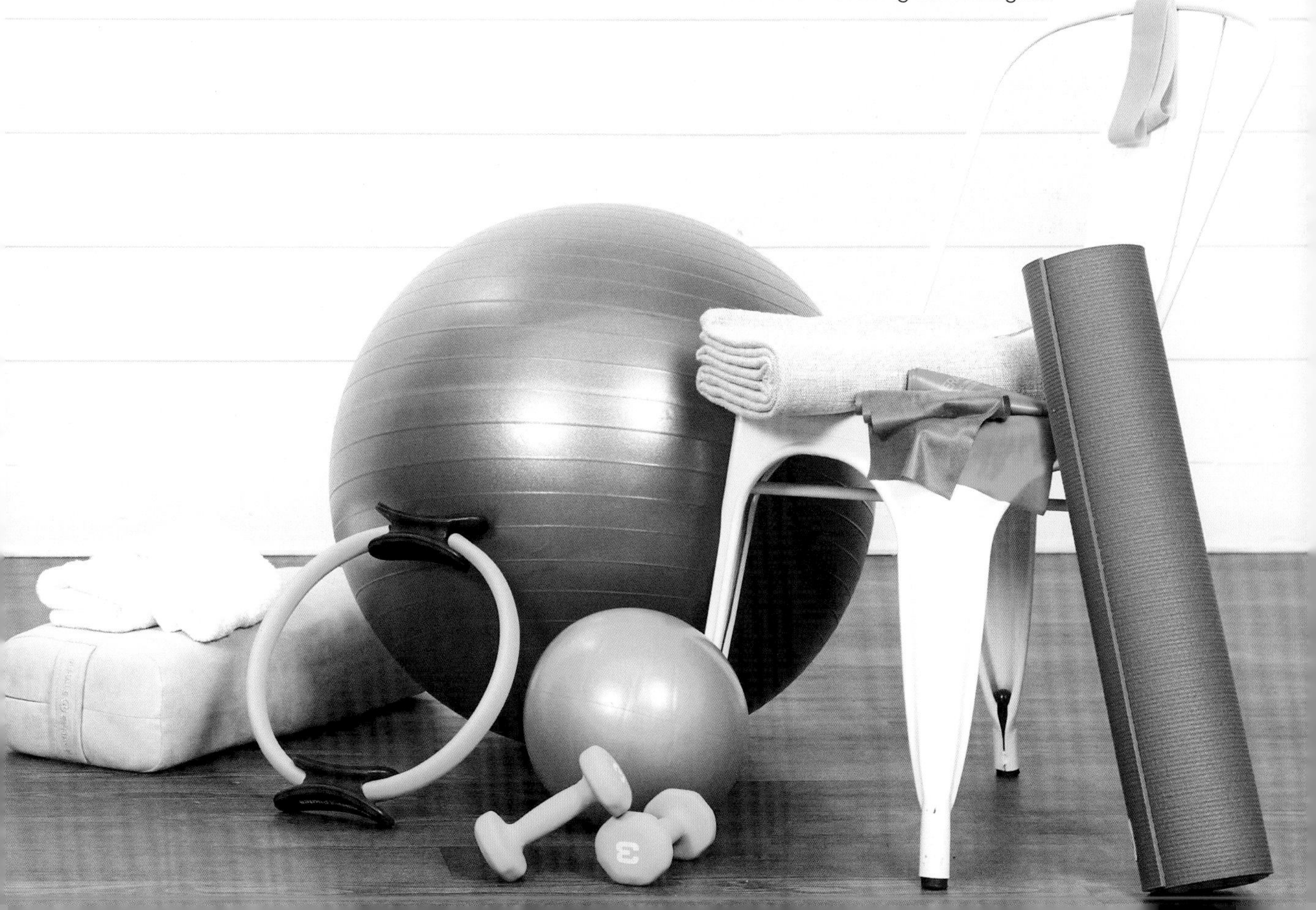

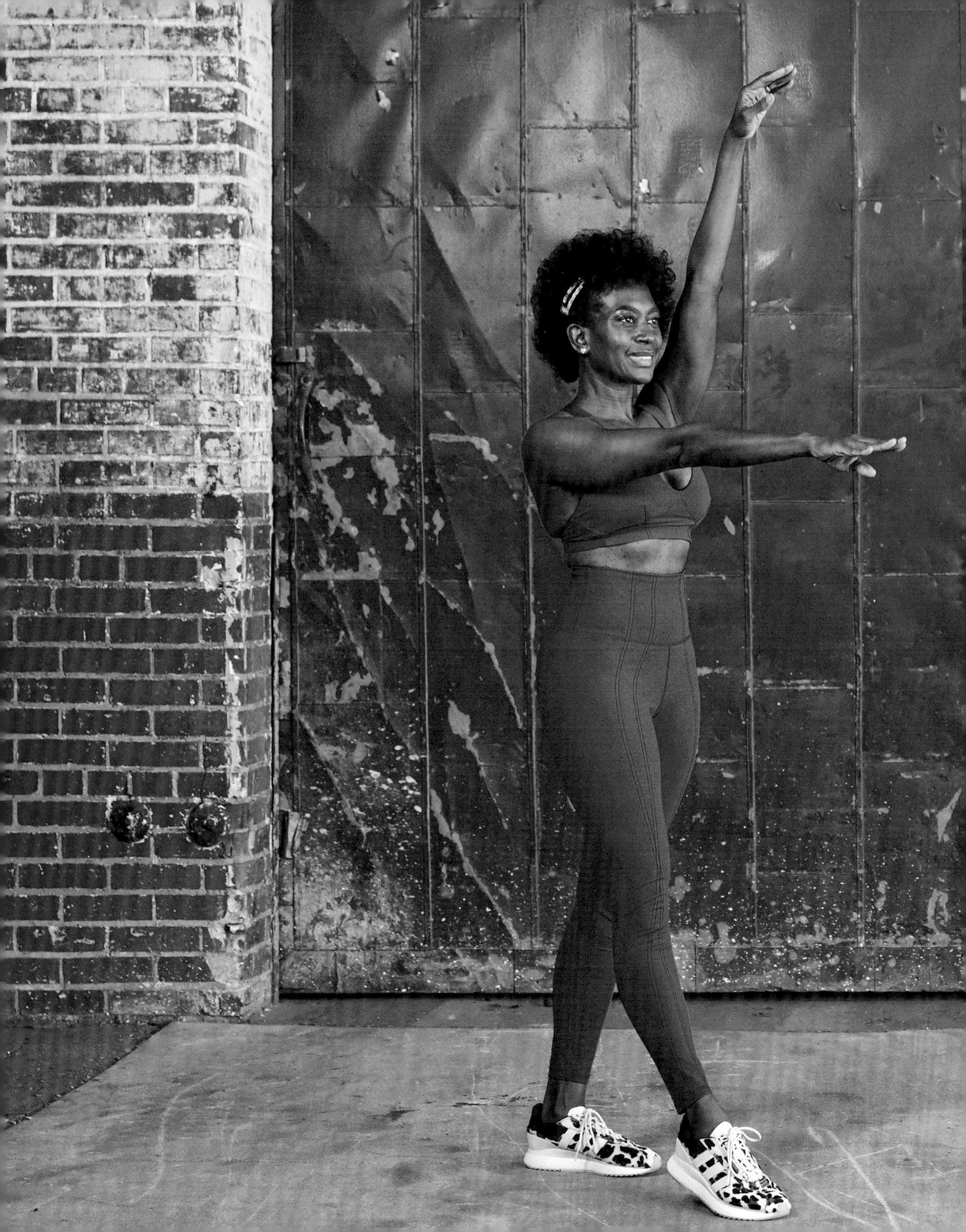

CHAPTER 2

Upper Body

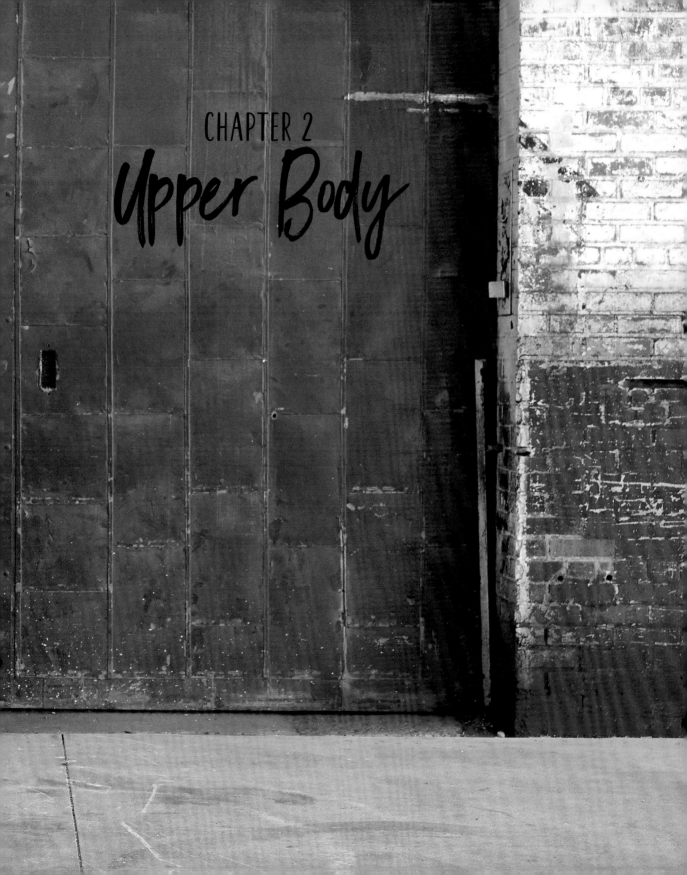

The Hundred

This breathing exercise simultaneously works your core muscles, legs, and arms. The movements get your blood flowing, warm the body for Pilates matwork, and help aid with breath control. The modifications are equally suitable for different fitness levels, body types, and needs.

1 Lie flat on your back on the floor and raise your legs to form a 90-degree angle with the floor. Relax your arms at your sides and place your hands flat on the floor.

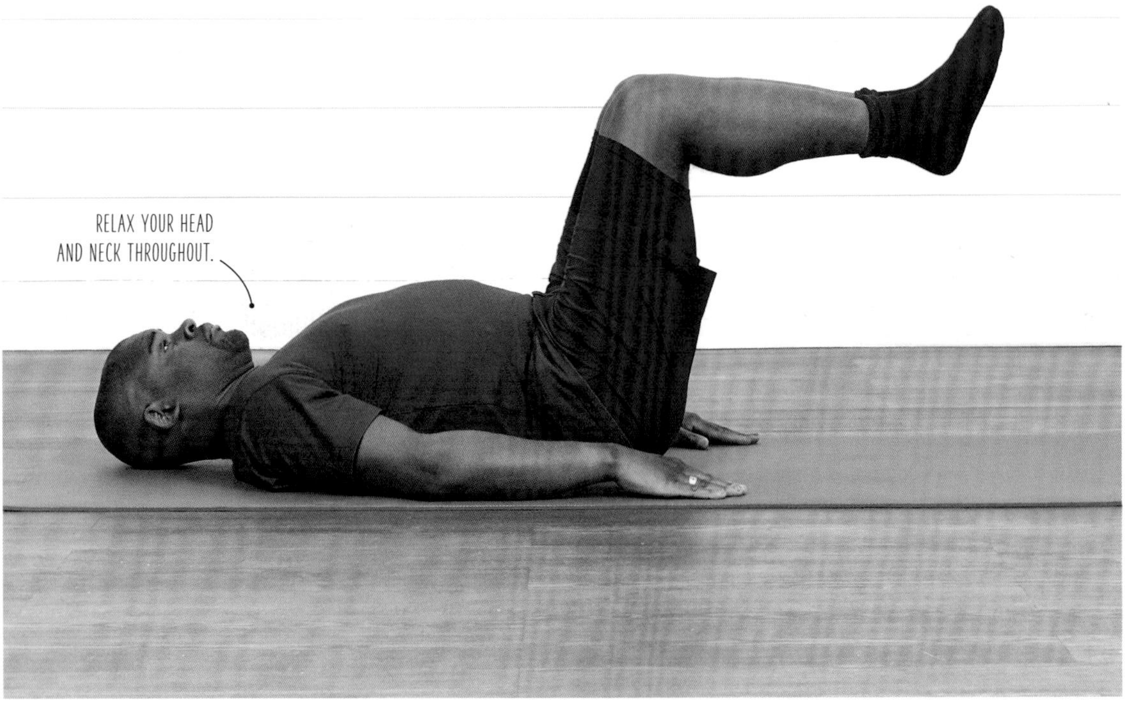

RELAX YOUR HEAD AND NECK THROUGHOUT.

2 Lift your head off the floor and bring your chin toward your chest. Engage your abdominal muscles as you curl your upper spine off the floor and raise your shoulder blades.

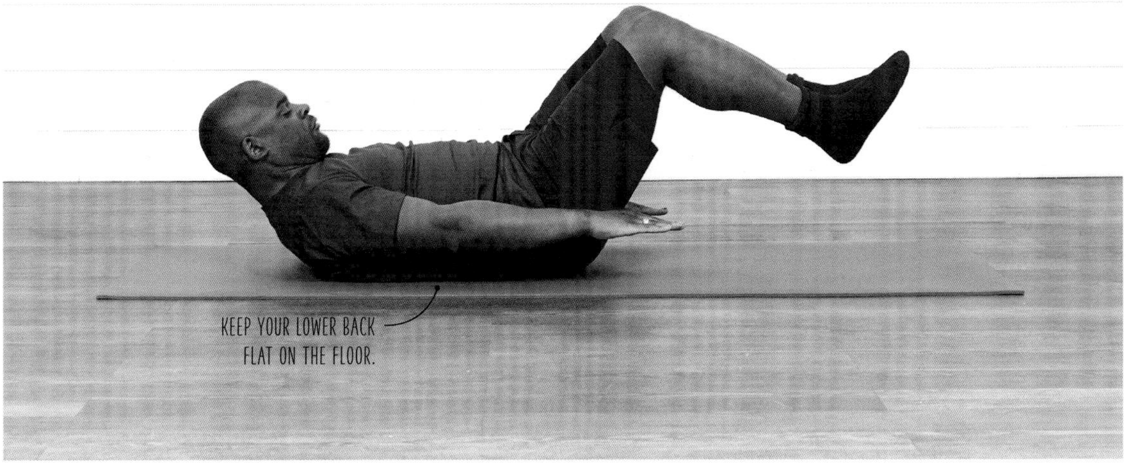
KEEP YOUR LOWER BACK
FLAT ON THE FLOOR.

3 As you inhale, raise your arms off the floor and quickly pulse them in an up-and-down motion for 5 seconds. As you exhale, quickly pulse your arms in an up-and-down motion for 5 seconds. Perform this step 10 times.

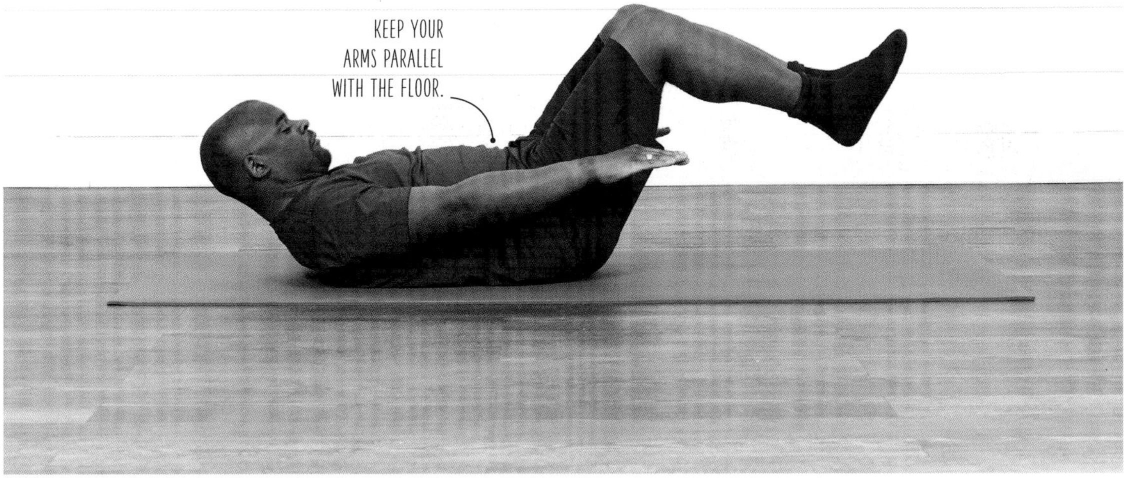
KEEP YOUR
ARMS PARALLEL
WITH THE FLOOR.

THE HUNDRED

VARIATIONS

If you're experiencing neck pain or have a delicate neck, modifying this exercise by keeping your head on the floor can be beneficial. If your abdominal or upper back muscles are weak, bending your legs, keeping them on the floor, or placing a small Pilates ball under your back can assist in performing this exercise.

WITH LEGS STRAIGHT UP

In step 1, raise your legs straight up to form a 90-degree angle with your upper body. Continue with the remaining text.

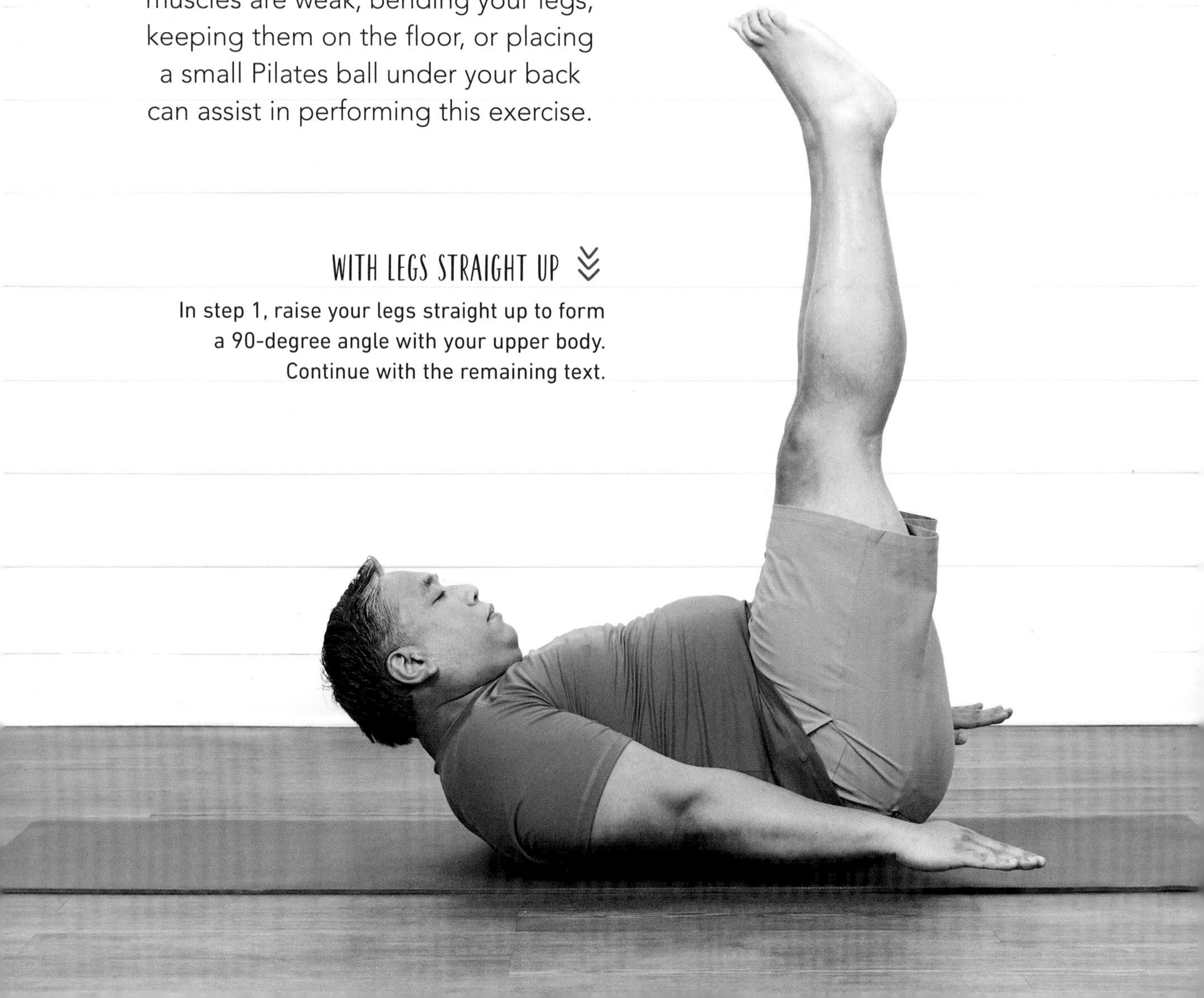

WITH FEET ON THE FLOOR AND KNEES BENT

In step 1, bend your knees to form a 45-degree angle with your legs. Keep your feet flat on the floor. Continue with the remaining text.

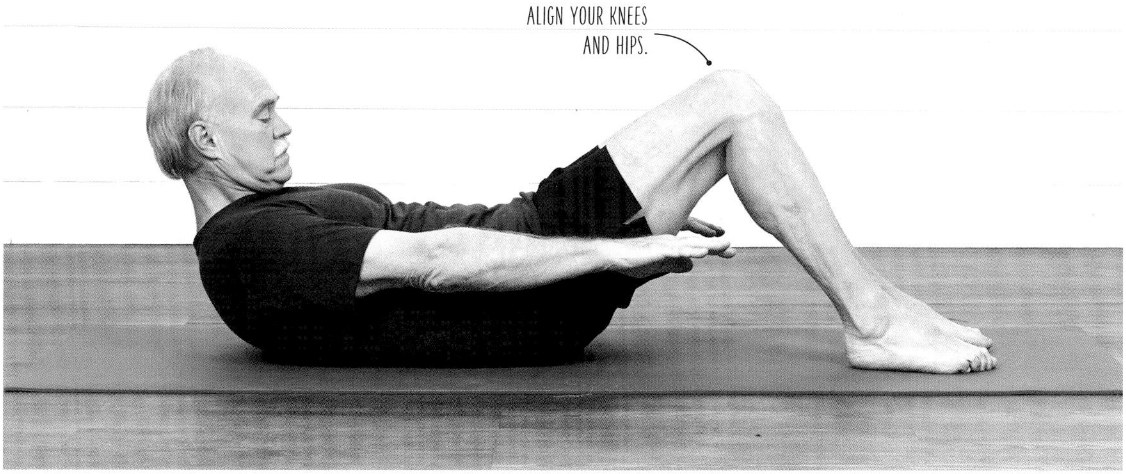
ALIGN YOUR KNEES
AND HIPS.

WITH A SMALL PILATES BALL

In step 1, place a small Pilates ball at your lower back. Bend your knees to form a 45-degree angle with your legs. Keep your feet flat on the floor. Continue with the remaining text.

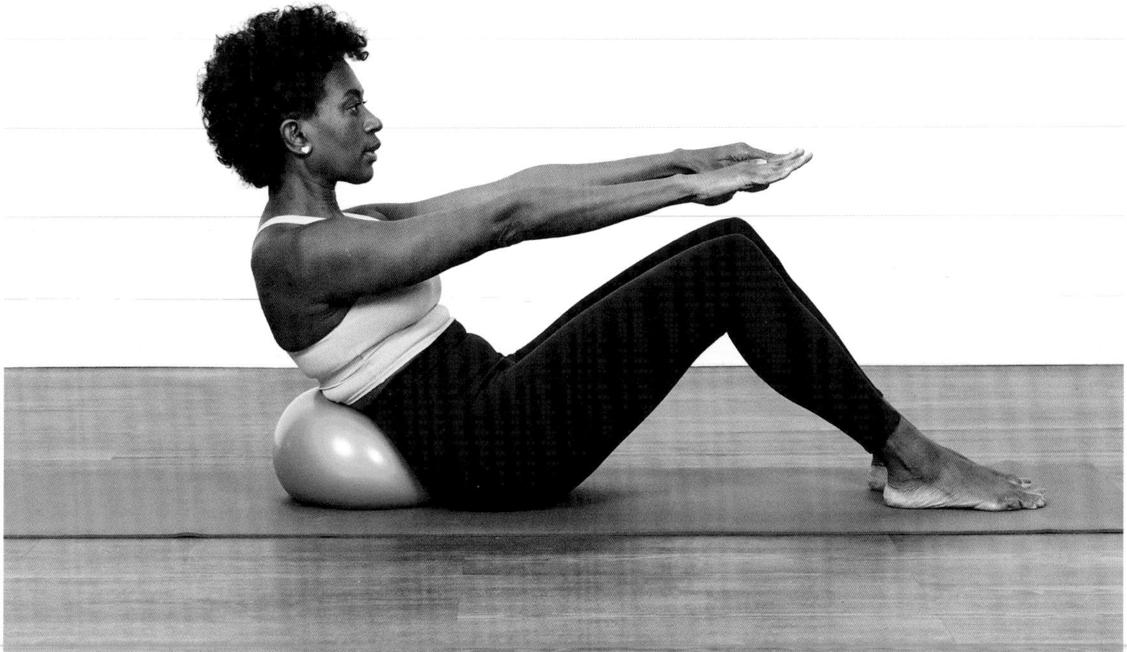

Roll-Ups

Performing the movements of this exercise strengthens your abs, stretches your spine, and increases spinal articulation (moving one vertebra at a time). The latter is a foundational movement in Pilates. It wakes up your core and develops awareness of the connection between your abs and your spine.

1 Lie flat on your back on the floor with your legs together and your feet flexed toward your body. Raise your arms toward the ceiling, facing your hands toward your toes.

PRESS YOUR GLUTES AND INNER THIGHS TOGETHER.

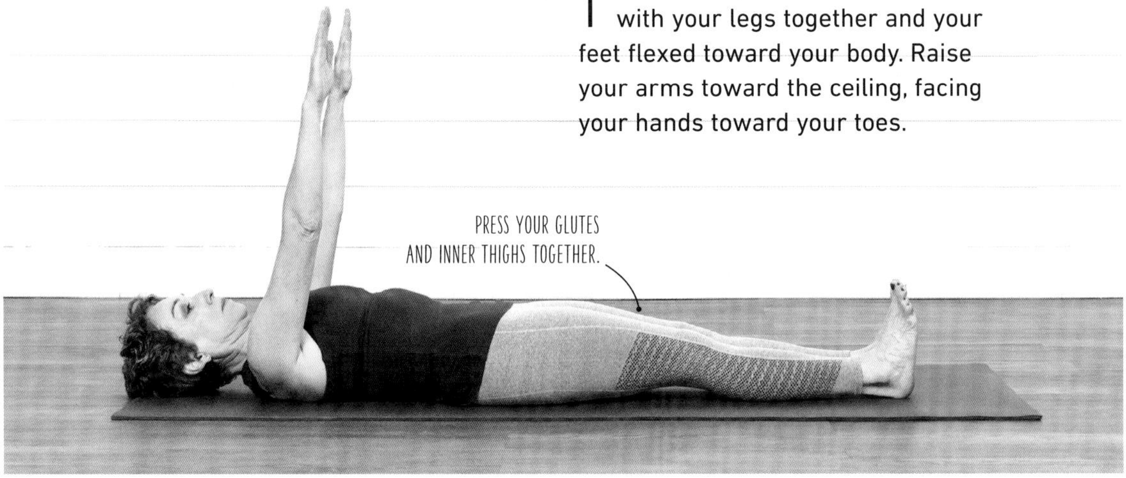

2 Lift your head and shoulders off the floor and bring your chin toward your chest.

KEEP YOUR ARMS AND HEAD PARALLEL.

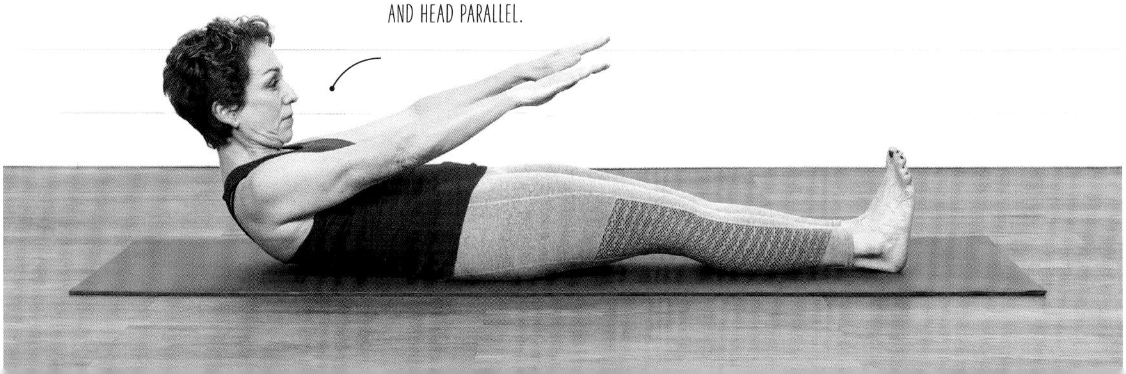

3 Continue rounding forward, lifting your upper body off the floor, and reach your hands toward your toes. Pull your navel toward your spine as you reverse your movements one vertebra at a time until you return to your starting position. Perform these steps 5 times.

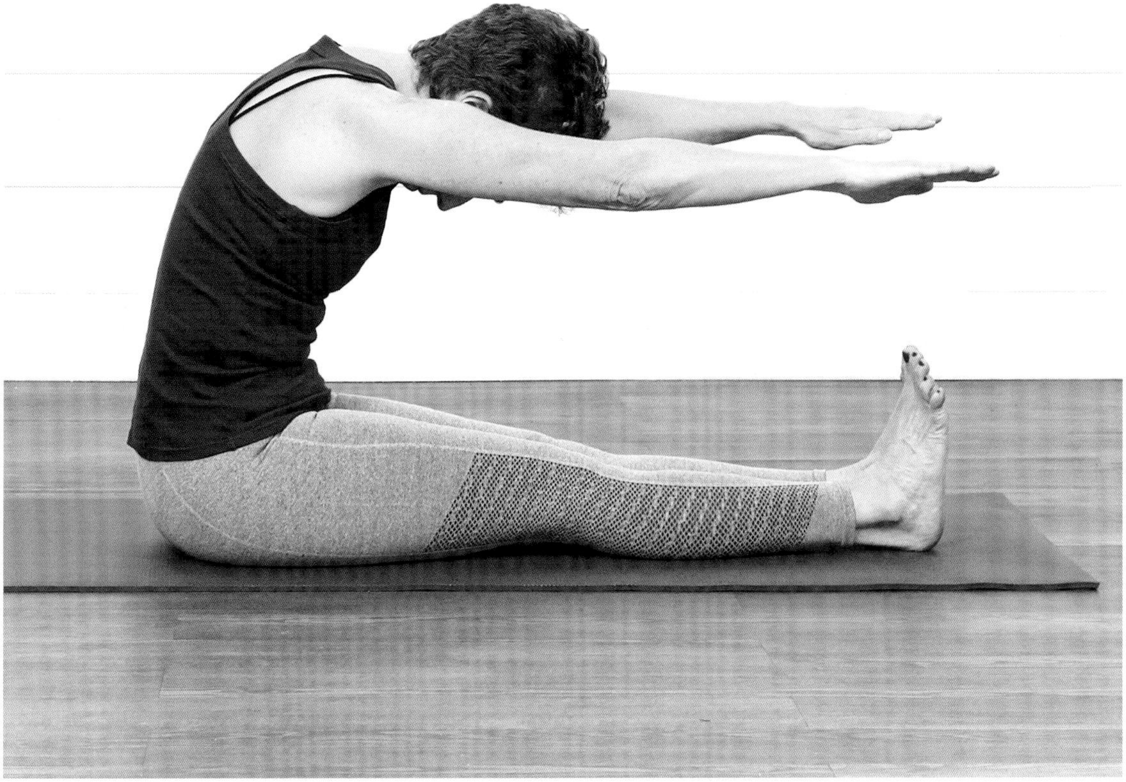

ROLL-UPS

VARIATIONS

Lacking lower back and hamstring flexibility and/or core strength might require you to modify this exercise by bending your knees. The addition of the Magic Circle can assist you with the proper shoulder alignment required to perform this exercise while giving your core muscles the feedback to fire up properly.

WITH BENT KNEES

In step 1, bend your knees to form a 45-degree angle with your legs. Place your feet flat on the floor shoulder width apart. Continue with the remaining text.

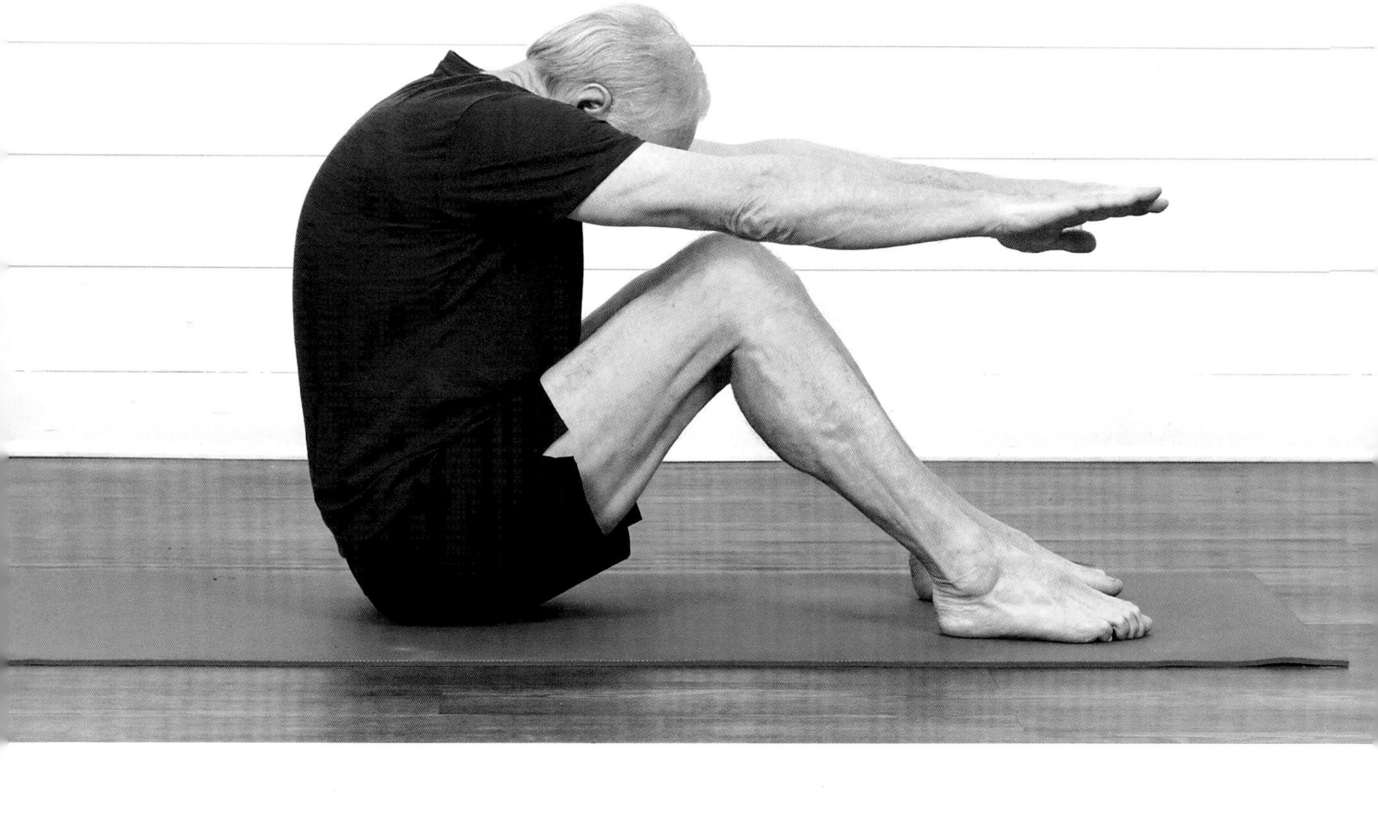

WITH THE MAGIC CIRCLE >>>

In step 1, hold the Magic Circle with the heels of your hands.

In step 2, as you start to roll forward, press the heels of your hands into the pads of the Magic Circle. Continue with the remaining text.

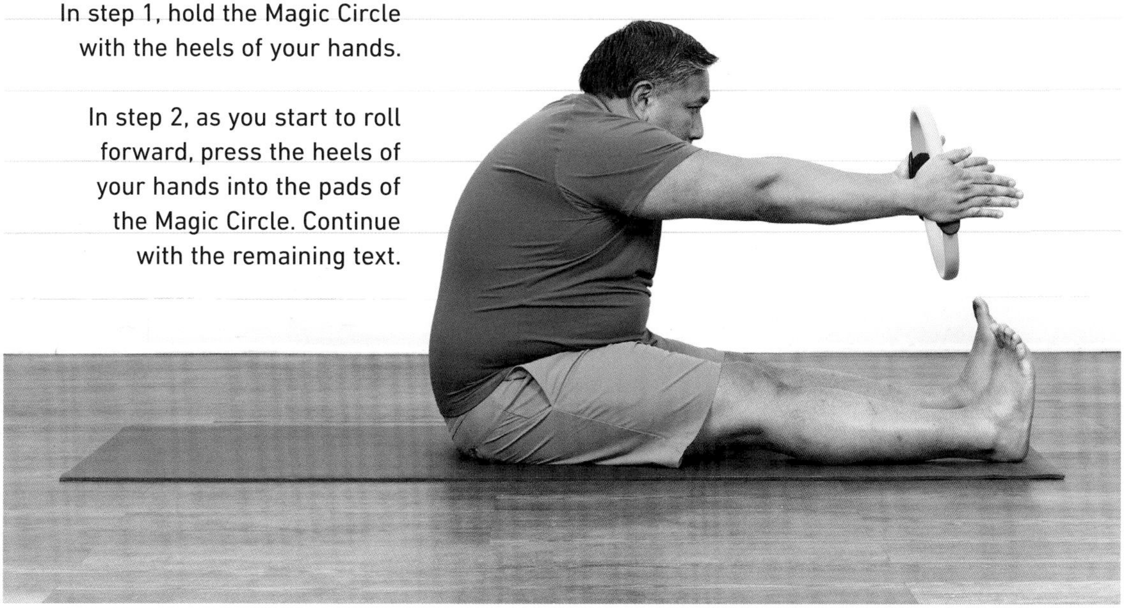

<<< SITTING ON THE FLOOR

1. Sit on the floor with your knees bent to form a 45-degree angle with your legs. Place your feet flat on the floor. Place your hands on your thighs just above the back of your knees.

2. Pull your lower abs toward your spine. Round your back into a C shape while bringing your chin toward your chest, using your hands as support to lean as far forward as you can.

3. Reverse your movements to return to your starting position. Repeat these steps 4 to 6 times.

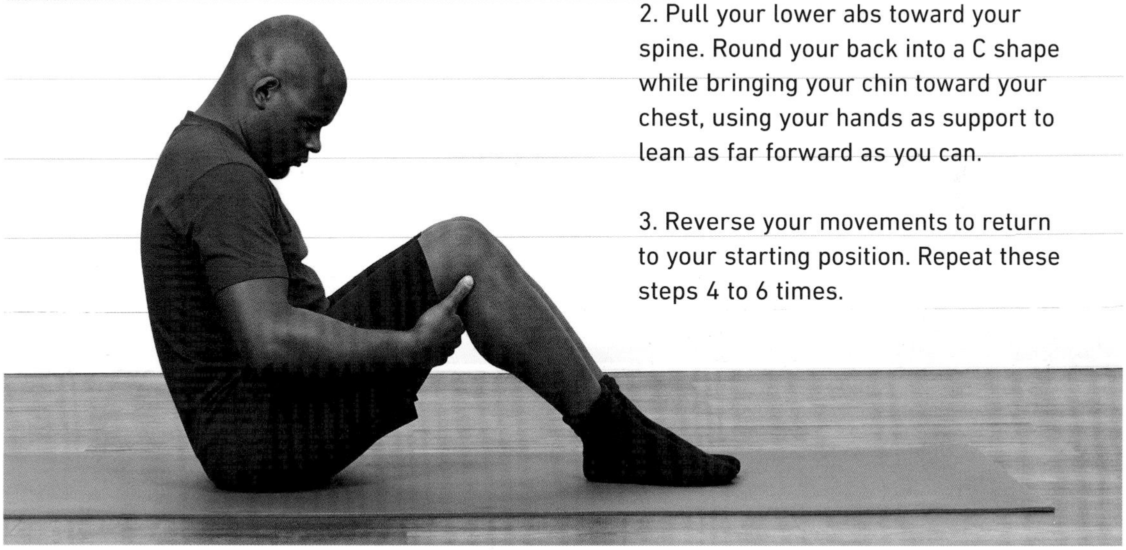

One-Leg Circles

This exercise can strengthen leg muscles, encourage body awareness, develop muscular control, and promote healthy hip joints. Performing these movements engages your core, glute, and hip muscles, improving pelvic stability. Leg circles are an isometric core exercise, requiring you to use your core muscles to support your raised leg.

1 Lie flat on your back on the floor and relax your arms at your sides. Pull your navel toward your spine and press your back into the floor.

ENGAGE YOUR CORE TO KEEP YOUR BACK ON THE FLOOR.

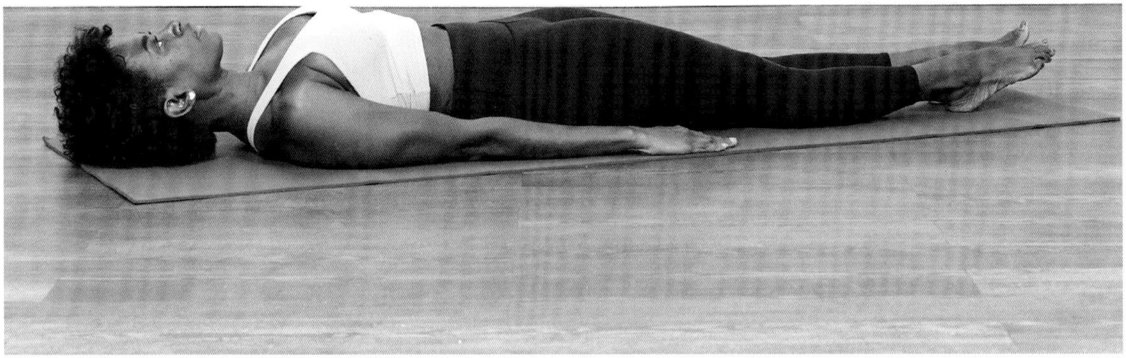

2 Raise your right leg toward the ceiling. Rotate your right leg in a circular motion (clockwise or counterclockwise) toward the floor and then back toward the ceiling. Perform this step 5 times. Repeat these steps with your left leg.

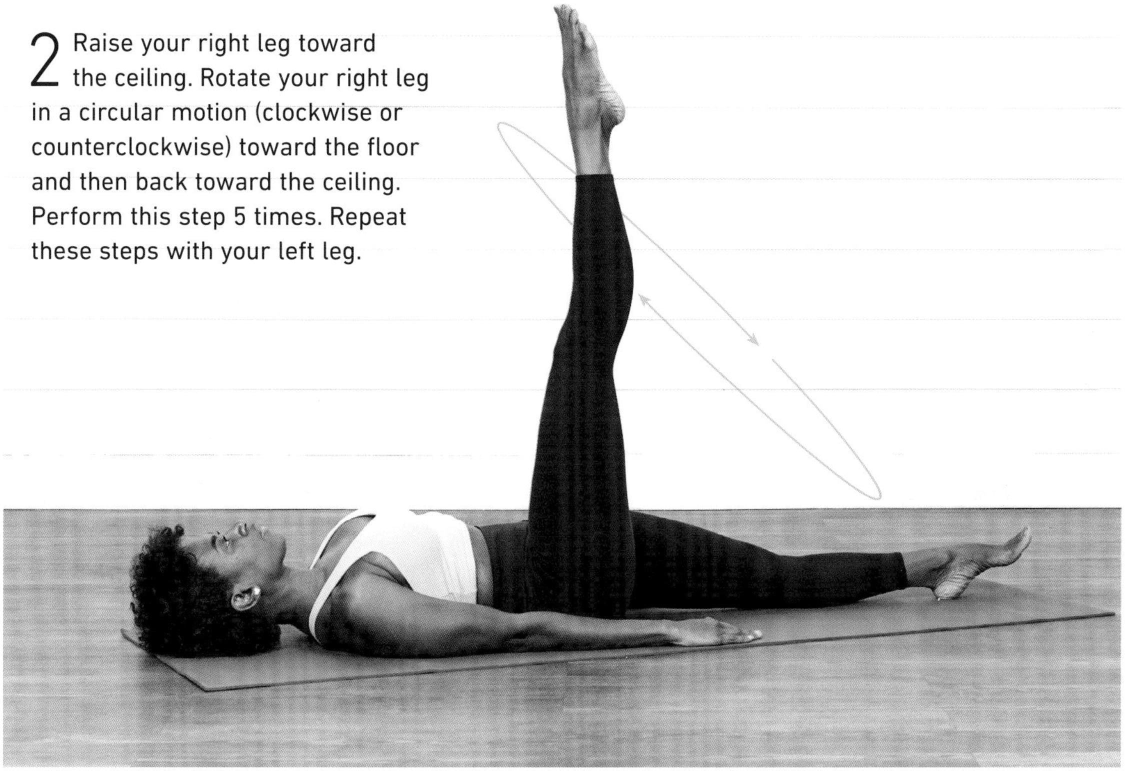

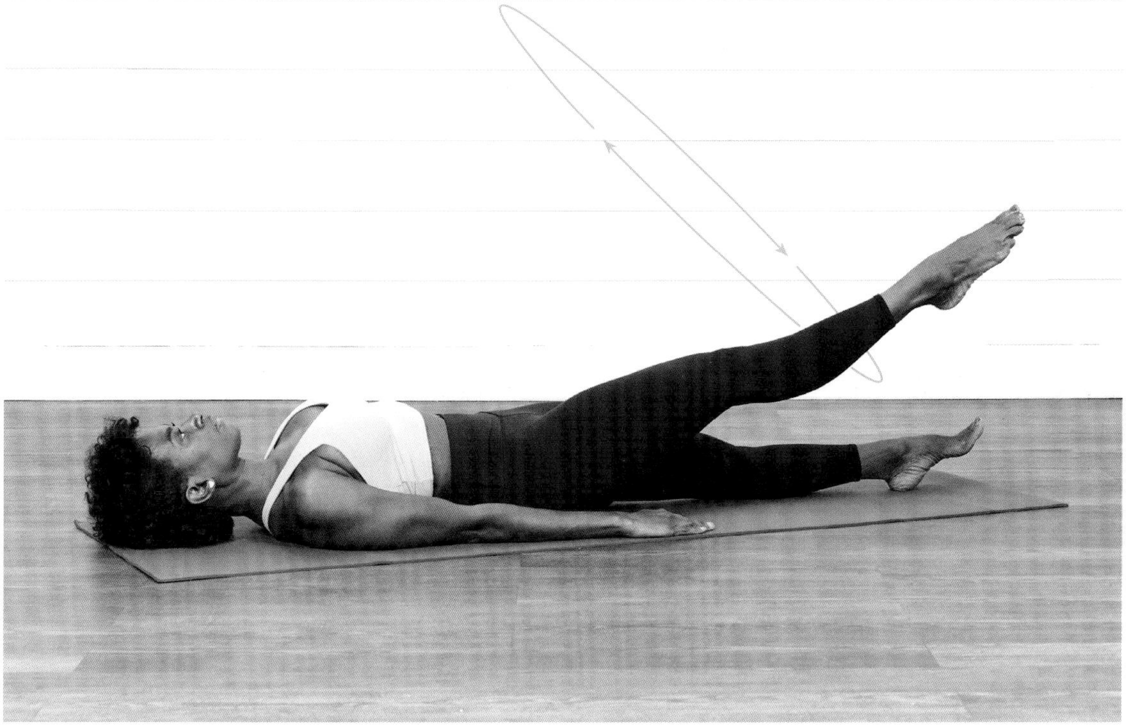

ONE-LEG CIRCLES

VARIATIONS

Performing this exercise with a bent knee or with a resistance band will decrease the core strength and stability required to execute the movements. Pregnant people or anyone who has difficulty coming to the floor will benefit from the standing variation.

WITH A RESISTANCE BAND

1. Lie flat on your back on the floor and extend your legs. Loop a resistance band around the bottom of your right foot, holding the ends of the band in both hands.

2. Extend your right leg and flex your right foot toward your body.

3. Rotate your right leg in a circular motion (clockwise or counterclockwise) toward the floor and then back toward the ceiling. Perform this step 5 times. Repeat these steps with your left leg and the resistance band around your left foot.

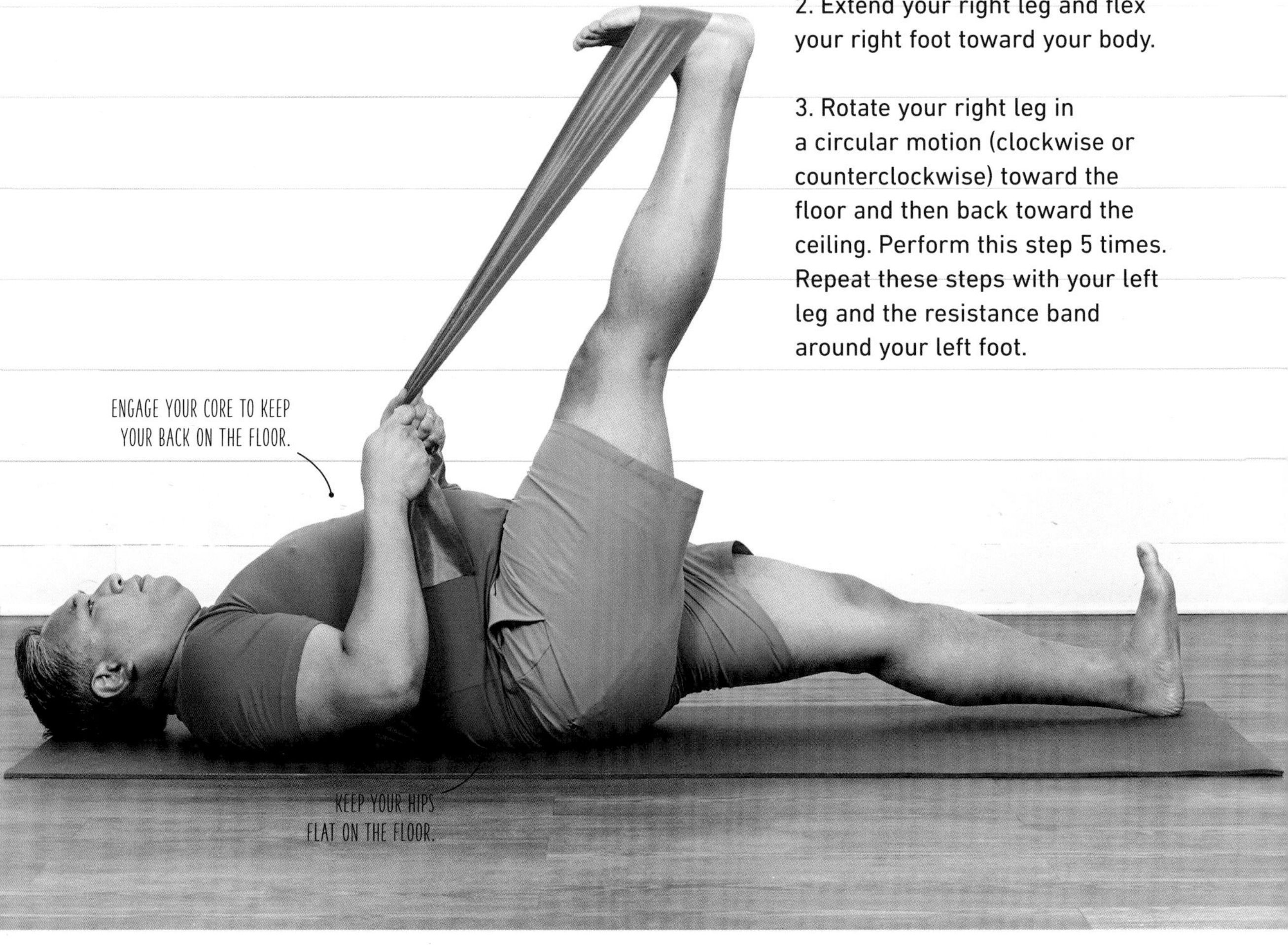
ENGAGE YOUR CORE TO KEEP YOUR BACK ON THE FLOOR.
KEEP YOUR HIPS FLAT ON THE FLOOR.

WITH A KNEE BENT

In step 1, bend your left leg and place your left foot flat on the floor. Bend your right knee and form a 90-degree angle with your right leg. Continue with the remaining text, keeping your knees bent.

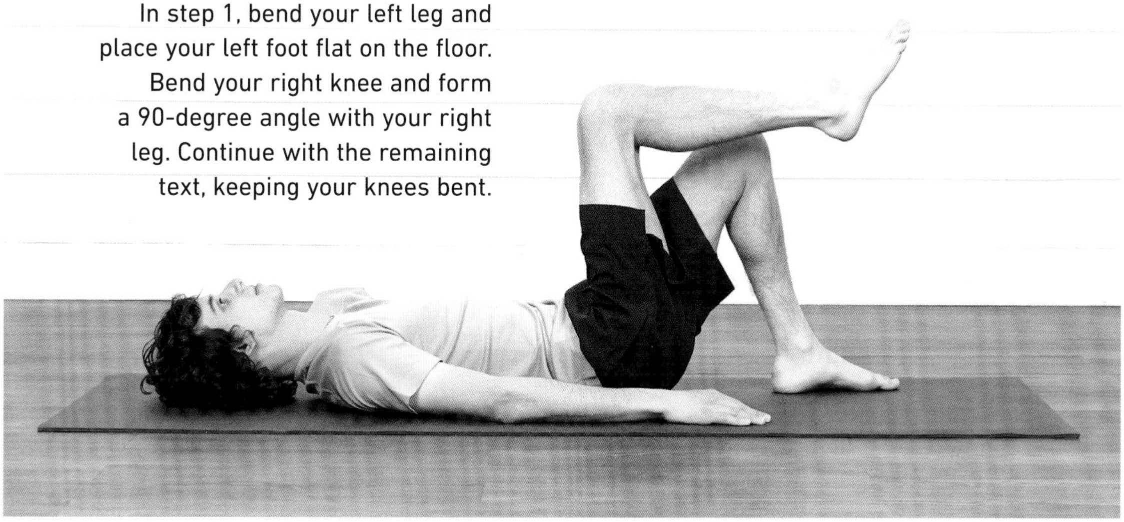

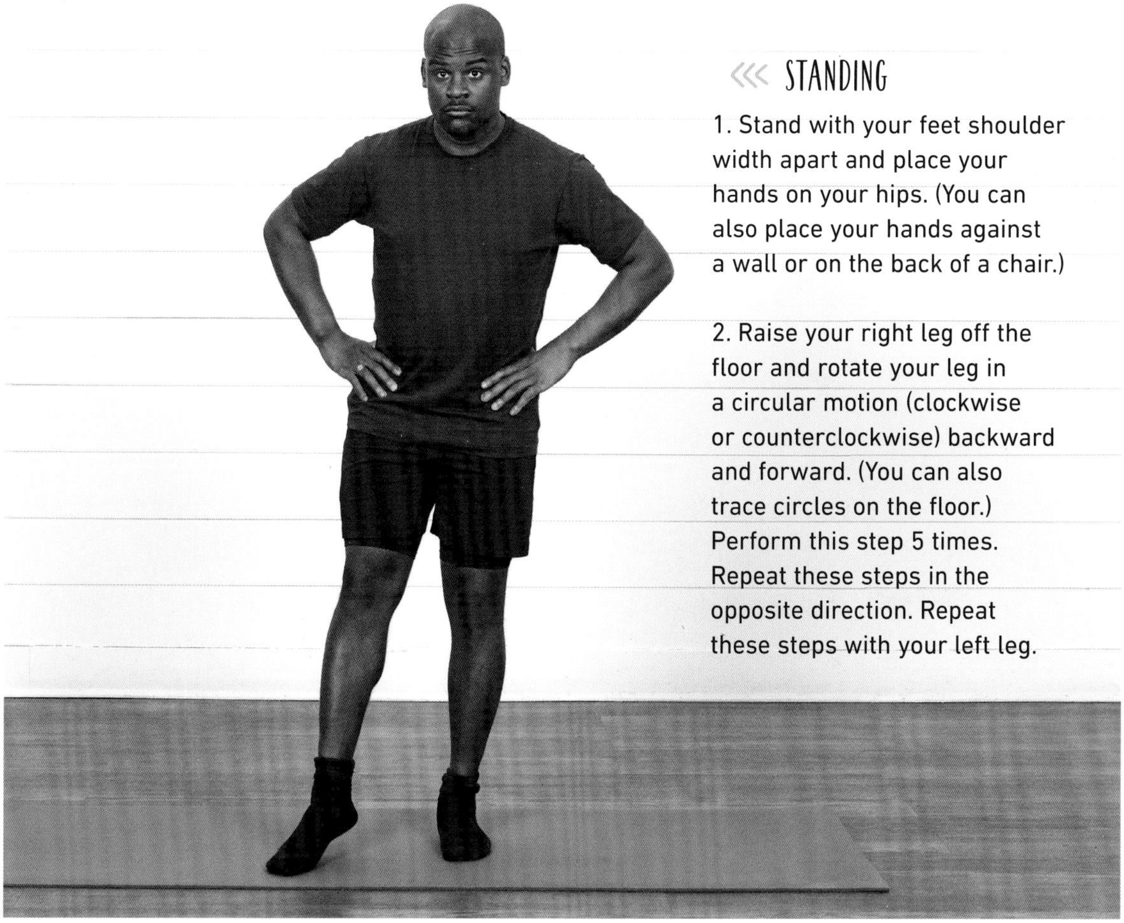

STANDING

1. Stand with your feet shoulder width apart and place your hands on your hips. (You can also place your hands against a wall or on the back of a chair.)

2. Raise your right leg off the floor and rotate your leg in a circular motion (clockwise or counterclockwise) backward and forward. (You can also trace circles on the floor.) Perform this step 5 times. Repeat these steps in the opposite direction. Repeat these steps with your left leg.

Rolling Like a Ball

To improve balance, strengthen your abs, and enhance spinal articulation (moving one vertebra at a time), and massage your spine, try this exercise. These movements can also help with spinal mobility, back flexibility, and balance. Rolling like a ball trains your upper and lower abs, which can help prevent back injuries and back pain.

1 Sit at the bottom of the mat. Bring your knees toward your chest and lower your head toward your chest. Place your hands on your shins and raise your feet off the floor.

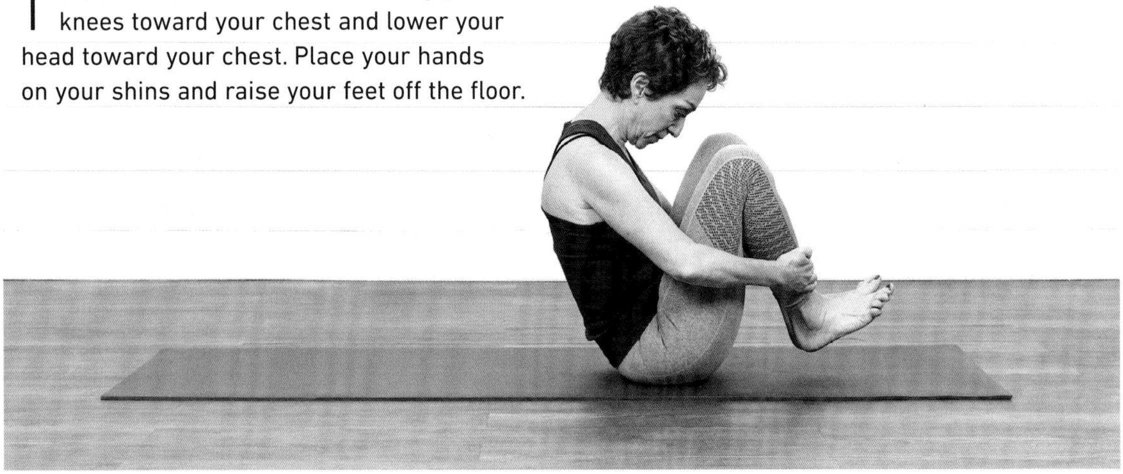

2 Begin to roll backward one vertebra at a time until your feet are parallel with the ceiling and your head is flat on the floor.

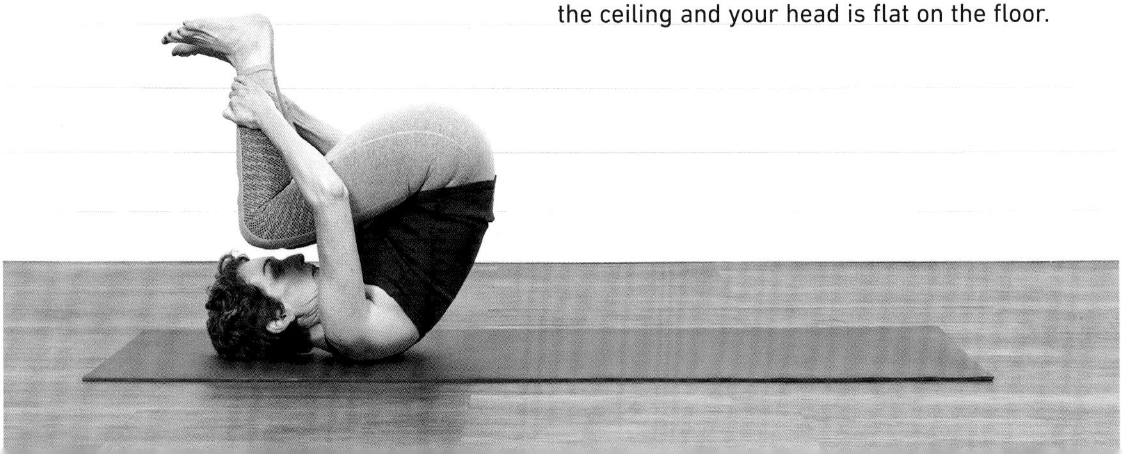

3 Lift your head and upper back off the floor as you begin to roll forward one vertebra at a time.

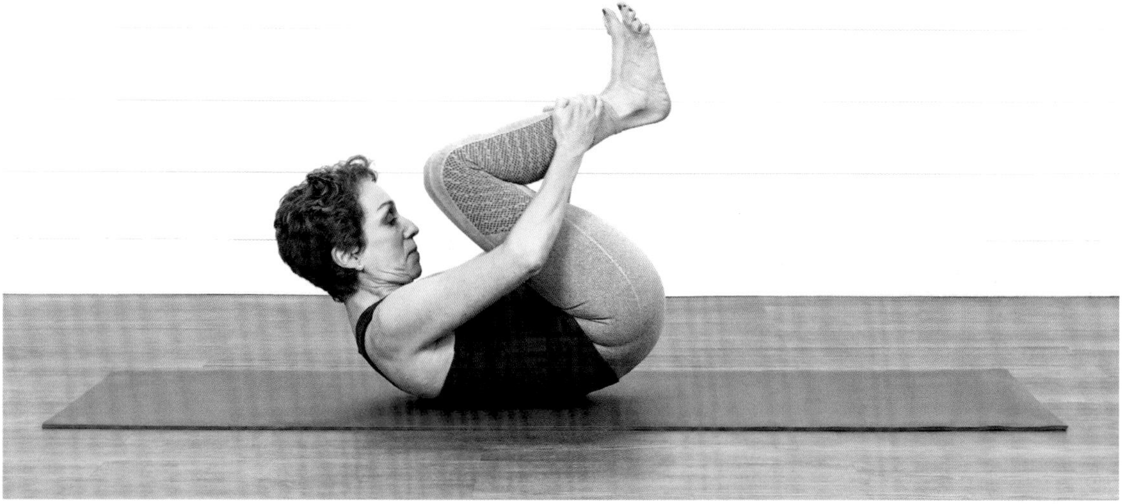

4 Continue to roll forward until you're sitting on your tailbone. Perform the last two steps 5 times.

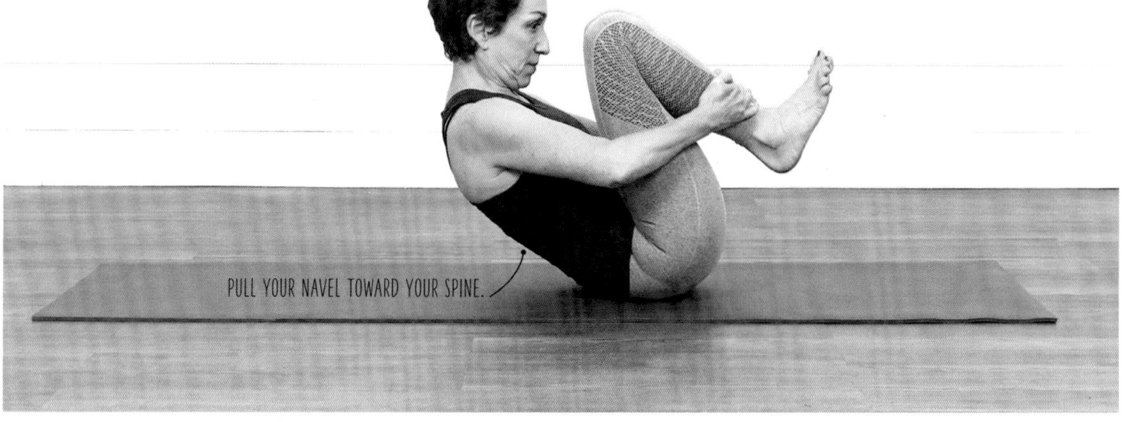
PULL YOUR NAVEL TOWARD YOUR SPINE.

ROLLING LIKE A BALL

VARIATIONS

Try these modifications if you have back or neck problems, osteoporosis, or herniated discs. If you have difficulty connecting to your abs, using a Pilates prop can help establish a greater core connection.

WITH THE MAGIC CIRCLE

In step 1, place the Magic Circle over your knees. Place your hands around the backs of your thighs. Continue with the remaining text.

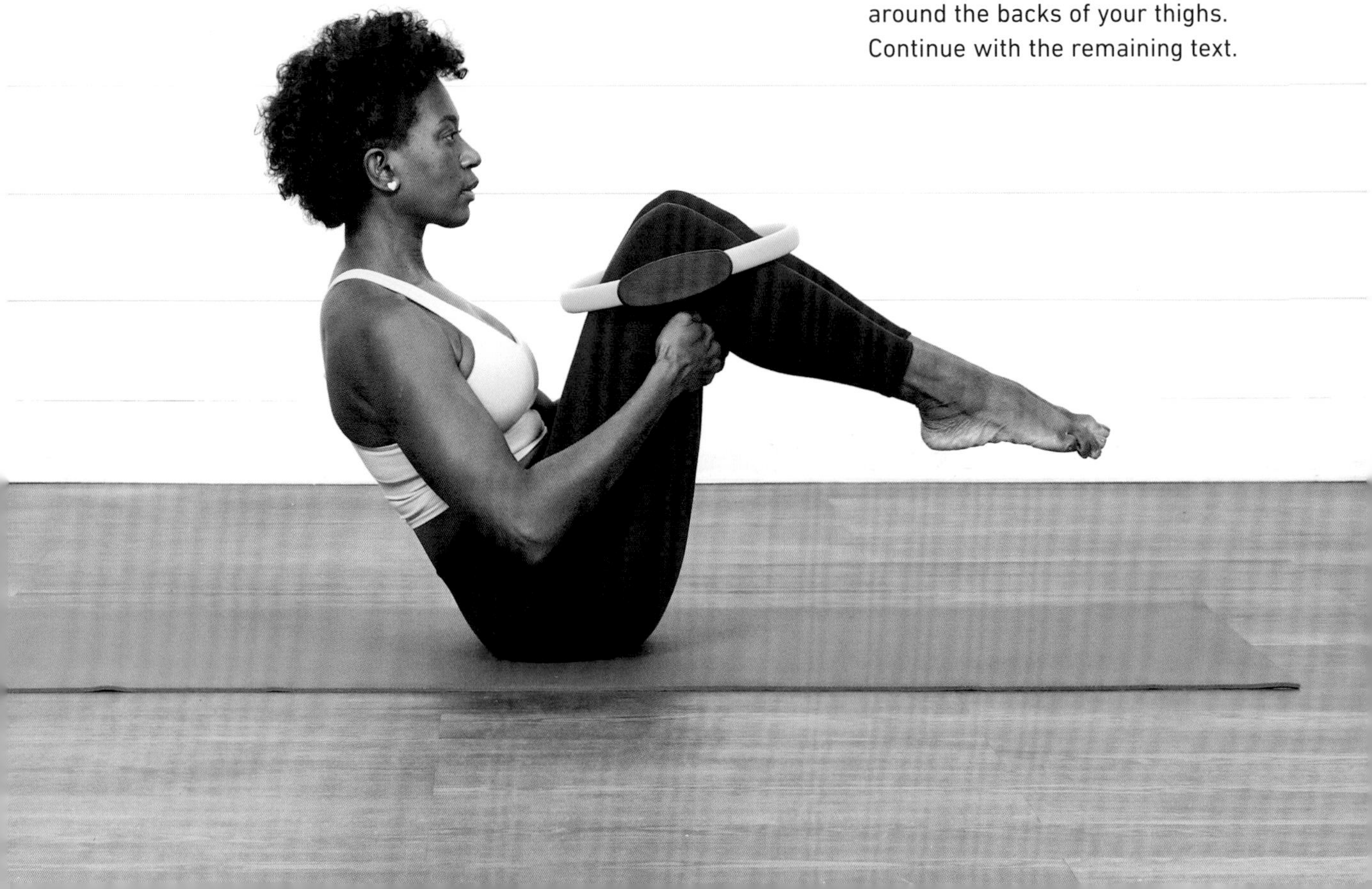

WITH A SMALL PILATES BALL

In step 1, place a small Pilates ball between your knees. Hold the ball in place throughout the exercise. Continue with the remaining text.

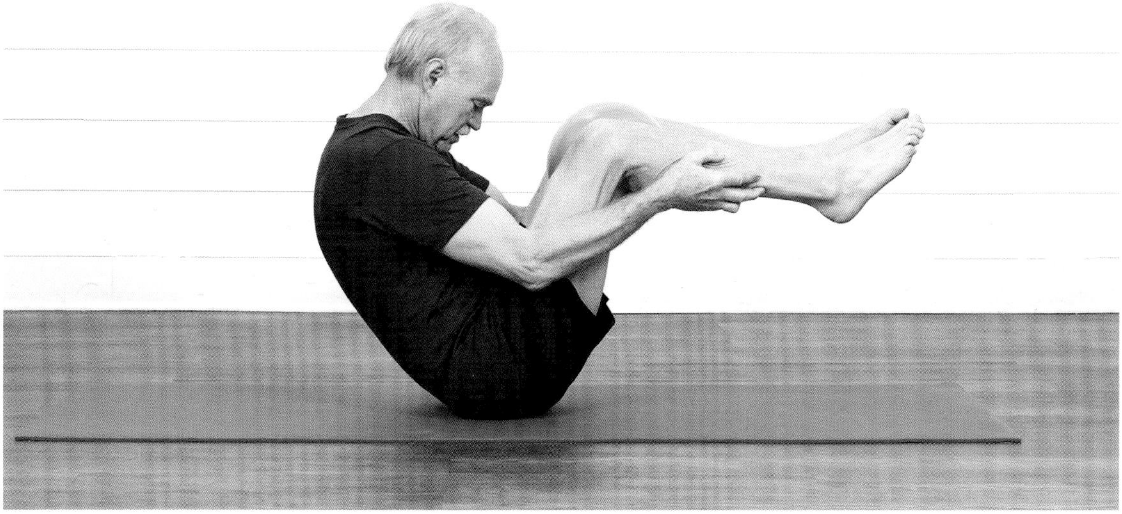

BALANCING

1. Sit at the top of the mat with your knees bent toward your chest. Place your hands under your thighs.

2. Raise your feet off the floor and balance your body just behind your sit bones. Hold this position for 3 seconds. Reverse your movements to return to your starting position. Perform these steps 5 times.

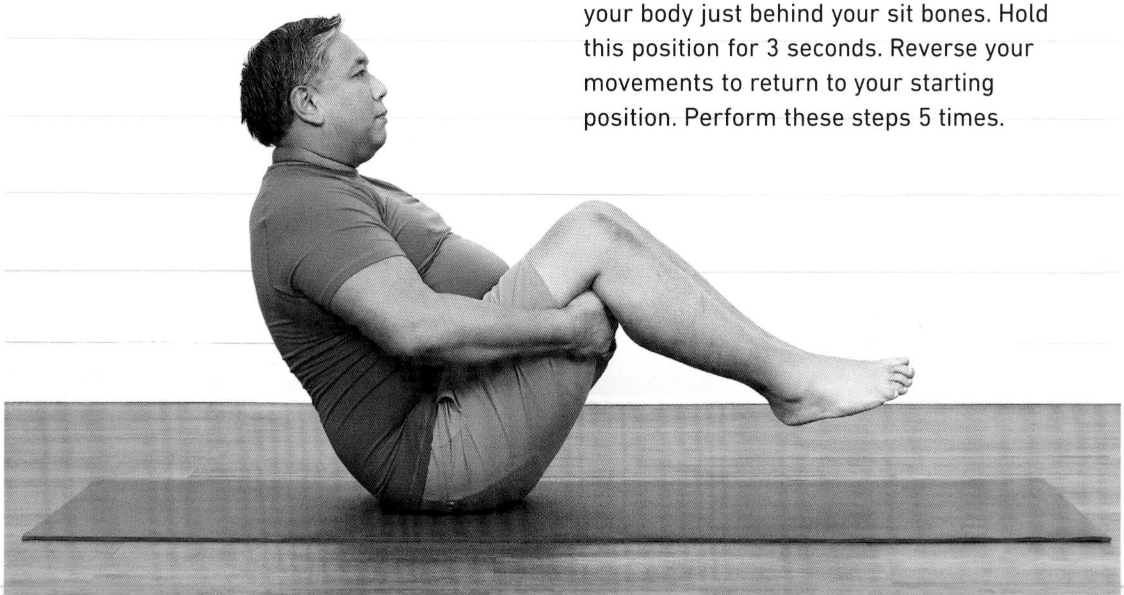

Forearm Kicks

Performing these kicks can improve strength in your hip flexors, abs, lower back, and shoulders. This exercise can also help you achieve greater core and shoulder stability while aiding in balance and proprioception (the awareness of movement of your body).

1 Sit on the floor with your knees bent to form a 45-degree angle with your legs. Lean backward and place your forearms and hands flat on the floor.

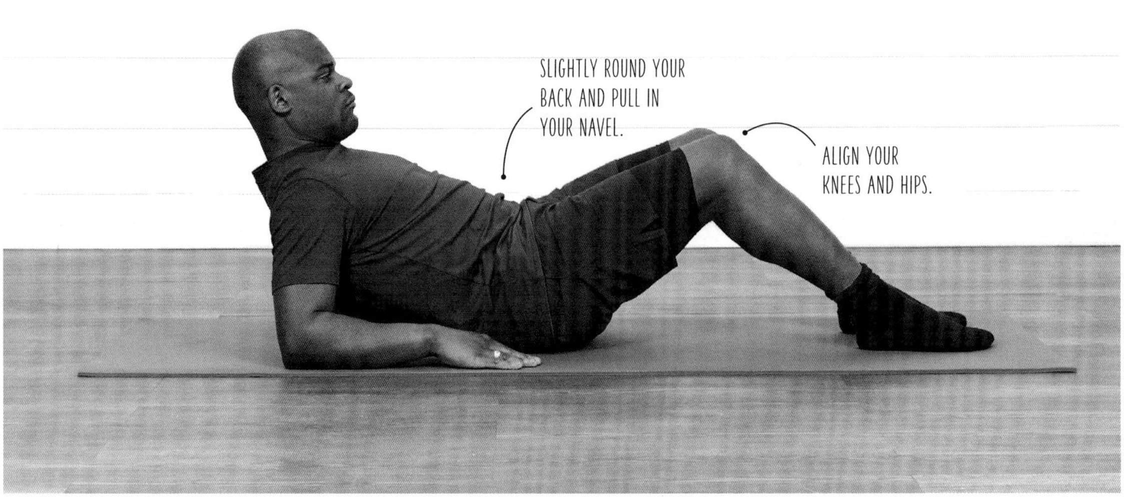

SLIGHTLY ROUND YOUR BACK AND PULL IN YOUR NAVEL.
ALIGN YOUR KNEES AND HIPS.

2 Raise your legs to form a 90-degree angle with the floor.

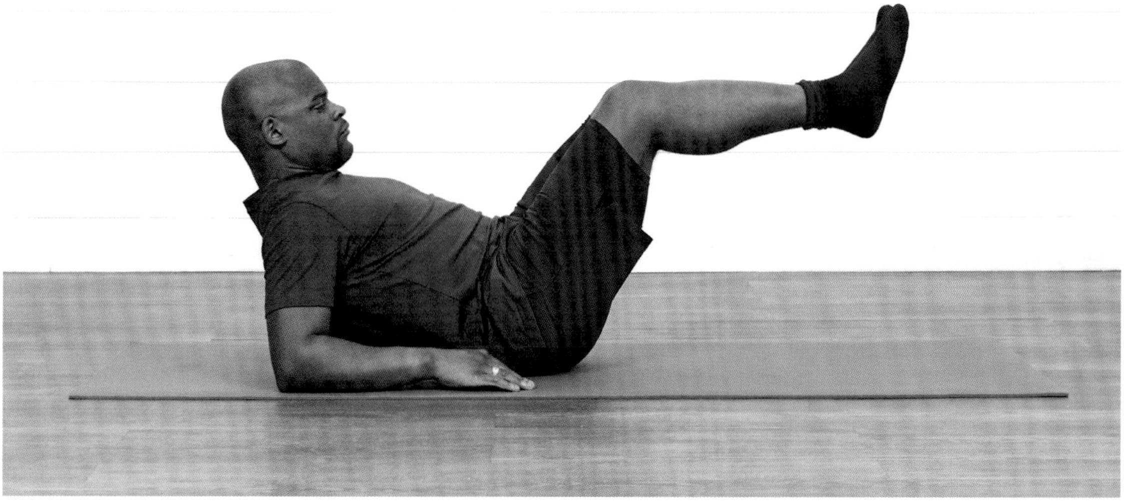

3 Straighten your right leg to form a 45-degree angle with the floor. Reverse your movements to return to your starting position. Perform these steps 5 times. Repeat these steps with your left leg straightened.

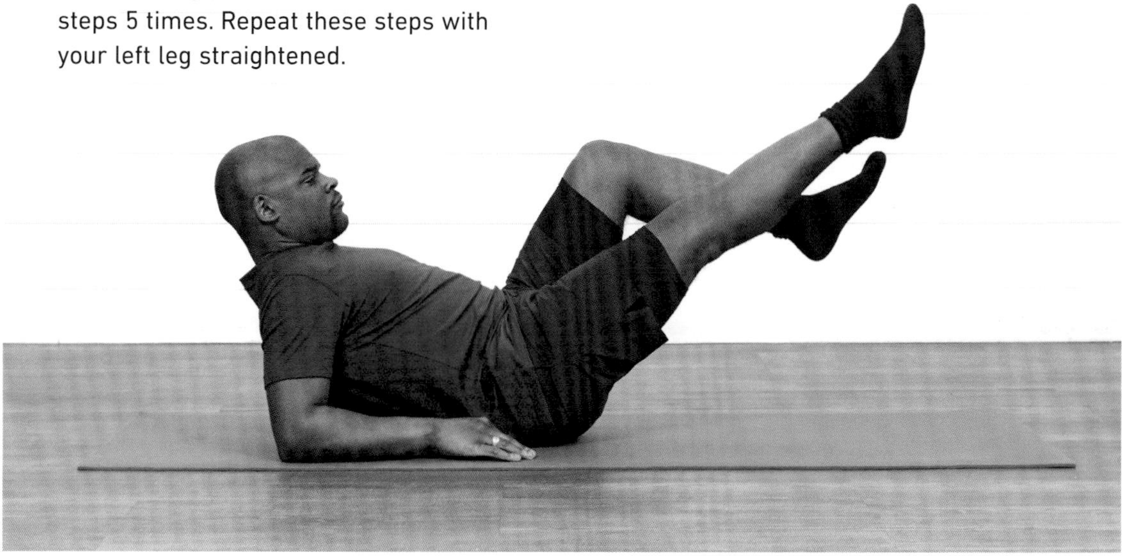

FOREARM KICKS

VARIATIONS

Lacking flexibility in your hamstrings or strength in your hip flexors and/or core might require you to modify this exercise. Using a prop might help with alignment, making the movements less challenging to perform.

WITH DIFFERENT LEG ANGLES

In step 2, keep your knees bent at a 45-degree angle.

In step 3, keep your bent knee at a 45-degree angle. Continue with the remaining text.

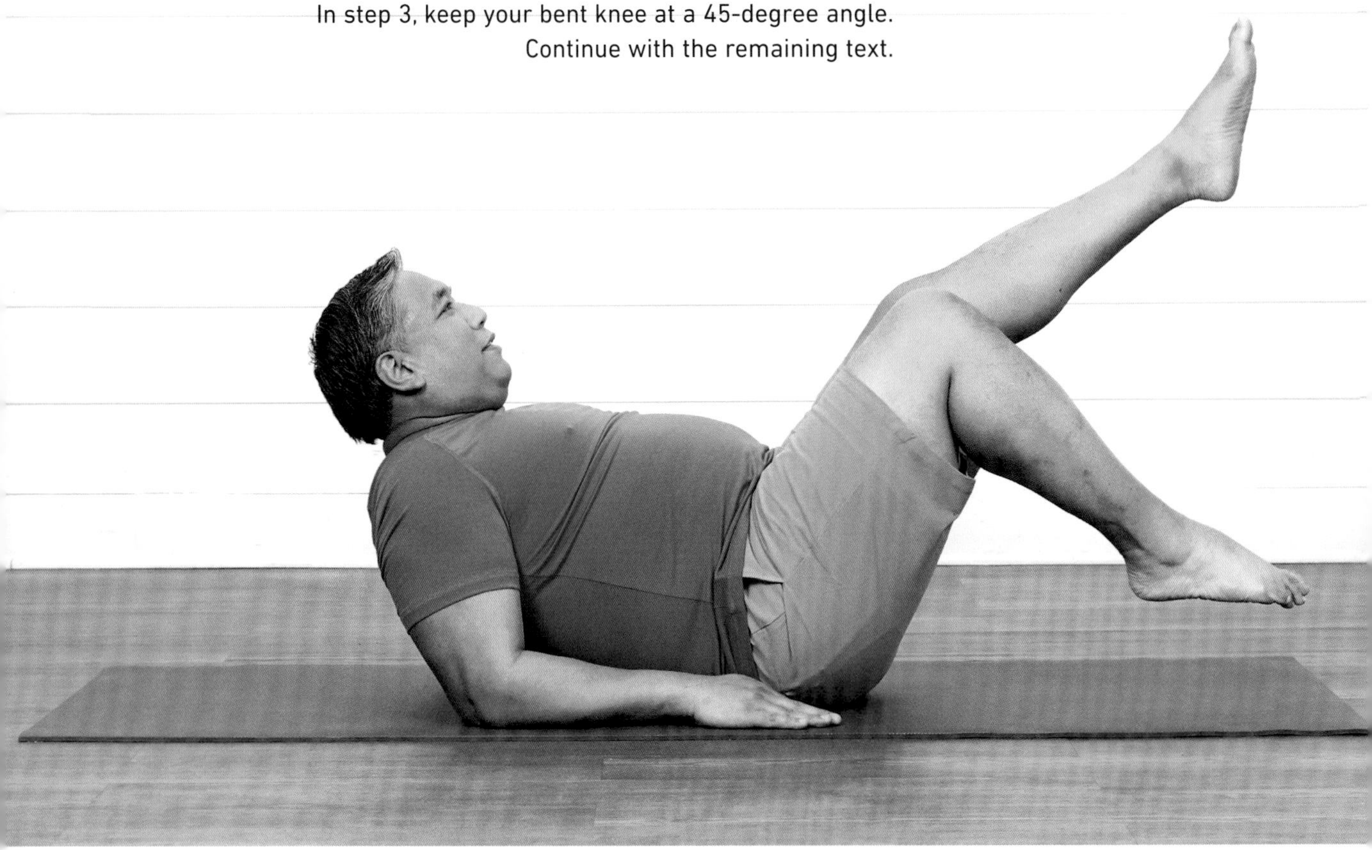

WITH A LOOP BAND »»

In step 1, place a loop band around your ankles.

In step 3, push against the band to create tension. Hold this position for 3 seconds. Continue with the remaining text.

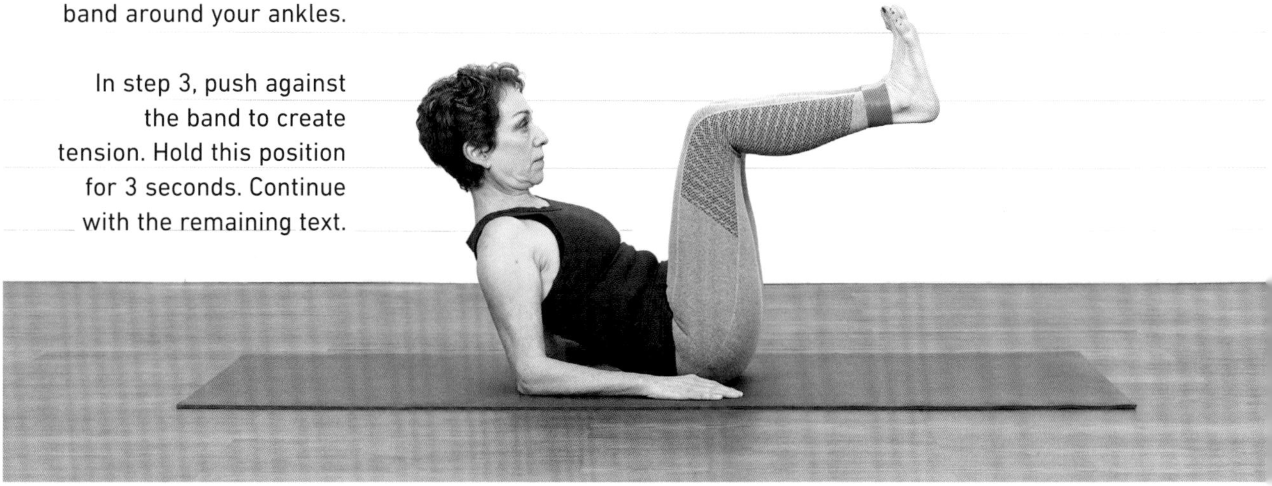

«« SITTING IN A CHAIR

1. Sit in a chair with your hands on the sides of the chair. Place your feet flat on the floor.

2. Extend your left leg until it's parallel with the floor. Reverse your movements to lower your left leg to the floor. Perform this step 6 times. Repeat these steps with your right leg extended.

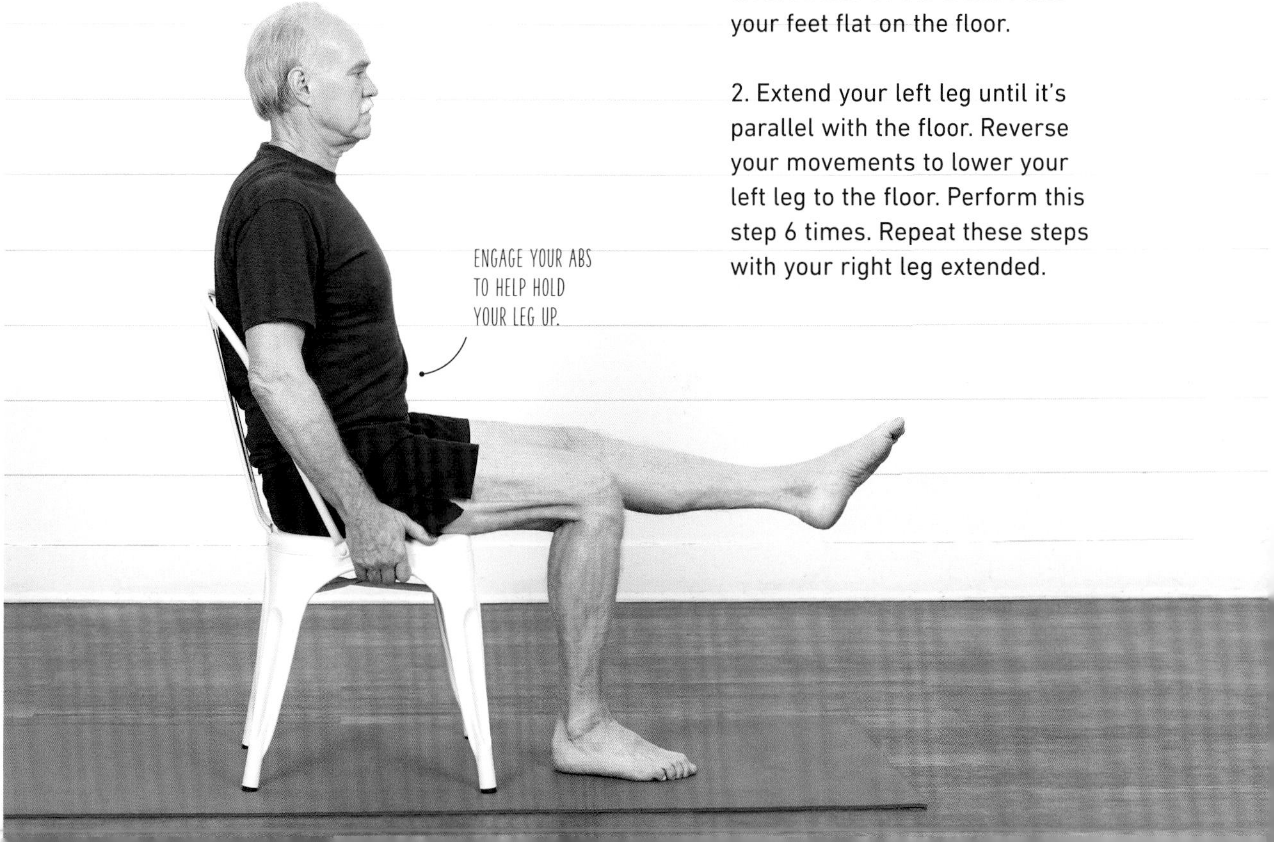

ENGAGE YOUR ABS TO HELP HOLD YOUR LEG UP.

JILLIAN PETERSON

It was late in my 20s that my fitness journey began. What started out as video workouts in my living room soon turned into live instruction of Pilates and yoga at a local studio. It wasn't long before I realized that my love for fitness would become a passion I wanted to share with others.

I decided to get my certification in yoga, and for the last five years, I've been teaching at various gyms around town. My mission has always been to welcome all students and ability levels and to meet each individual where they are in their personal fitness journey.

I enjoy creating an environment in my classes that helps foster a love and passion for the many benefits that fitness brings. I strive to make class accessible for all by using modifications and cues during instruction. By personally using these modifications, I've been able to maintain strength and flexibility throughout three pregnancies.

I've begun incorporating Pilates into my personal fitness routines to better help my body recover postdelivery and to provide core stability and strength for years to come.

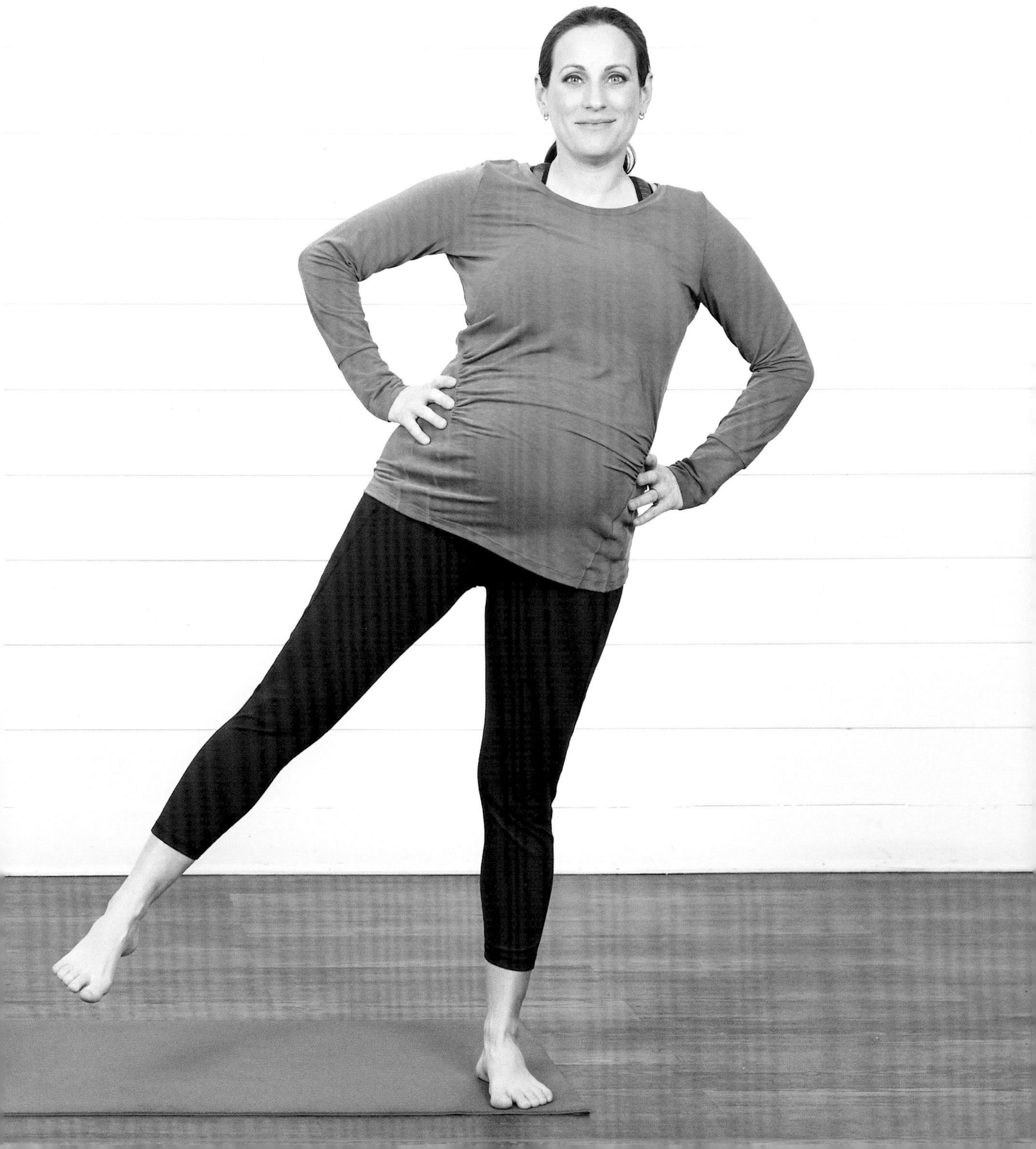

Push-Ups

This exercise is beneficial for building upper- and lower-body strength, working your chest, shoulder, arm, upper back, leg, and gluteal muscles. When you simultaneously engage large muscle groups, your heart must work harder to deliver oxygen-rich blood to muscle tissue, making this an effective cardiovascular exercise.

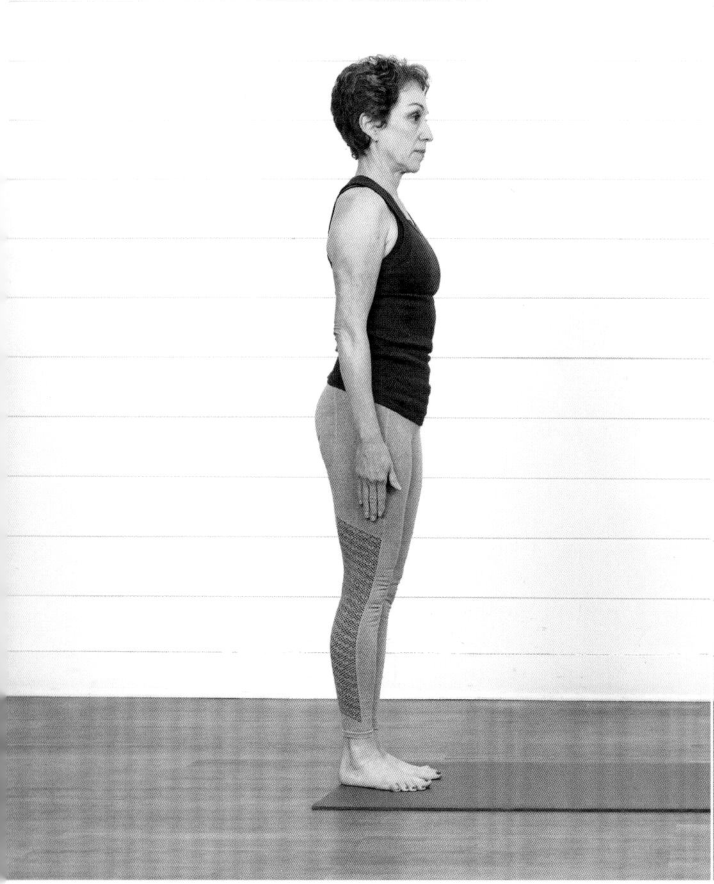

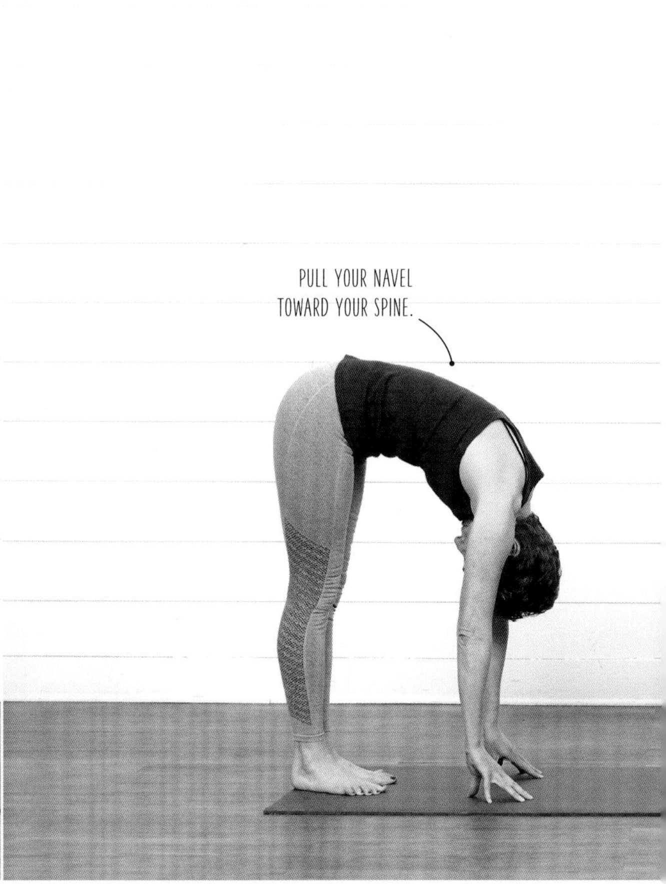
PULL YOUR NAVEL
TOWARD YOUR SPINE.

1 Stand at the back of the mat with your feet together. Relax your arms at your sides.

2 Walk your hands down the front of your legs and place your fingertips on the mat.

3 Walk your hands forward until they're under your shoulders and your heels are over your toes, forming a plank.

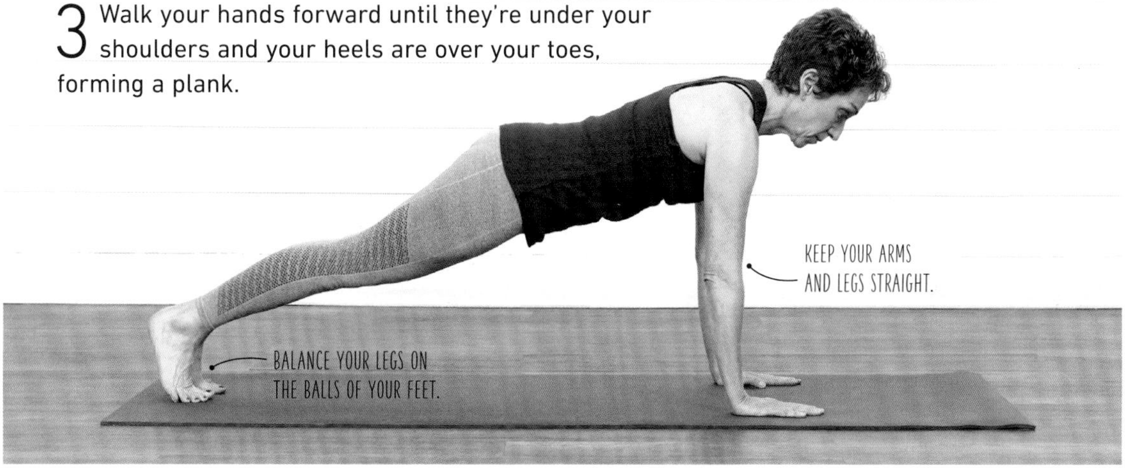

KEEP YOUR ARMS AND LEGS STRAIGHT.
BALANCE YOUR LEGS ON THE BALLS OF YOUR FEET.

4 Bend your elbows and lower your chest toward the floor.

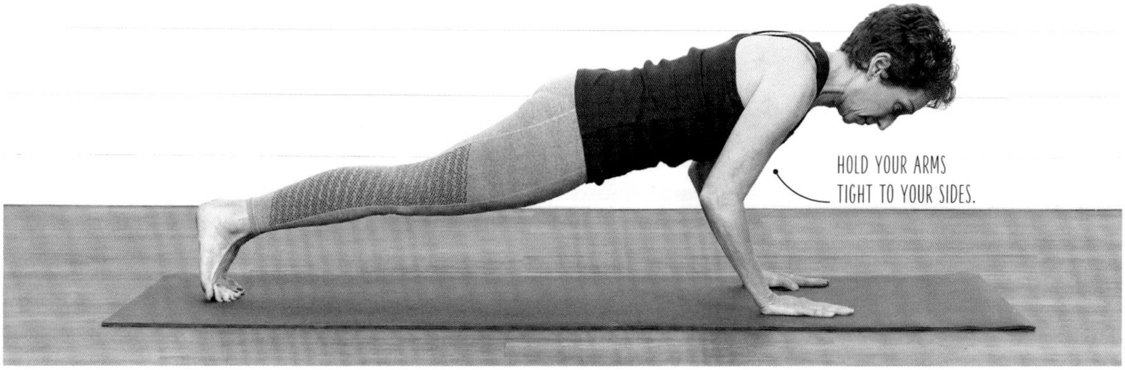

HOLD YOUR ARMS TIGHT TO YOUR SIDES.

5 Straighten your elbows and return to a plank. Perform the last three steps 2 times. Walk your hands toward your feet to return to your starting position. Repeat these steps 3 times.

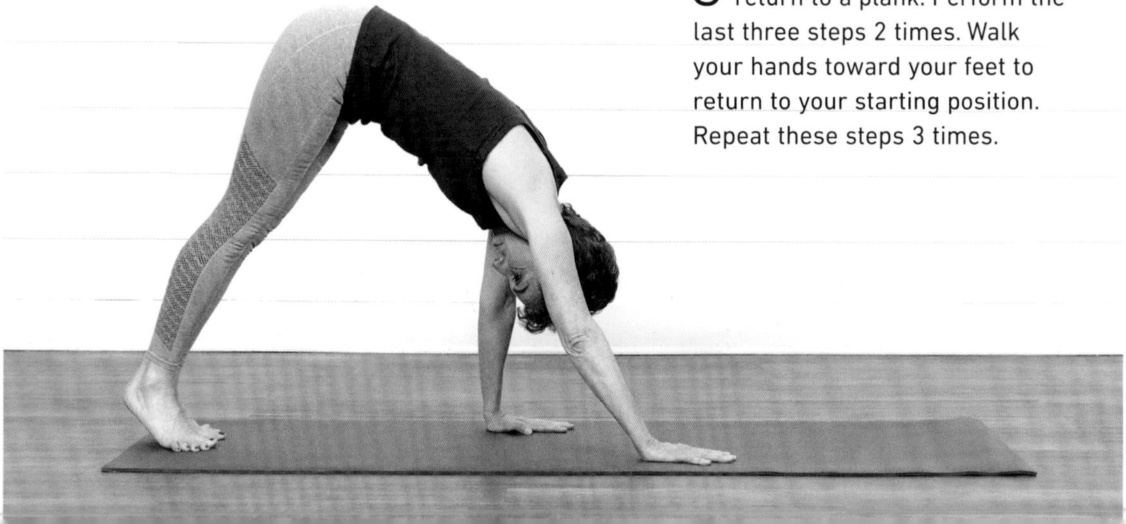

PUSH-UPS

VARIATIONS

If you can't completely support your own body weight or have suffered a shoulder injury, one of these variations might better suit you. You'll push less of your own body weight in each of the modifications.

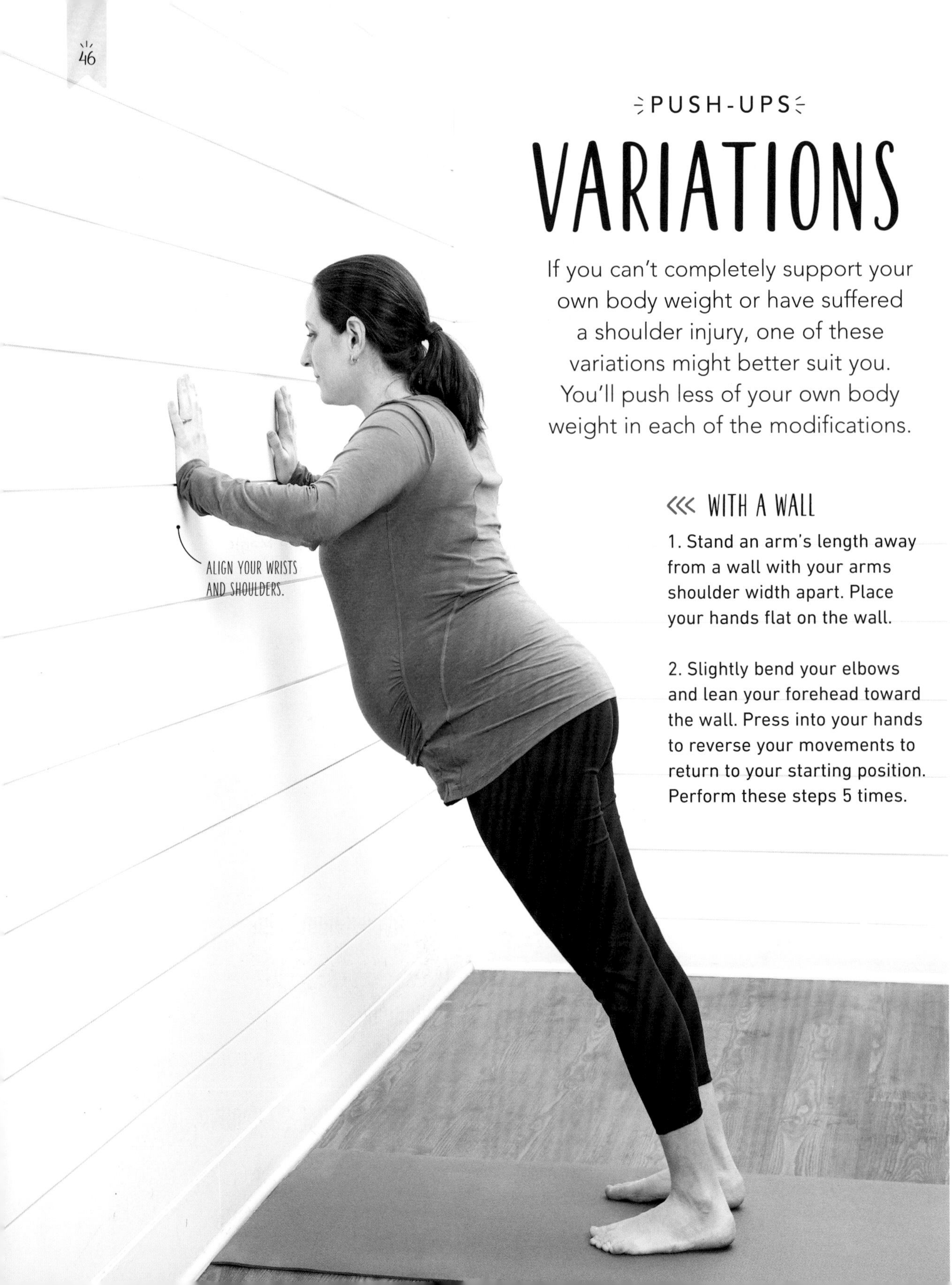
ALIGN YOUR WRISTS AND SHOULDERS.

WITH A WALL

1. Stand an arm's length away from a wall with your arms shoulder width apart. Place your hands flat on the wall.

2. Slightly bend your elbows and lean your forehead toward the wall. Press into your hands to reverse your movements to return to your starting position. Perform these steps 5 times.

ON YOUR KNEES >>>

In step 3, place your knees flat on the floor. Continue with the remaining text.

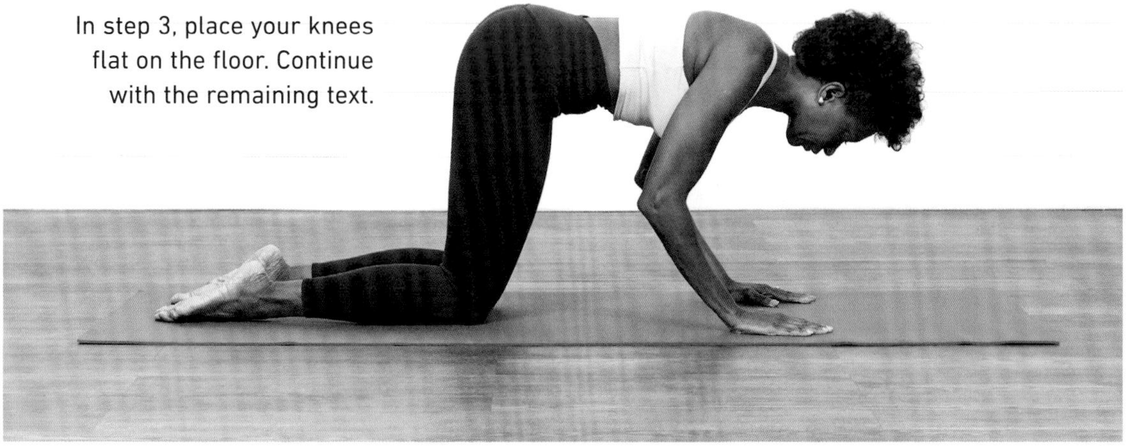

WITH THE MAGIC CIRCLE

1. Place your hands and knees flat on the floor. Place the Magic Circle vertically under your chest, with the outer pad pushing against the floor and the other side against your sternum.

2. Bend your elbows and lower your body toward the floor, slightly depressing the circle.

3. Slowly straighten your arms, resisting the circle as you return to your position in step 2. Perform the last two steps 6 times.

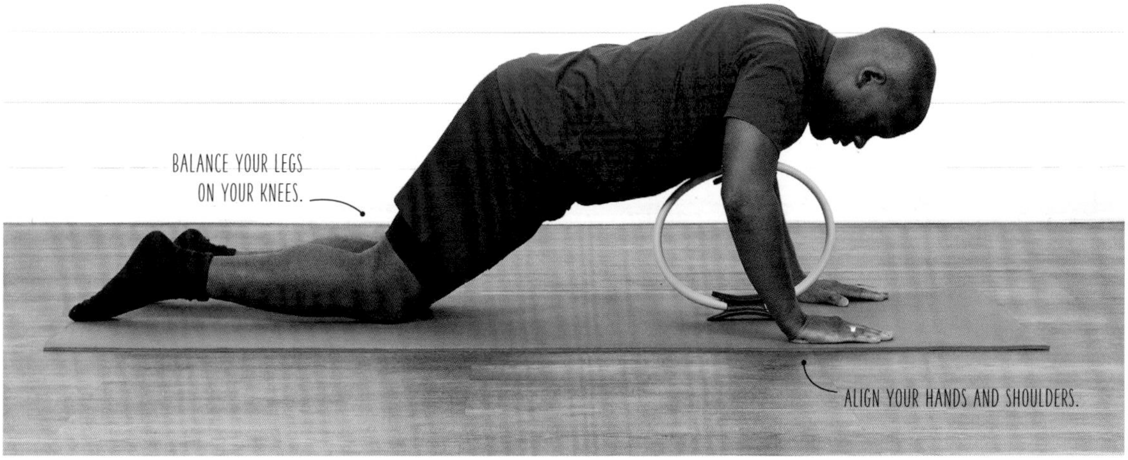

BALANCE YOUR LEGS ON YOUR KNEES.
ALIGN YOUR HANDS AND SHOULDERS.

Criss-Cross

This exercise works your entire core, with an emphasis on your obliques and lower abdominal muscles. Performing these movements can help improve overall posture and back strength. This exercise can also help prevent injuries and pain, especially that associated with the lower back.

1 Lie on your back on the floor with your hands behind your head. Raise your legs and bend your knees to form a 90-degree angle with the floor.

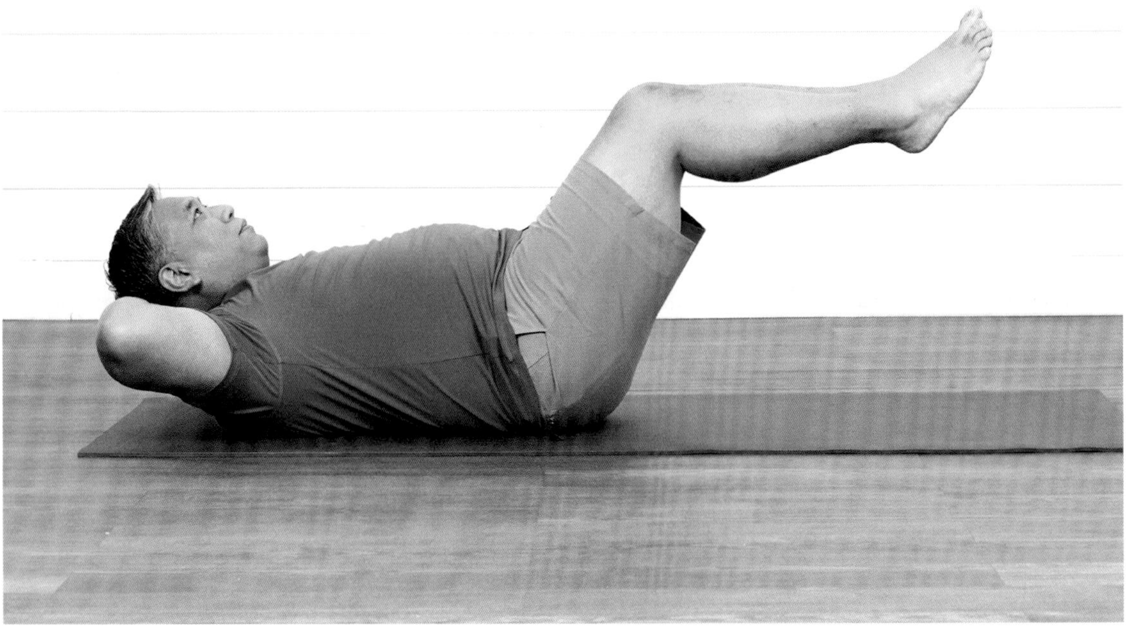

2 Straighten your left leg while rotating your upper body toward your right knee.

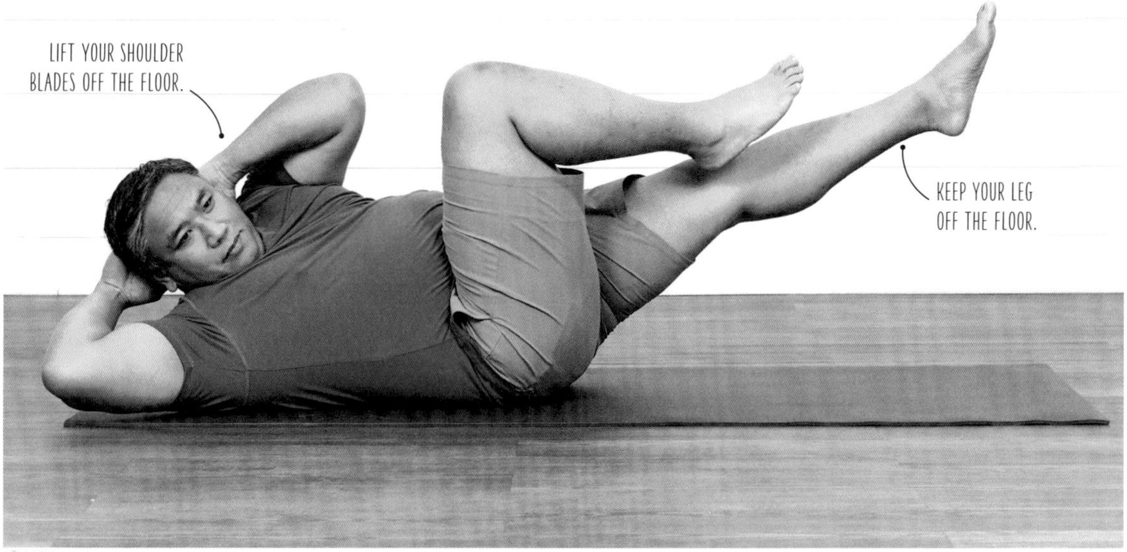

LIFT YOUR SHOULDER
BLADES OFF THE FLOOR.
KEEP YOUR LEG
OFF THE FLOOR.

3 Reverse your movements to bend your left knee and straighten your right leg while rotating your upper body toward your left knee. Perform the last two steps 10 times.

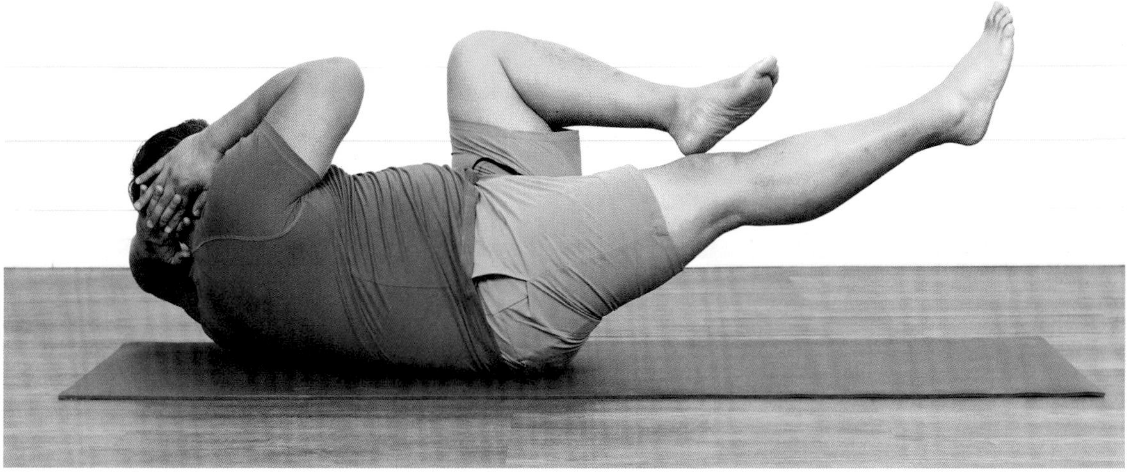

CRISS-CROSS

VARIATIONS

Modifying this exercise can stabilize your hips and trunk while allowing you to develop a better oblique and abdominal connection. You'll also stabilize your hips when moving your legs.

WITH A STRAIGHT LEG

In step 2, extend your right leg toward the ceiling.

In step 3, extend your left leg toward the ceiling. Continue with the remaining text.

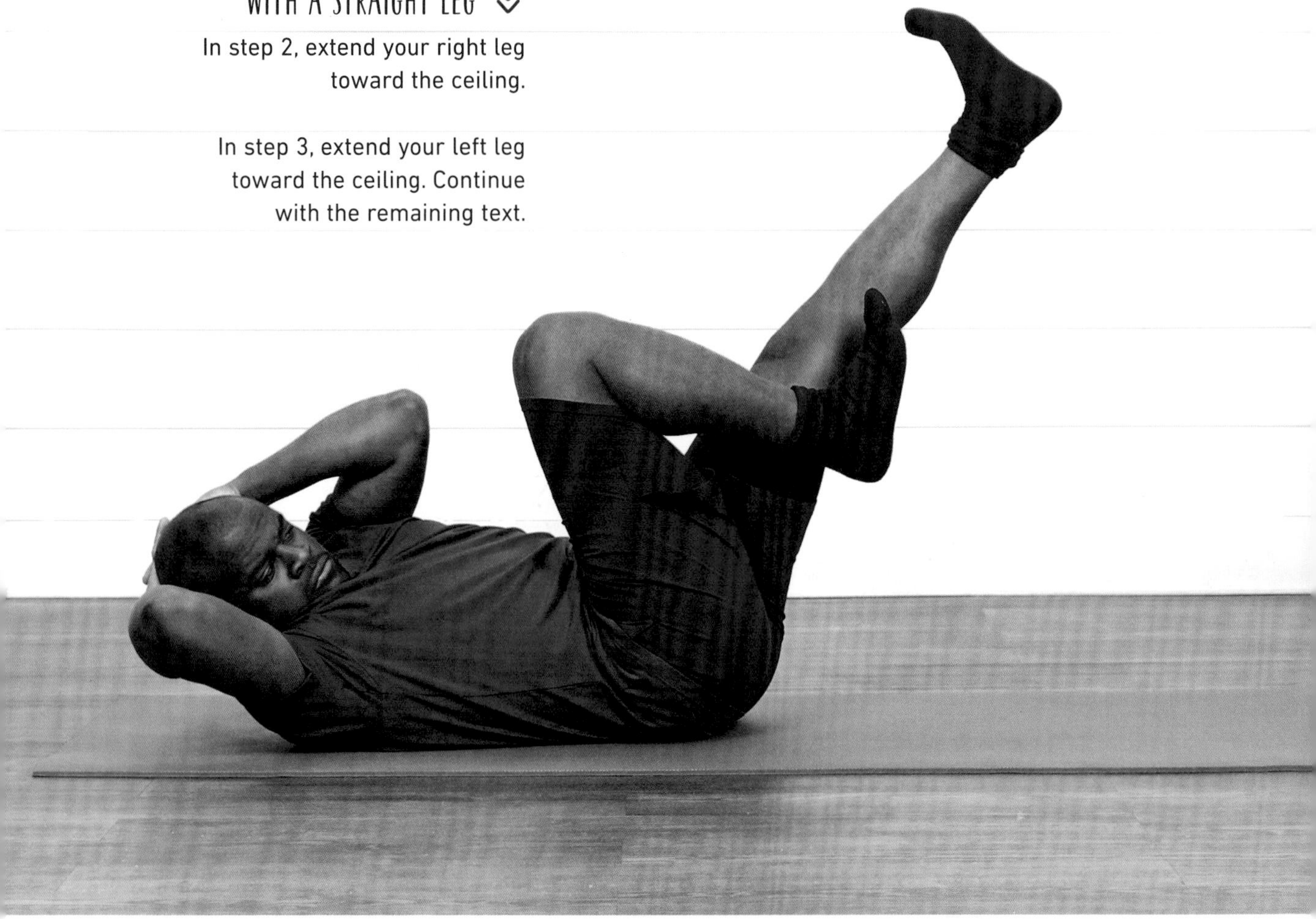

WITH THE MAGIC CIRCLE

In step 1, place one pad of the Magic Circle around the base of your head and hold the opposite pad with both hands. Continue with the remaining text. (You can either rotate or stay stationary.)

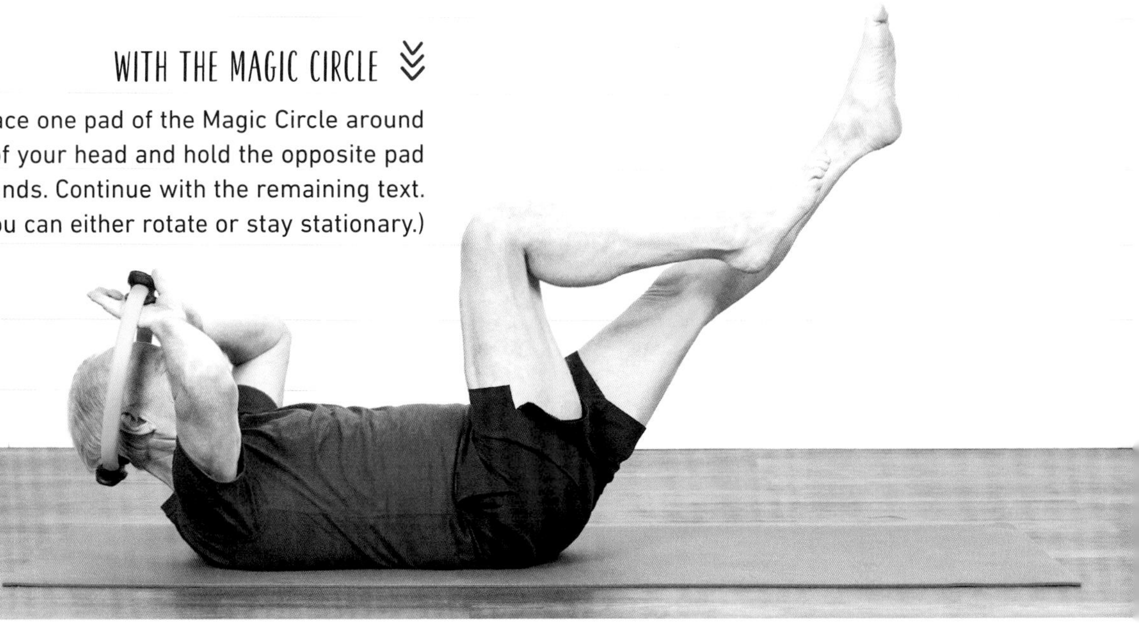

SITTING IN A CHAIR

1. Sit in a chair with your hands behind your head and your feet flat on the floor.

2. Raise your left leg to parallel with the floor while rotating your torso toward your left side. Reverse your movements to lower your left leg to the floor.

3. Raise your right leg to parallel with the floor and rotate your upper body toward your right side. Reverse your movements to lower your right leg to the floor. Perform the last two steps 10 times—one at a time or in a continuous motion.

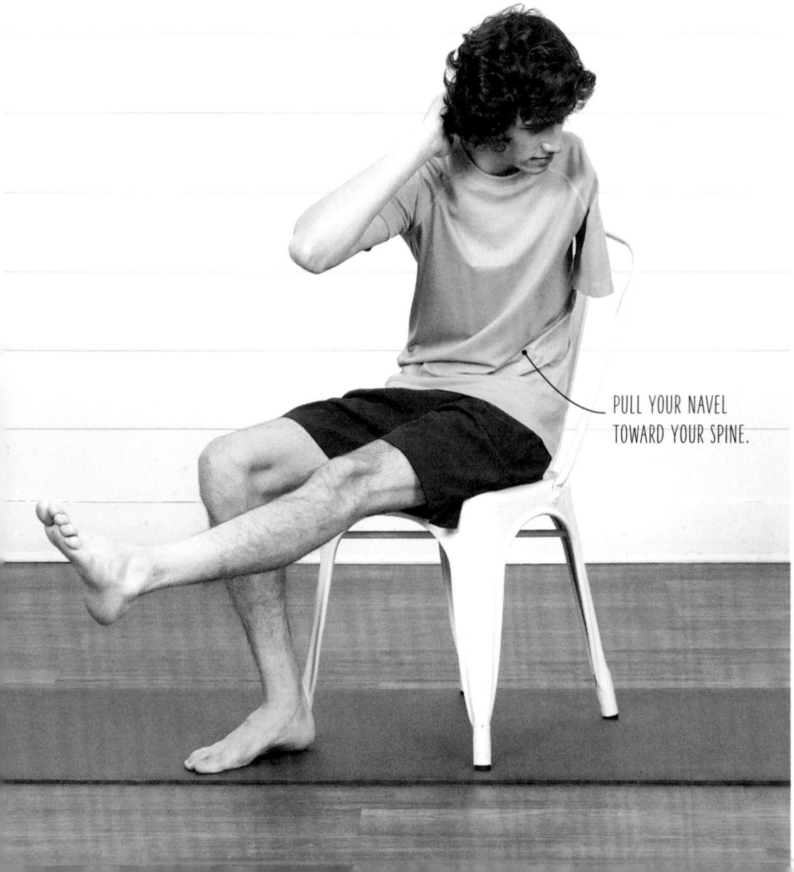
PULL YOUR NAVEL
TOWARD YOUR SPINE.

Scissors

These movements can strengthen your abdominal and shoulder muscles while increasing hip and hamstring flexibility. This exercise is great for challenging your torso stability and balance. You have to keep everything steady in your hips and torso as you move your legs with control.

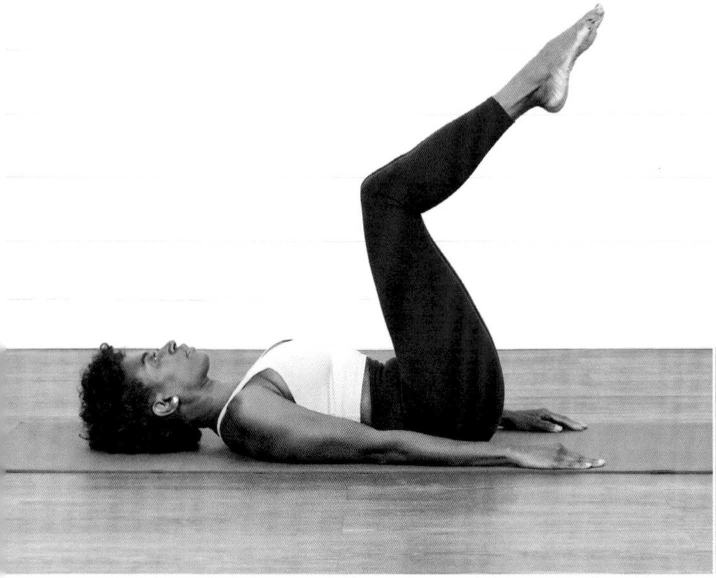

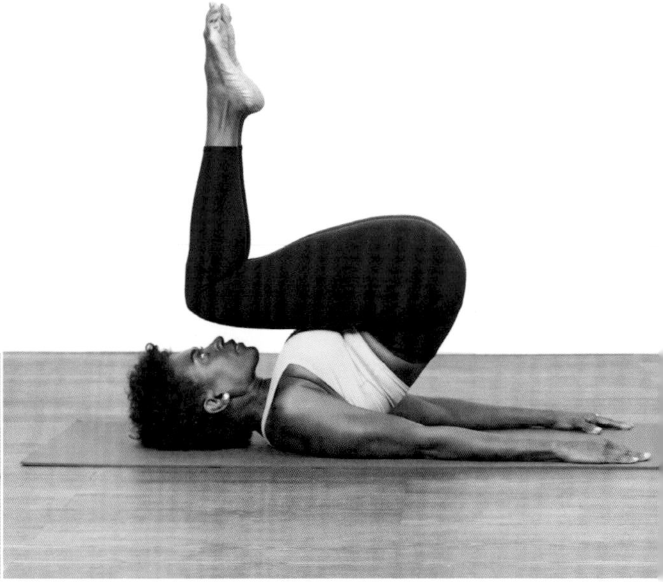

1 Lie on your back on the floor with your knees bent toward your chest. Relax your arms at your sides and place your hands flat on the floor.

2 Bring your knees toward your head until your legs form a 90-degree angle. Keep your head and upper back flat on the floor.

3 Place your hands on your buttocks. Keep your upper arms flat on the floor.

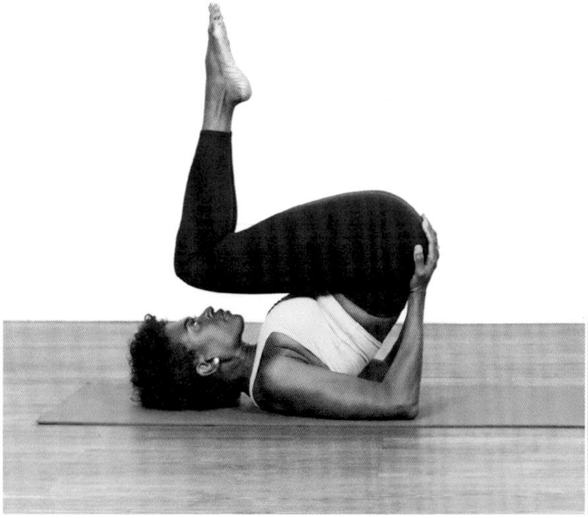

4 Extend your legs toward the ceiling, using your hands to support your body weight.

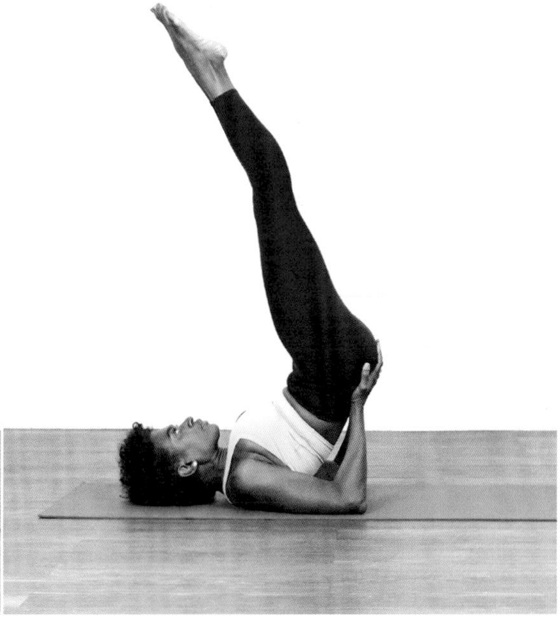

5 Extend your right leg toward the top of the mat, stopping a few inches from the floor above your head. Pulse your right leg 2 times. End with your right leg in its starting position. Perform the last two steps 6 times. Repeat these steps with your left leg extended.

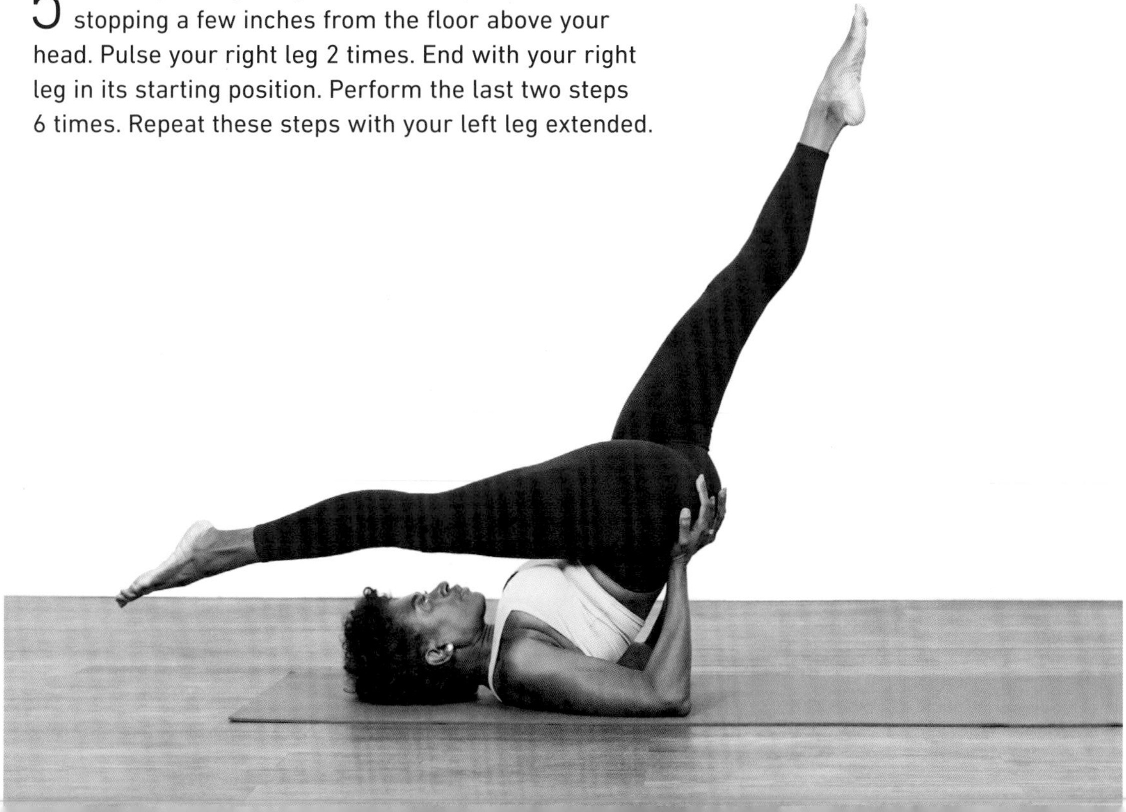

SCISSORS

VARIATIONS

Avoid the main exercise if you have back or neck problems, osteoporosis, or herniated discs. If you have difficulty connecting to your abs, performing this exercise on your back or in a chair will prove beneficial.

WITH YOUR BACK ON THE FLOOR

1. Lie on your back on the floor. Relax your arms at your sides and extend your legs toward the ceiling.

2. Lower your left leg toward the floor, stopping about one foot away. Hold this position for 2 to 3 seconds. Reverse your movements to return to your starting position. Perform these steps 8 times. Repeat these steps with your right leg lowered.

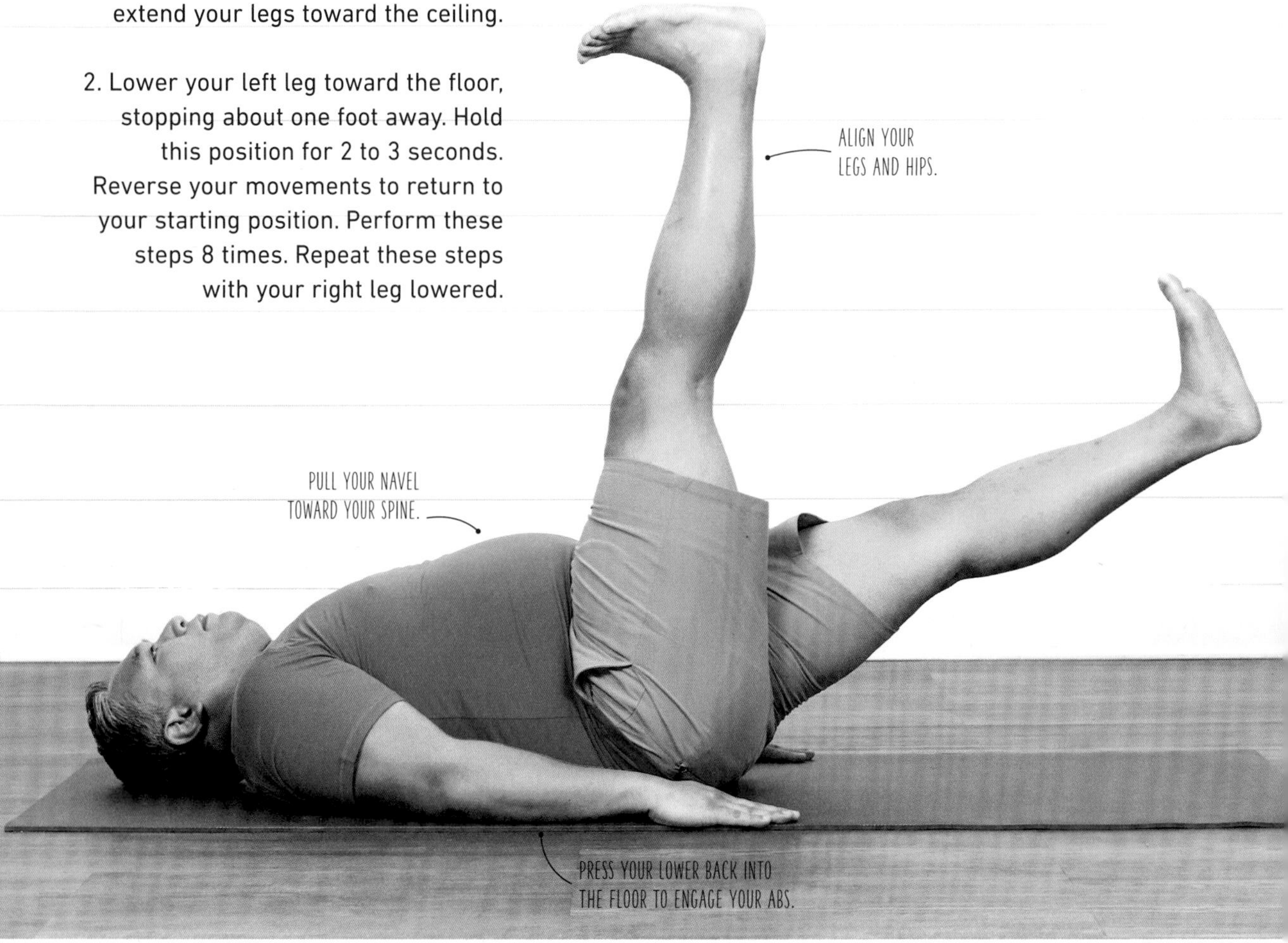
ALIGN YOUR LEGS AND HIPS.
PULL YOUR NAVEL TOWARD YOUR SPINE.
PRESS YOUR LOWER BACK INTO THE FLOOR TO ENGAGE YOUR ABS.

WITH A LOOP BAND

1. Lie on your back on the floor with a loop band around your ankles. Relax your arms at your sides.

2. Raise your right leg as high as possible while pressing your left leg into the floor. Reverse your movements to lower your right leg to the floor. Perform these steps 8 times. Repeat these steps with your left leg lifted.

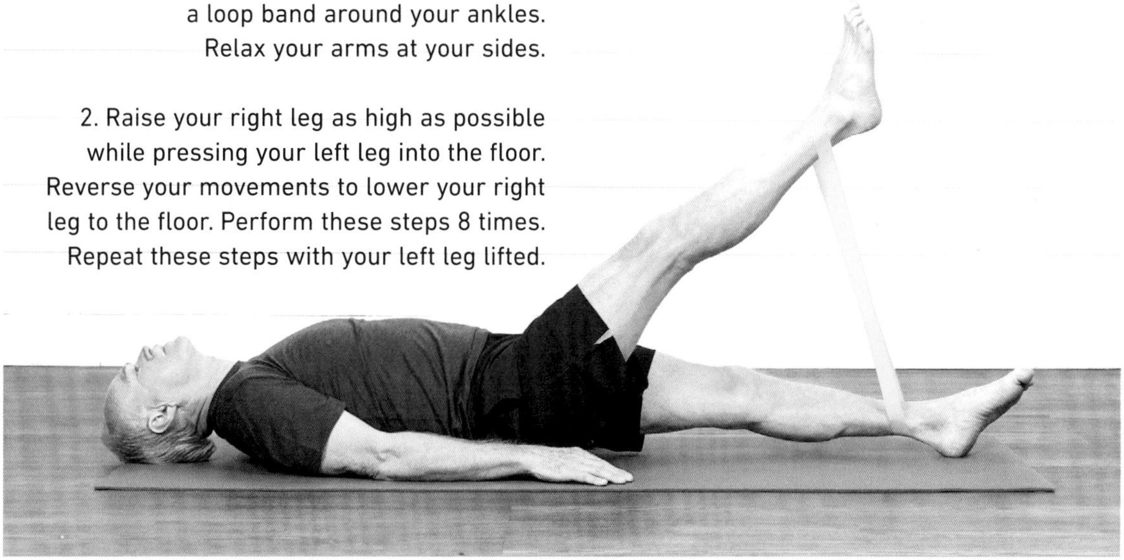
FLEX YOUR FEET TOWARD YOUR BODY.

SITTING IN A CHAIR

1. Sit in a chair with your legs extended forward and your hands behind your head or on the sides of the chair.

2. Lower your right leg toward the floor and tap your toes on the floor. Reverse your movements to return to your starting position. Perform these steps 5 times. Repeat these steps with your left leg lowering.

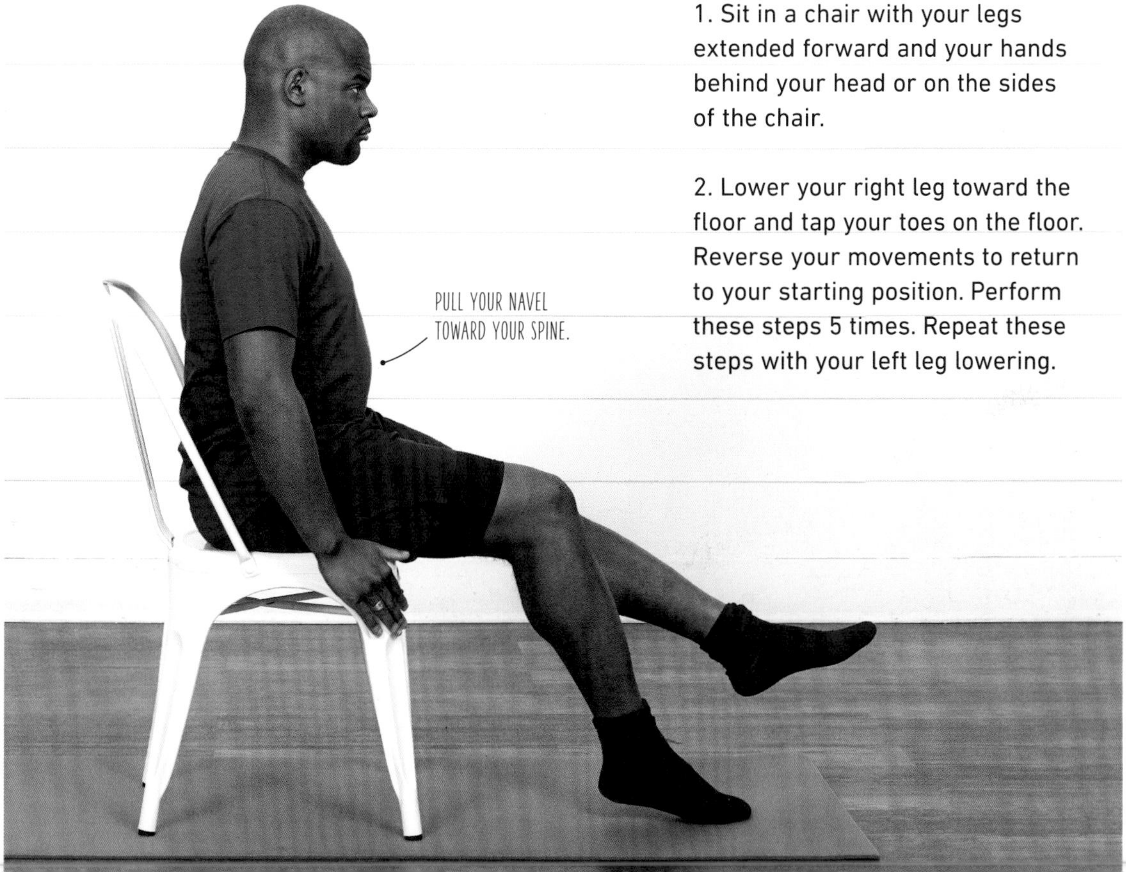
PULL YOUR NAVEL TOWARD YOUR SPINE.

Bicycle

This exercise challenges your core and shoulder stability while stretching your hip flexors and hamstrings. These movements will simultaneously work your legs, buttocks, abs, shoulders, and arms. You must maintain torso stability with the leg movements, which can help improve balance.

1 Lie on your back on the floor with your knees bent toward your chest. Place your hands on your back just above your hips to support the weight of your pelvis.

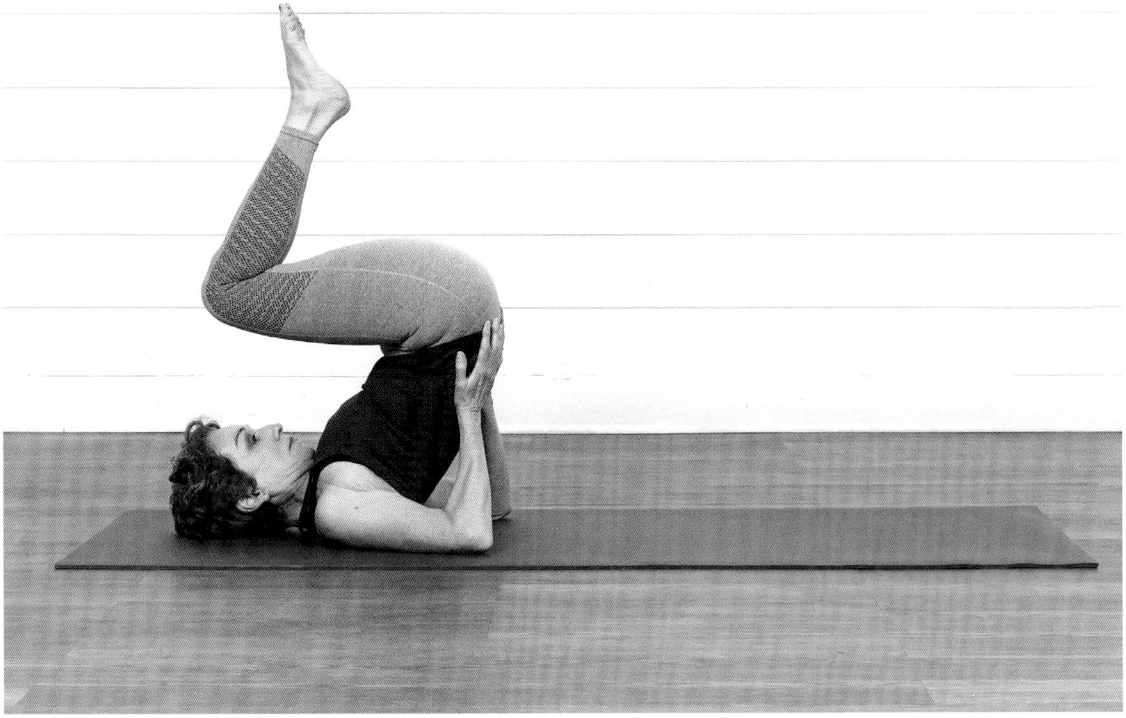

2 Extend your right leg toward the ceiling until aligned with your body.

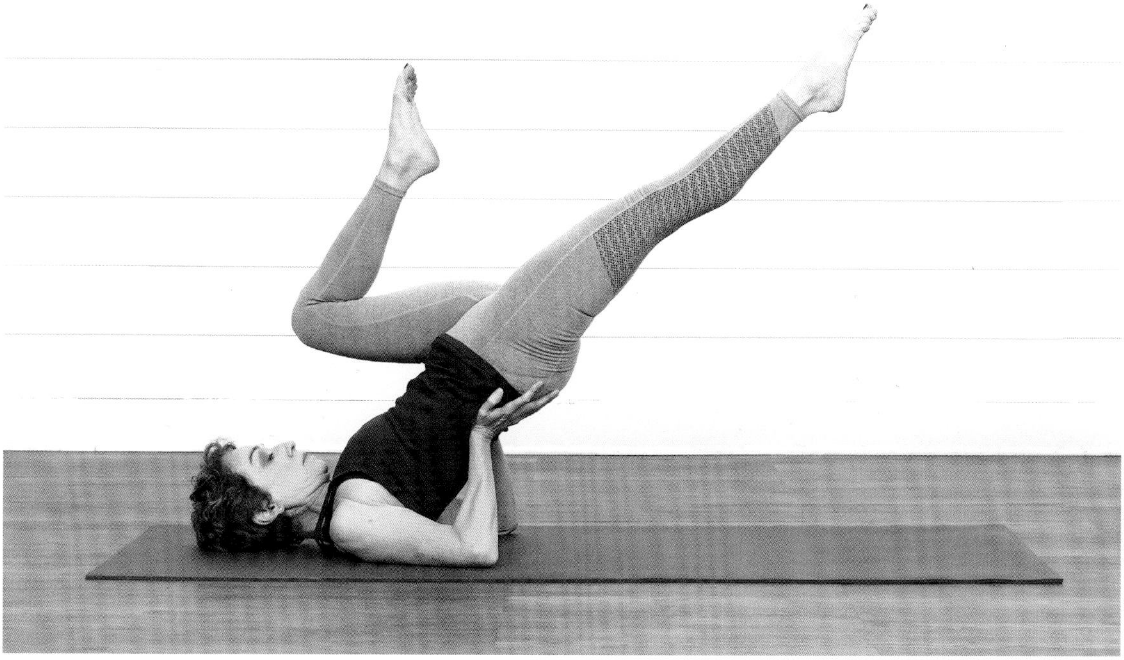

3 As you reverse your movements, extend your left leg toward the ceiling until aligned with your body. Perform the last two steps 10 times.

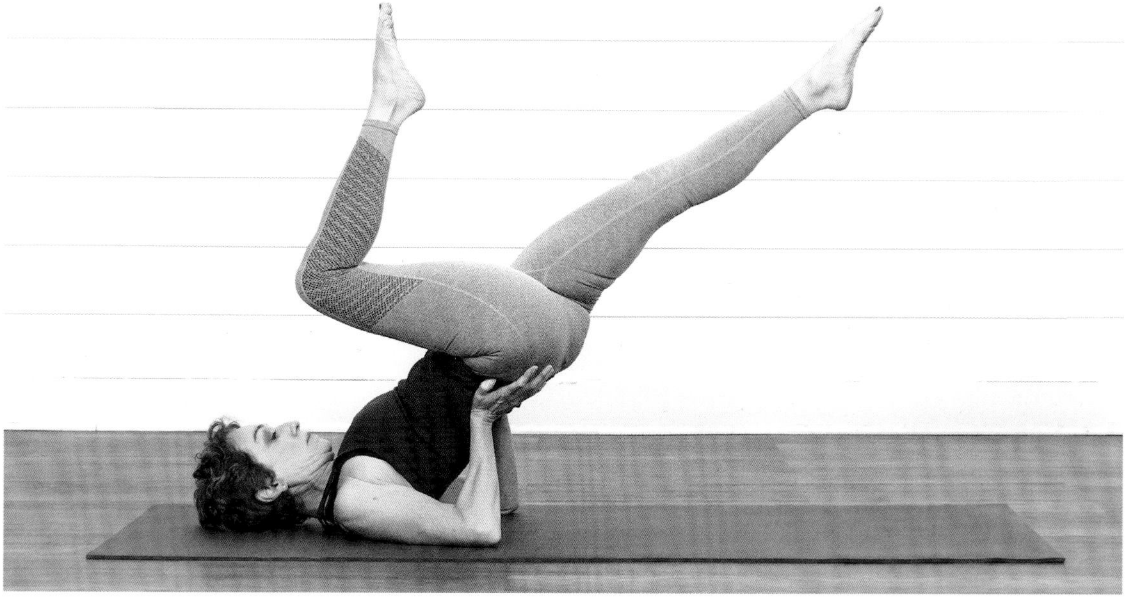

BICYCLE

VARIATIONS

If you lack the flexibility in your lower back or the strength to lift and support your body off the floor, the variations are good options. You can use these modifications to build the strength required to perform the main exercise.

WITH A SMALL PILATES BALL

1. Sit on the floor with your knees bent and place a small Pilates ball at your lower back. Relax your arms at your sides and place your hands flat on the floor.

2. Lean backward and place your forearms flat on the floor.

3. Extend your right leg at a 45-degree angle from the floor while bringing your left knee toward your chest.

4. Extend your left leg at a 45-degree angle from the floor while bringing your right knee toward your chest. Perform the last two steps 12 times.

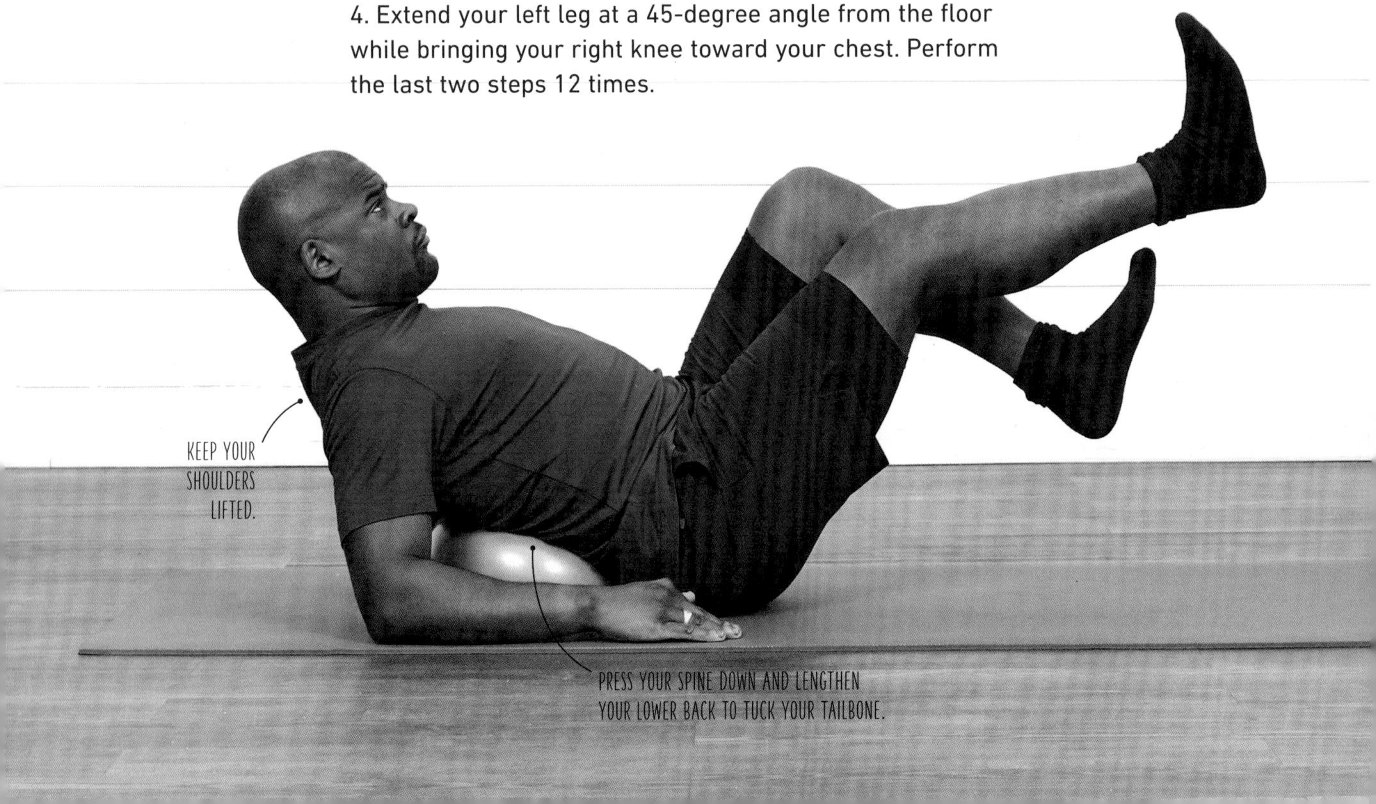

KEEP YOUR SHOULDERS LIFTED.
PRESS YOUR SPINE DOWN AND LENGTHEN YOUR LOWER BACK TO TUCK YOUR TAILBONE.

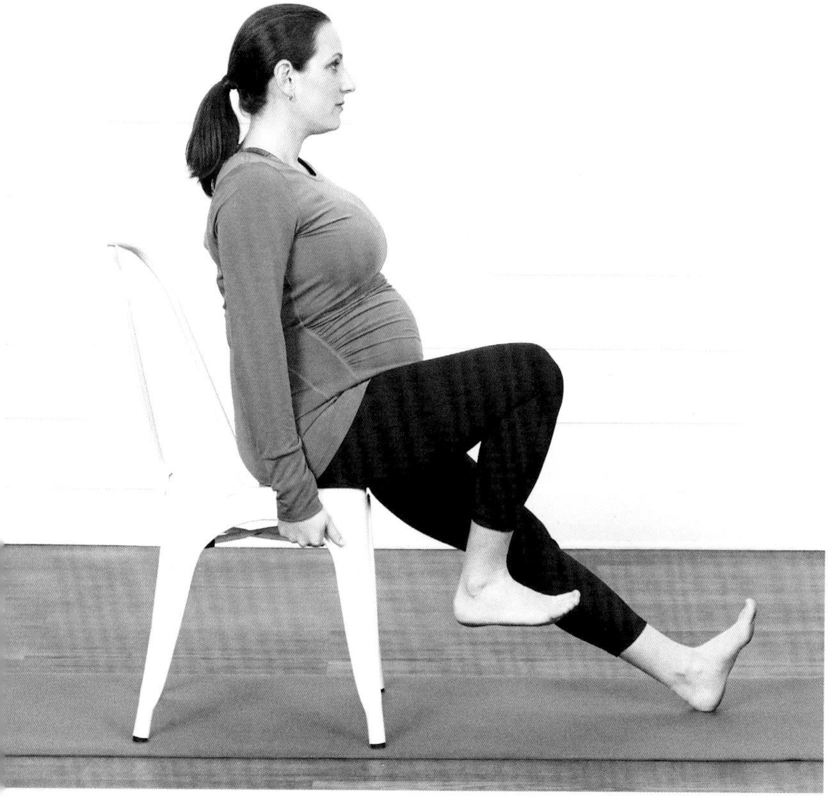

⋘ SITTING IN A CHAIR

1. Sit in a chair with your feet flat on the floor. Place your hands on the sides of the chair.

2. Raise your right leg and bring your right thigh toward your chest. Straighten your left leg, pressing through the heel of your left foot.

3. As you lower and straighten your right foot, raise your left leg and bring your left thigh toward your chest. Perform the last two steps 10 times.

BACK FLAT ON THE FLOOR

1. Lie on your back on the floor with your knees bent to form a 90-degree angle with your legs. Relax your arms at your sides.

2. Bring your left knee toward your chest and extend your right leg toward the ceiling.

3. Bring your right knee toward your chest and extend your left leg toward the ceiling. Perform the last two steps 12 times.

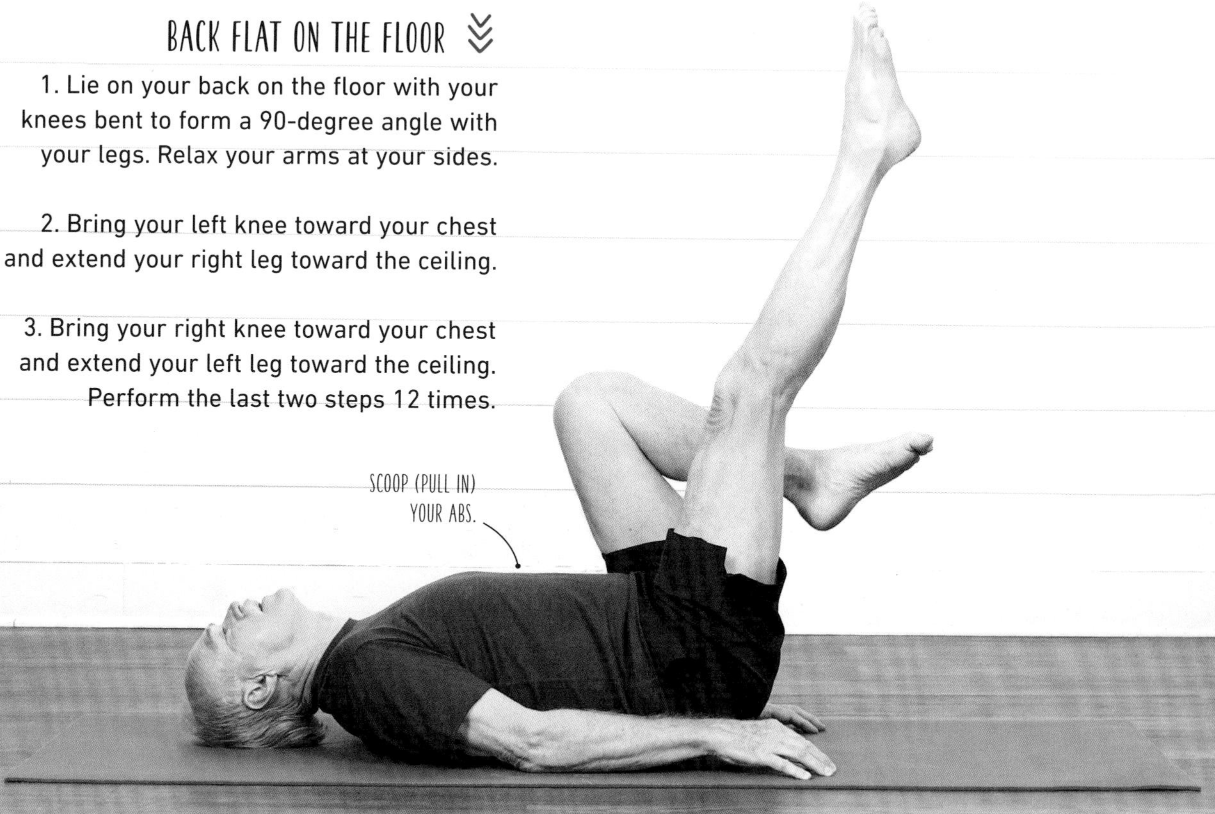

Forward Spine Stretches

This stretch is great for upper back, lower back, neck, and hamstring muscles. This exercise can improve spinal articulation (moving one vertebra at a time), decompression of the spine, and back tension. Plus, it can aid in lower back pain relief and help you develop better posture.

1 Sit on the floor with your legs extended and your feet shoulder width apart. Extend your arms forward and face your hands downward.

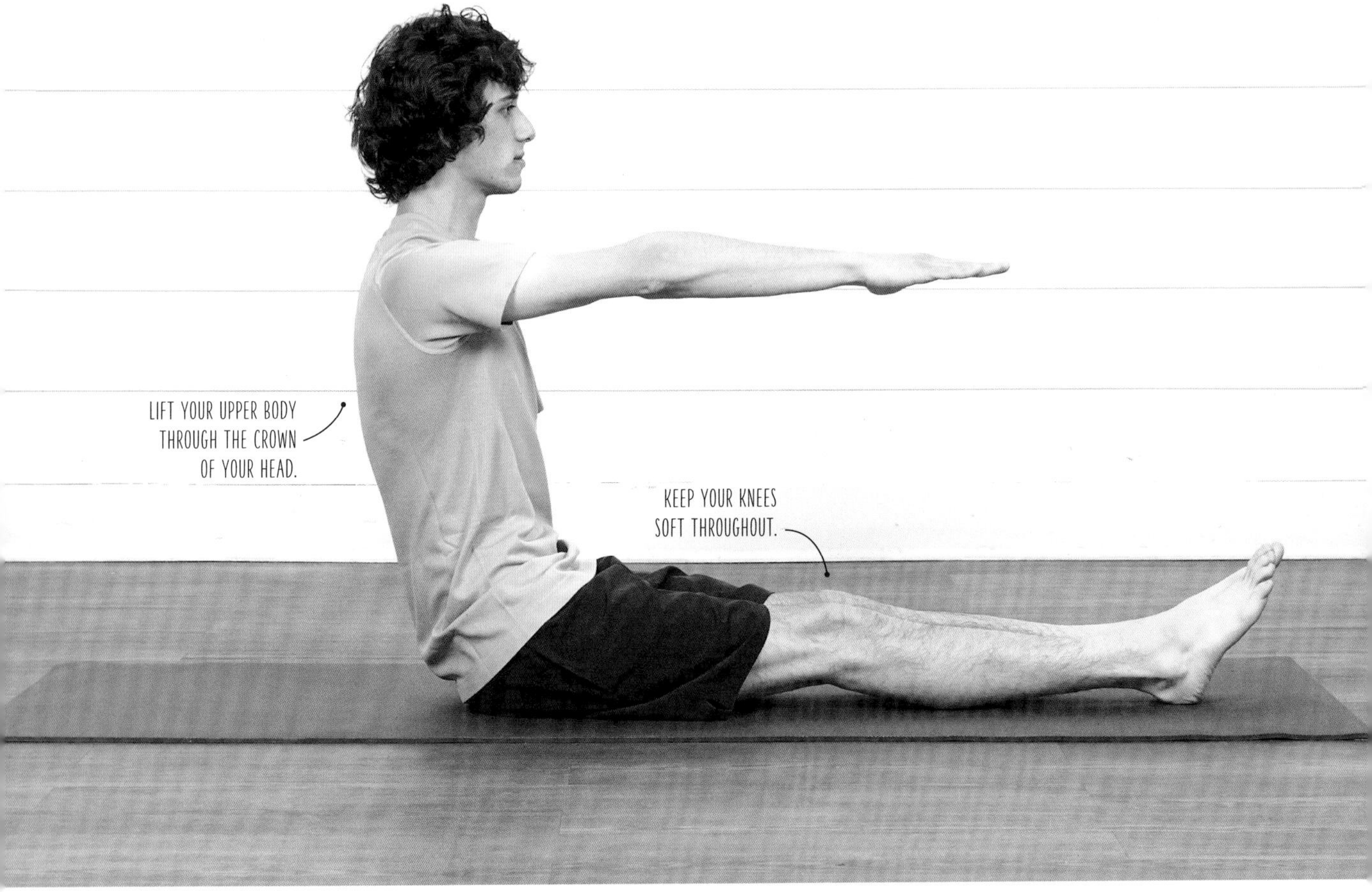

LIFT YOUR UPPER BODY THROUGH THE CROWN OF YOUR HEAD.
KEEP YOUR KNEES SOFT THROUGHOUT.

2 Bend at your waist and begin to lower your upper body toward your thighs.

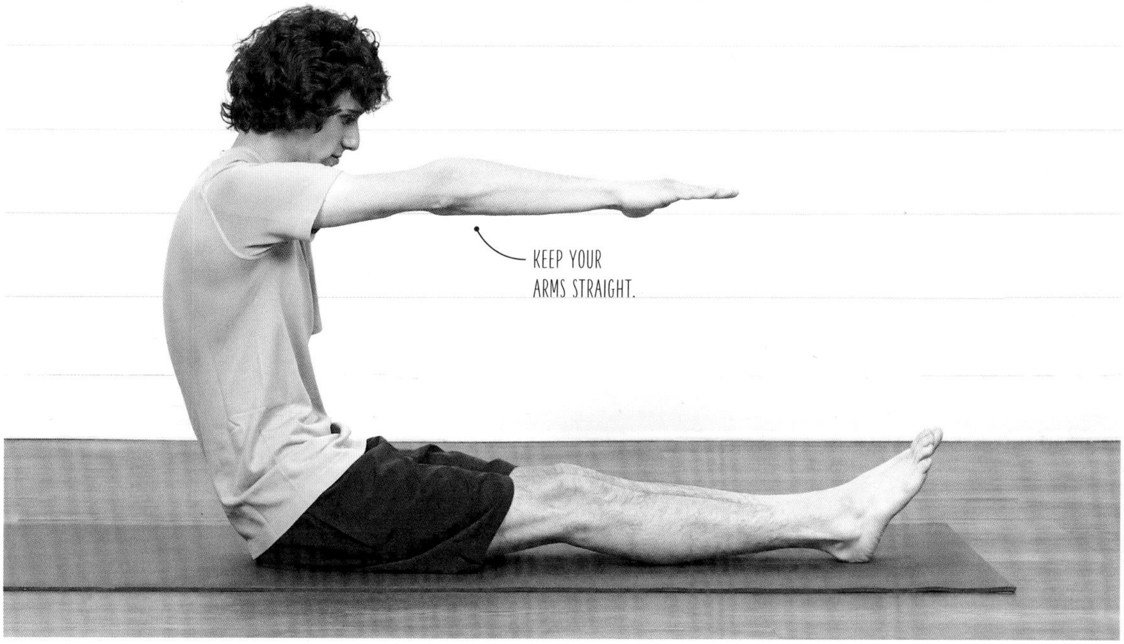
KEEP YOUR
ARMS STRAIGHT.

3 Continue leaning forward as you round your back into a C. Reverse your movements to roll through your spine and return to your starting position. Perform these steps 5 times.

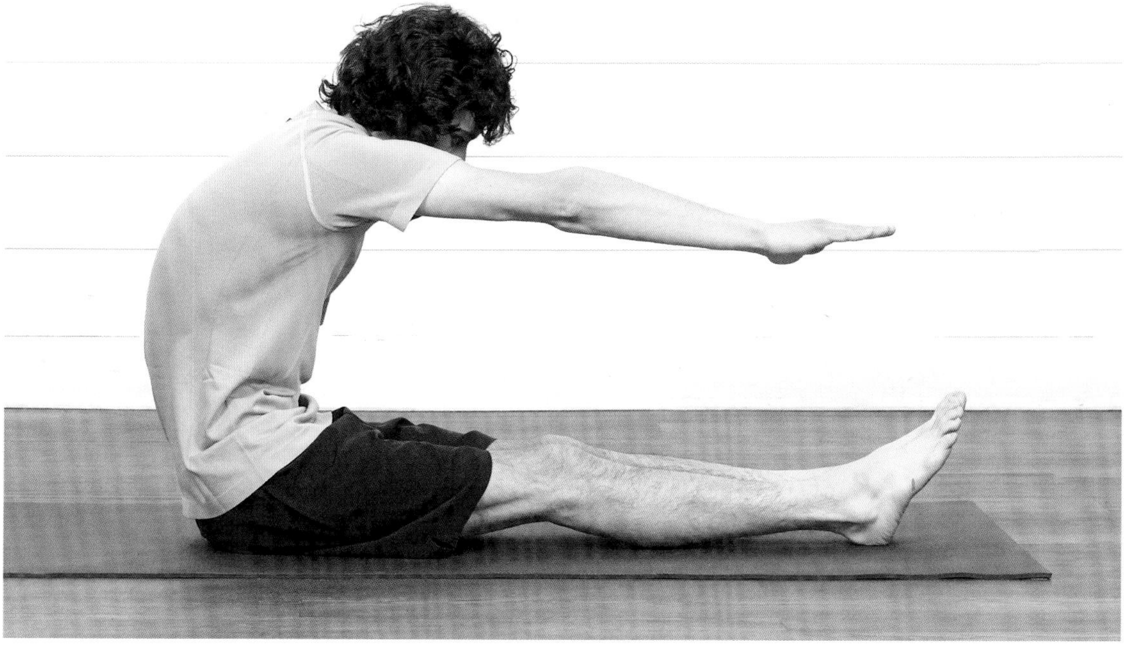

FORWARD SPINE STRETCHES

VARIATIONS

If you lack lower back, neck, and hamstring flexibility, bending your knees or using a stability ball can help you perform this exercise. The chair variation is a good option if you have difficulty getting down to or up from the floor.

WITH A STABILITY BALL

1. Sit on the floor with your legs extended and a little wider than shoulder width apart. Place a stability ball between your legs and place your hands on top of the ball.

2. Bend at your waist and lower your upper body toward your thighs while rolling the ball forward.

3. Roll the ball toward you as you reverse your movements and return to your starting position. Perform these steps 5 times.

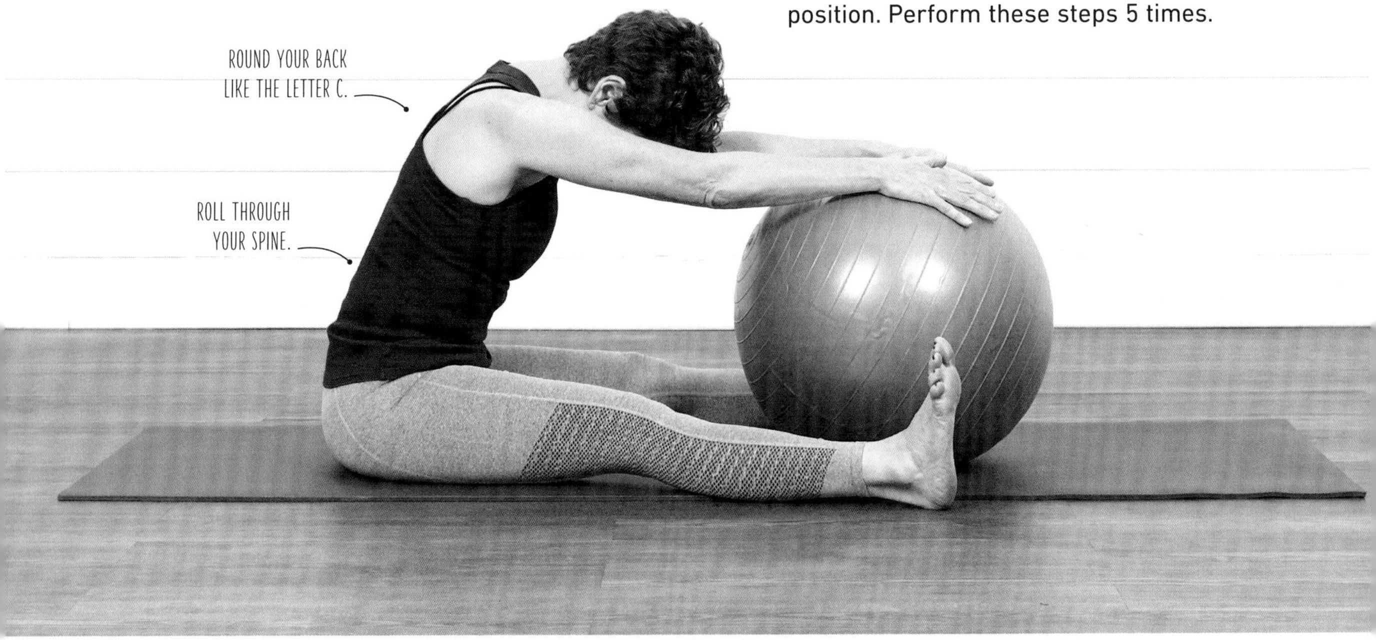
ROUND YOUR BACK LIKE THE LETTER C.
ROLL THROUGH YOUR SPINE.

WITH BENT KNEES

In step 1, bend your knees to form 45-degree angles with your legs. Continue with the remaining text.

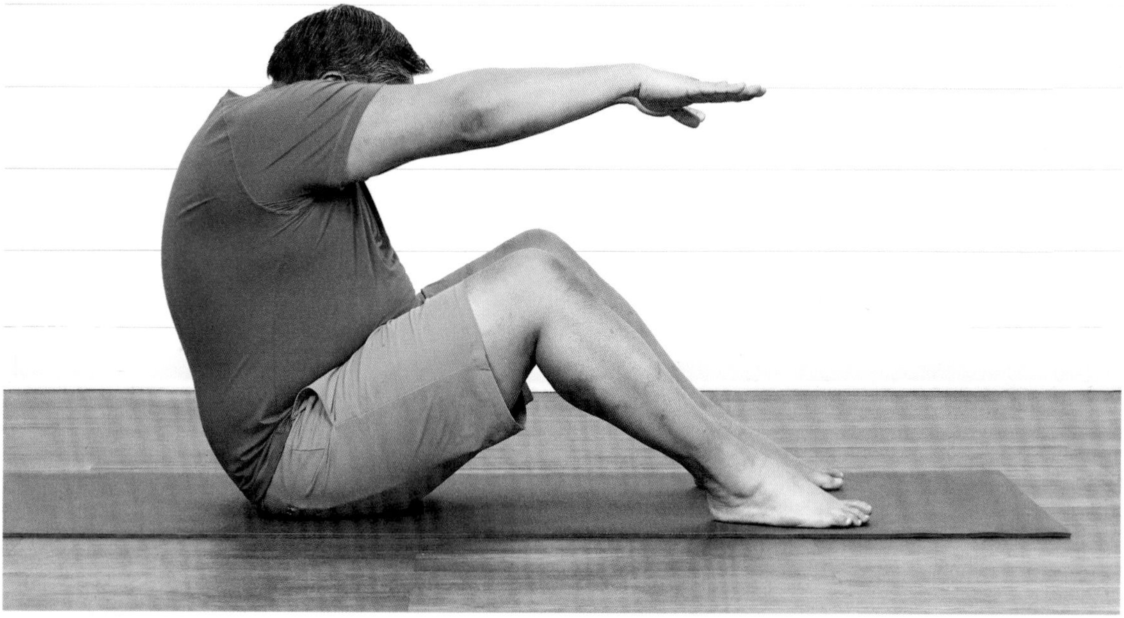

SITTING IN A CHAIR

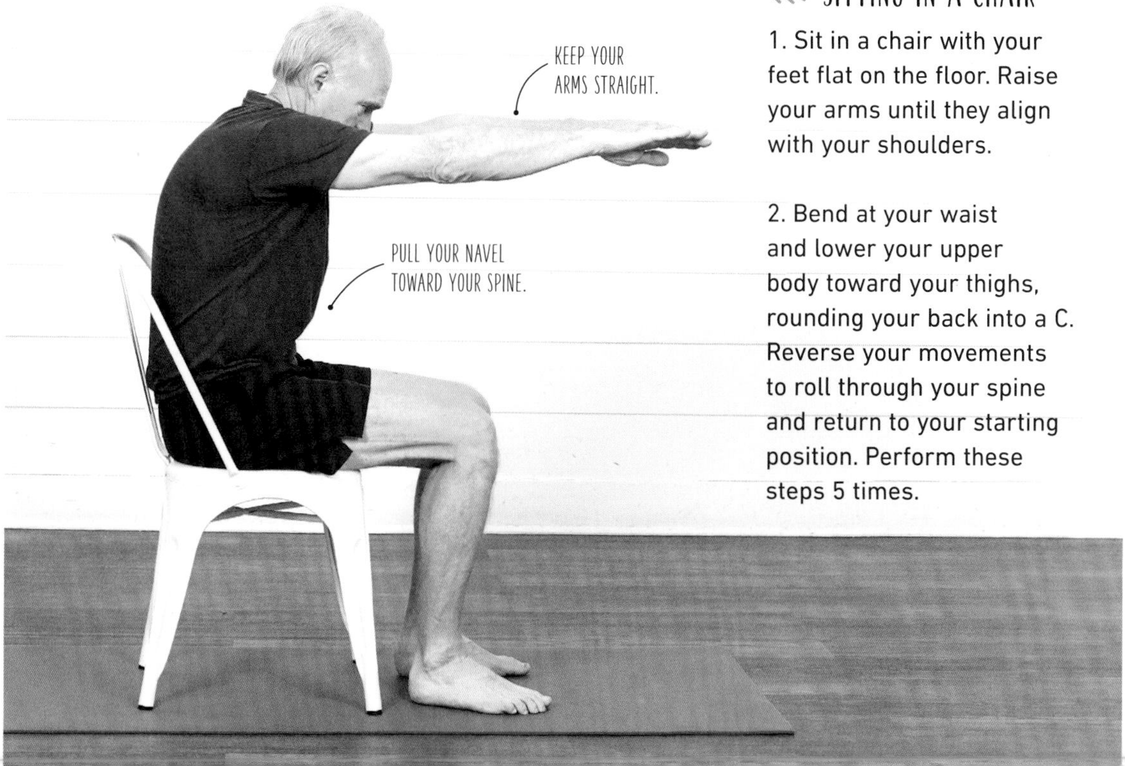
KEEP YOUR
ARMS STRAIGHT.
PULL YOUR NAVEL
TOWARD YOUR SPINE.

1. Sit in a chair with your feet flat on the floor. Raise your arms until they align with your shoulders.

2. Bend at your waist and lower your upper body toward your thighs, rounding your back into a C. Reverse your movements to roll through your spine and return to your starting position. Perform these steps 5 times.

Spinal Rotations

Rotating in this exercise challenges the stabilization of your spine, stretches your hamstrings, strengthens your back, and improves your posture. These movements use your deep abdominal muscles to pull your upper torso forward—a practice that helps you learn to initiate movement from your body's center.

1 Sit on the floor with your legs slightly wider than your shoulders and your feet flexed toward your body. Extend your arms to your sides at shoulder height.

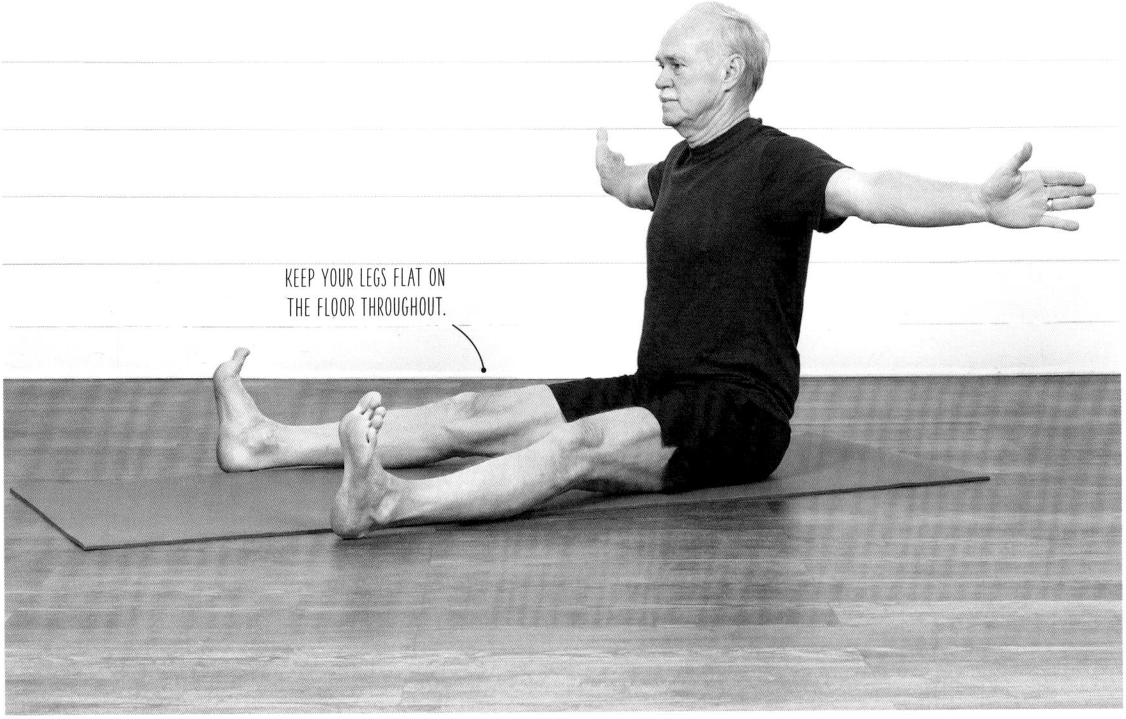
KEEP YOUR LEGS FLAT ON THE FLOOR THROUGHOUT.

2 As you inhale, rotate your torso to your left and extend your left arm behind you.

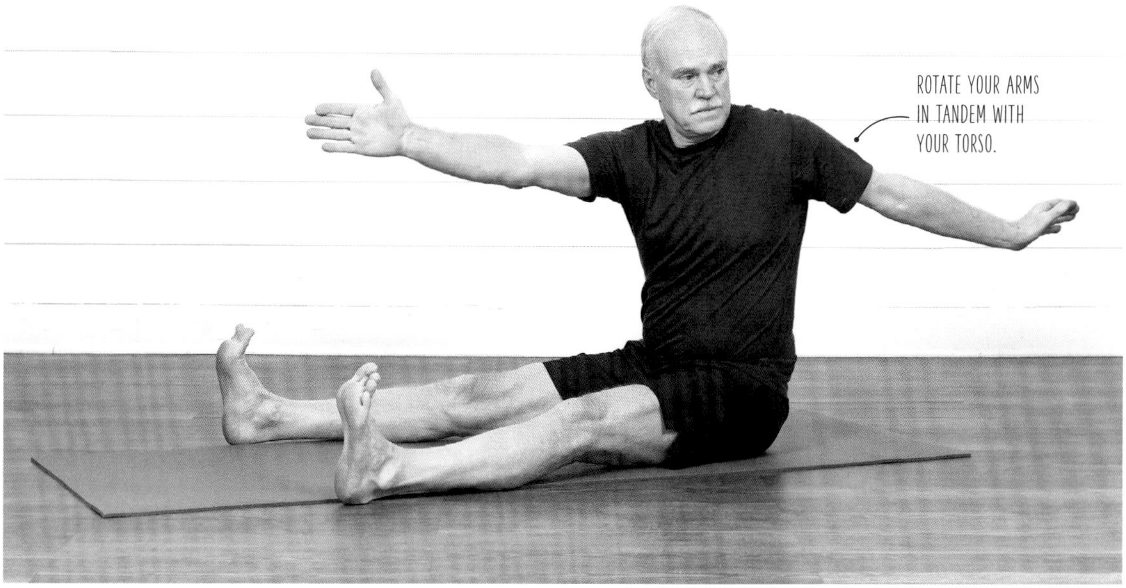

ROTATE YOUR ARMS IN TANDEM WITH YOUR TORSO.

3 As you exhale, lean toward your left leg and touch the inside of your left foot with your right hand. Reverse your movements to return to your starting position. Perform these steps 3 times. Repeat these steps rotating to your right.

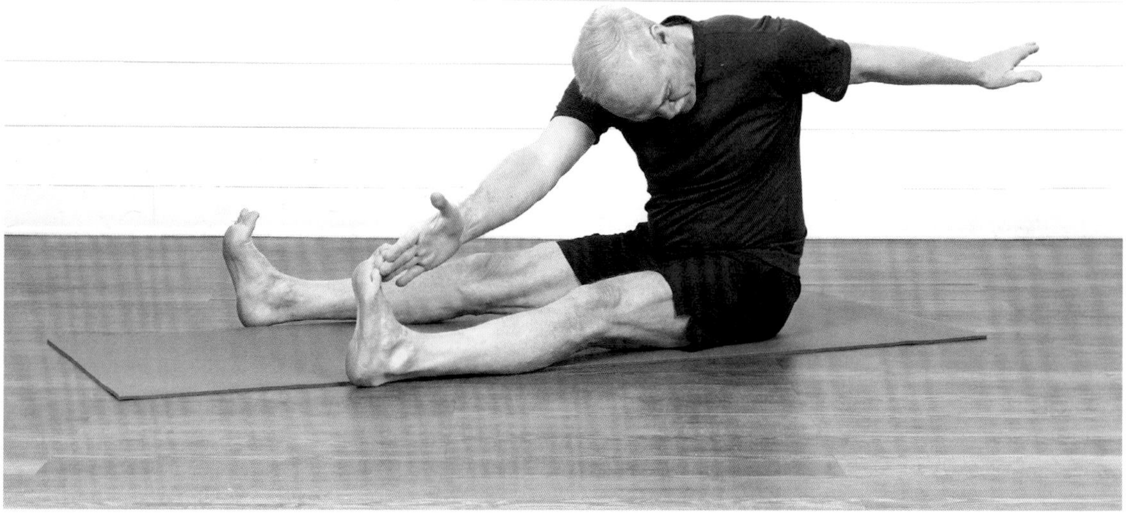

SPINAL ROTATIONS

VARIATIONS

Lacking flexibility in your hamstrings and upper and lower back might prevent you from performing this exercise. Bending your knees or sitting on a ball or in a chair can decrease your range of motion, making the movements less challenging.

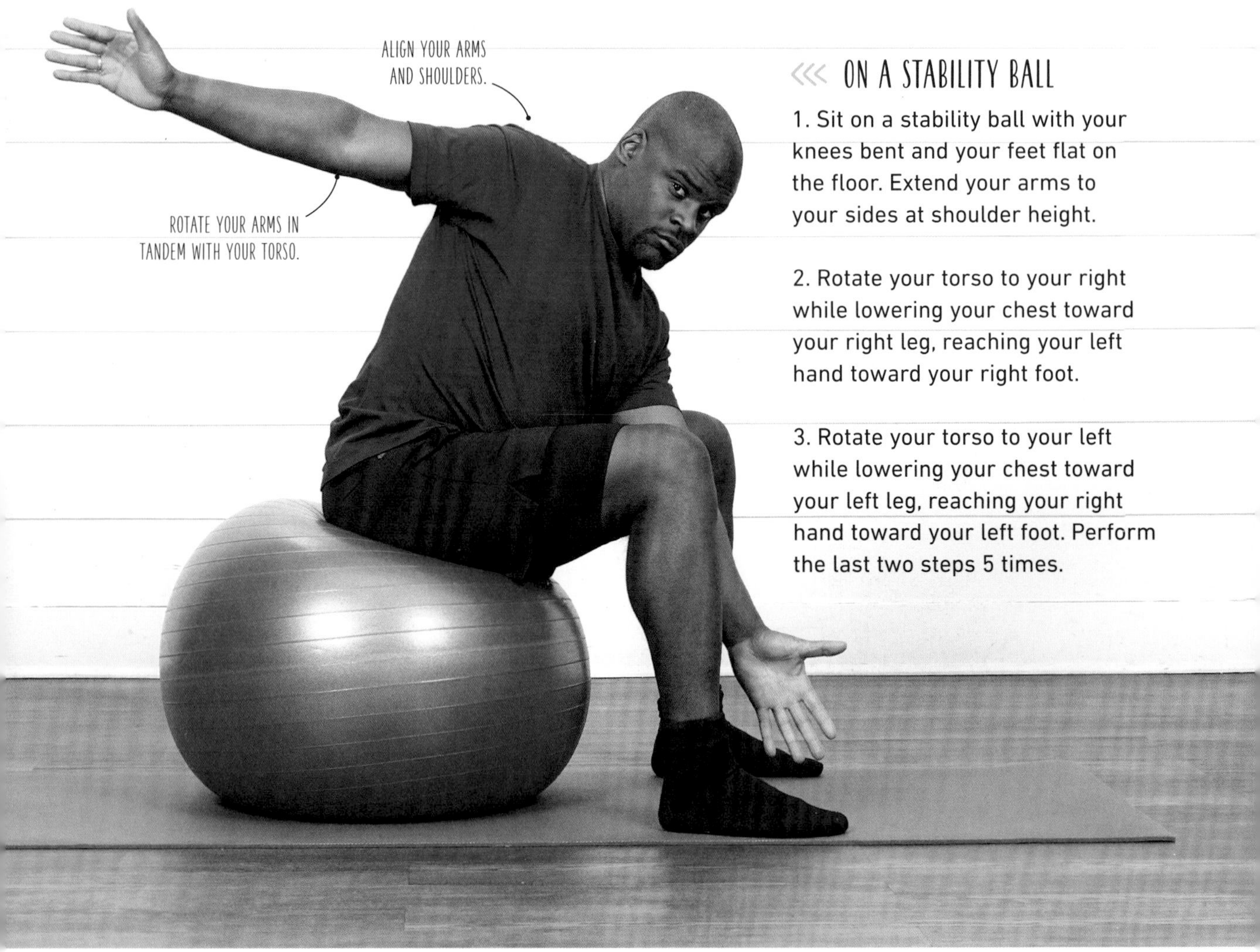

ALIGN YOUR ARMS AND SHOULDERS.
ROTATE YOUR ARMS IN TANDEM WITH YOUR TORSO.

ON A STABILITY BALL

1. Sit on a stability ball with your knees bent and your feet flat on the floor. Extend your arms to your sides at shoulder height.

2. Rotate your torso to your right while lowering your chest toward your right leg, reaching your left hand toward your right foot.

3. Rotate your torso to your left while lowering your chest toward your left leg, reaching your right hand toward your left foot. Perform the last two steps 5 times.

WITH BENT KNEES >>>

In step 1, bend your knees and curve your lower spine. Place your hands behind your head. Continue with the remaining text, reaching toward your bent knee with your elbow.

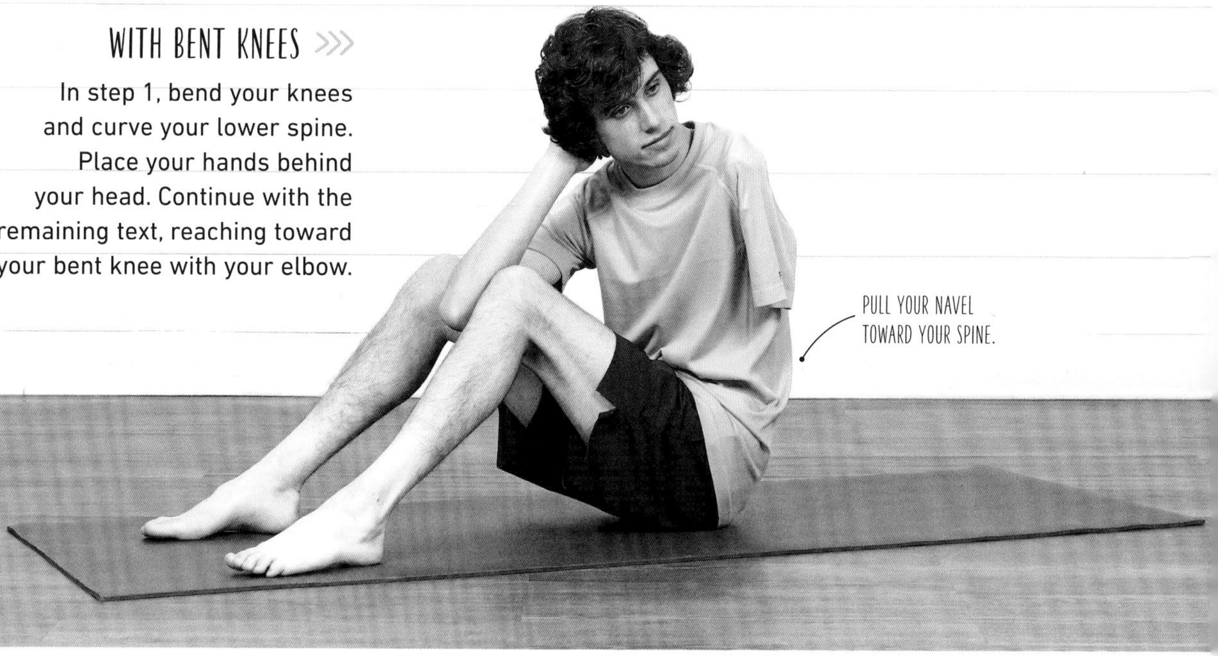
PULL YOUR NAVEL TOWARD YOUR SPINE.

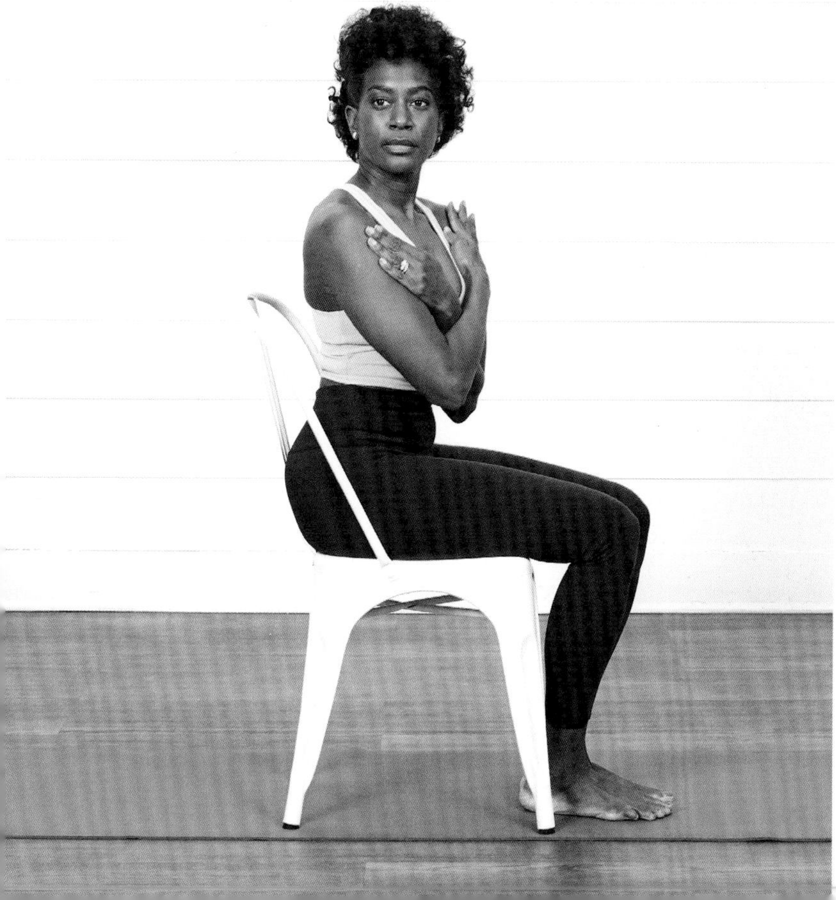

<<< SITTING IN A CHAIR

1. Sit in a chair with your feet flat on the floor. Cross your arms in front of your chest.

2. Rotate your torso to your right, keeping your legs as still as possible. Reverse your movements to return to your starting position.

3. Rotate your torso to your left, keeping your legs as still as possible. Reverse your movements to return to your starting position. Repeat these steps 6 times.

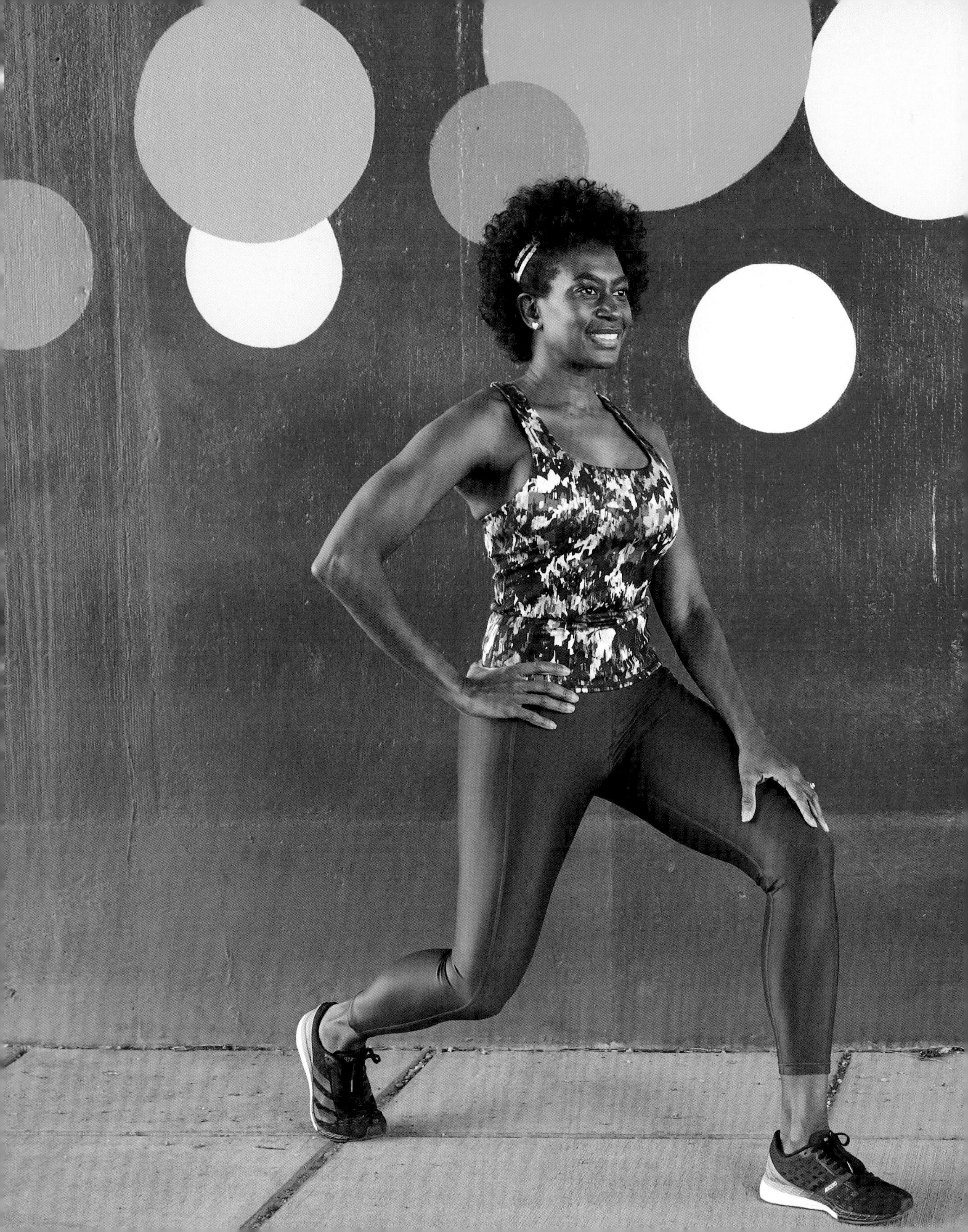

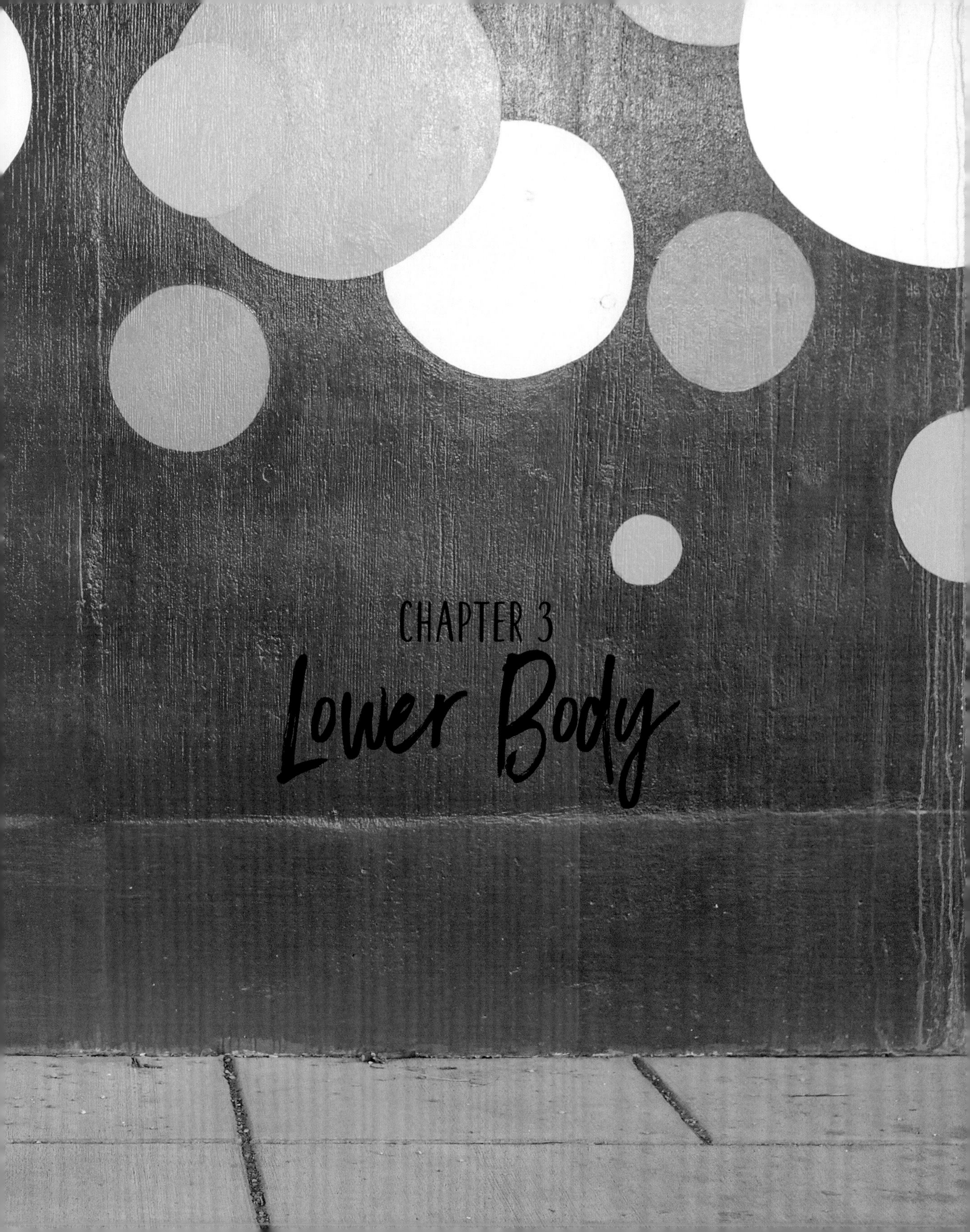

CHAPTER 3
Lower Body

Shoulder Bridge

This exercise isolates and strengthens your gluteus, hamstring, and lower back muscles. When done correctly, these movements can also enhance your core stability by targeting your abs and the muscles of your lower and middle back while challenging shoulder and pelvic stability.

1 Lie on your back on the floor with your feet shoulder width apart and your knees bent to form a 45-degree angle with your legs. Relax your arms at your sides and place your hands flat on the floor.

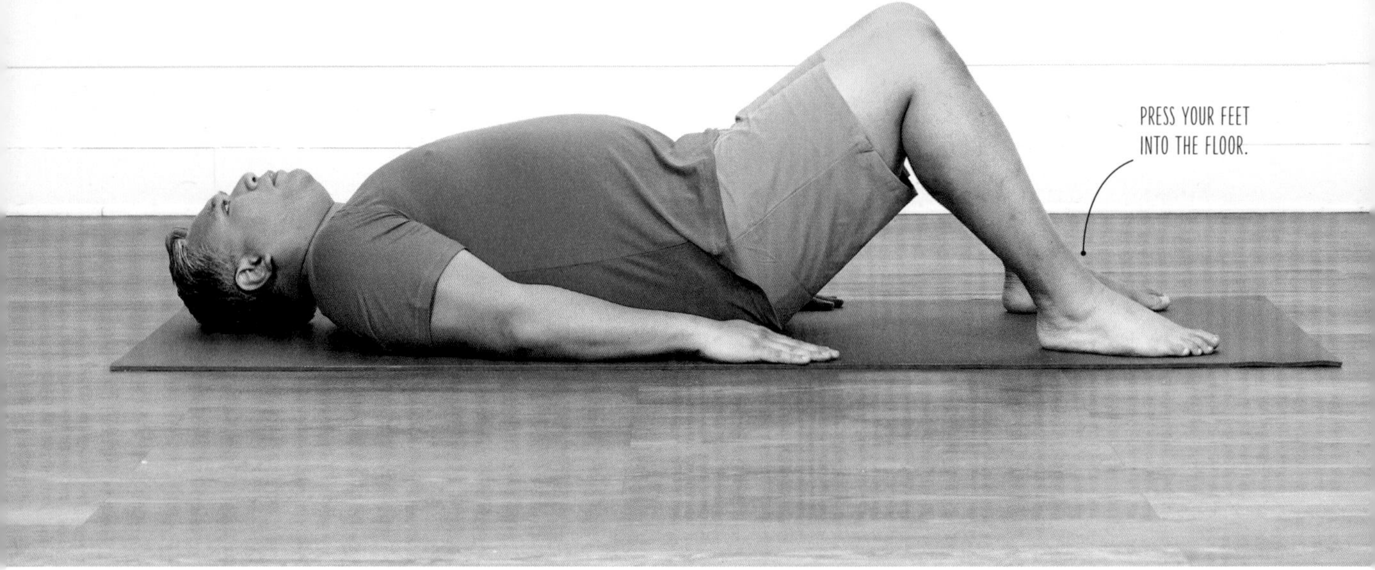
PRESS YOUR FEET INTO THE FLOOR.

2 Press your hands, feet, and shoulder blades into the floor to raise your glutes off the floor. Hold this position for 3 seconds. Reverse your movements to return to your starting position. Perform these steps 5 times.

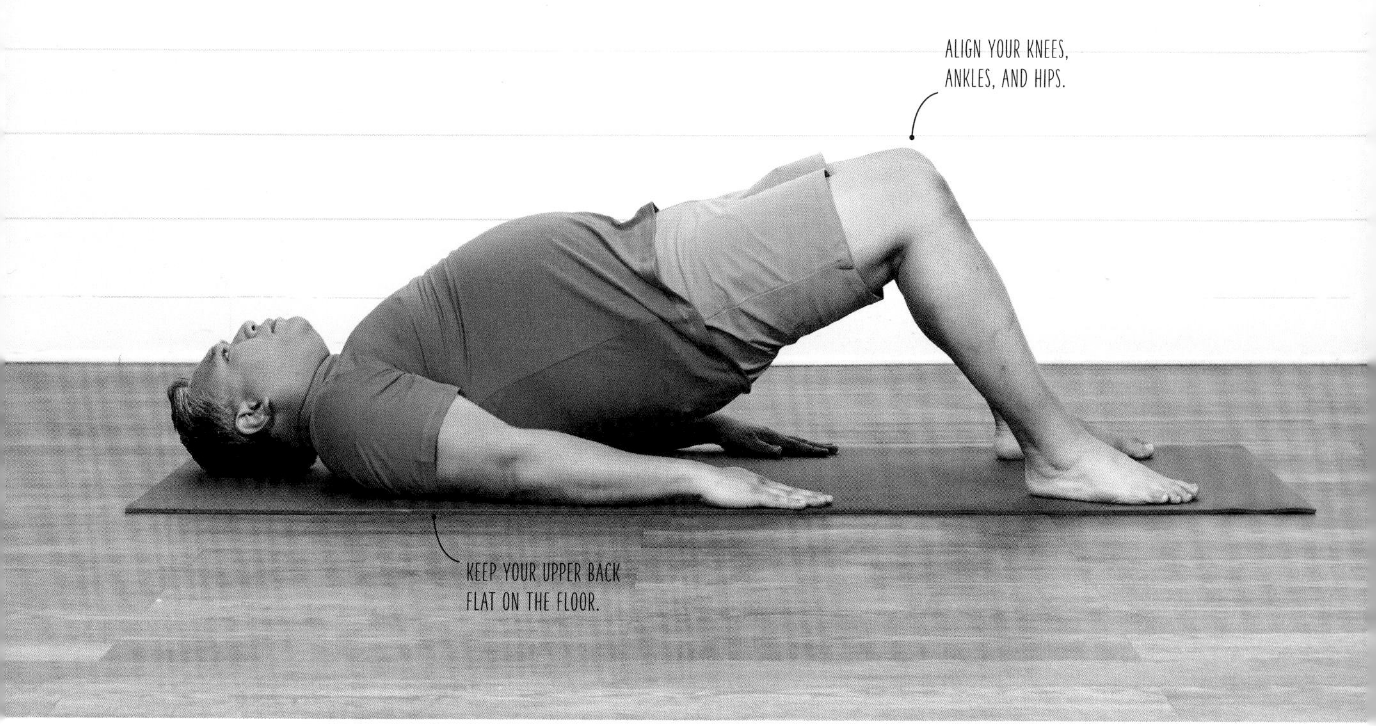
ALIGN YOUR KNEES,
ANKLES, AND HIPS.
KEEP YOUR UPPER BACK
FLAT ON THE FLOOR.

SHOULDER BRIDGE

VARIATIONS

Recruiting your gluteal muscles can be challenging because of tightness in your back extensors and hip flexors as well as weakness in your gluteal muscles (which can be caused by excessive sitting). Using props can help "wake up" those muscles and provide correct alignment.

WITH A SMALL PILATES BALL

In step 1, place a small Pilates ball between your knees.

In step 2, squeeze the ball as you raise and lower your glutes. Continue with the remaining text.

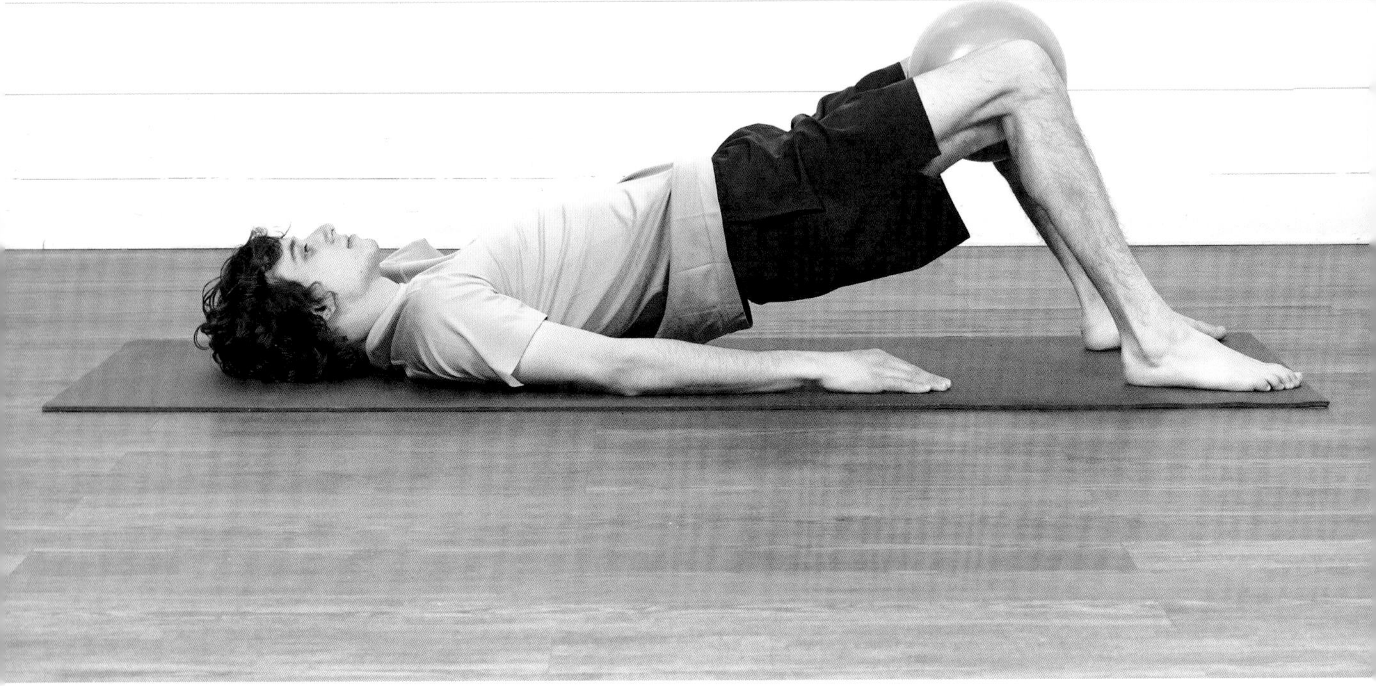

WITH A LOOP BAND

In step 1, place a loop band around your thighs above your knees.

In step 2, press your outer thighs against the band as you reverse your movements. Continue with the remaining text.

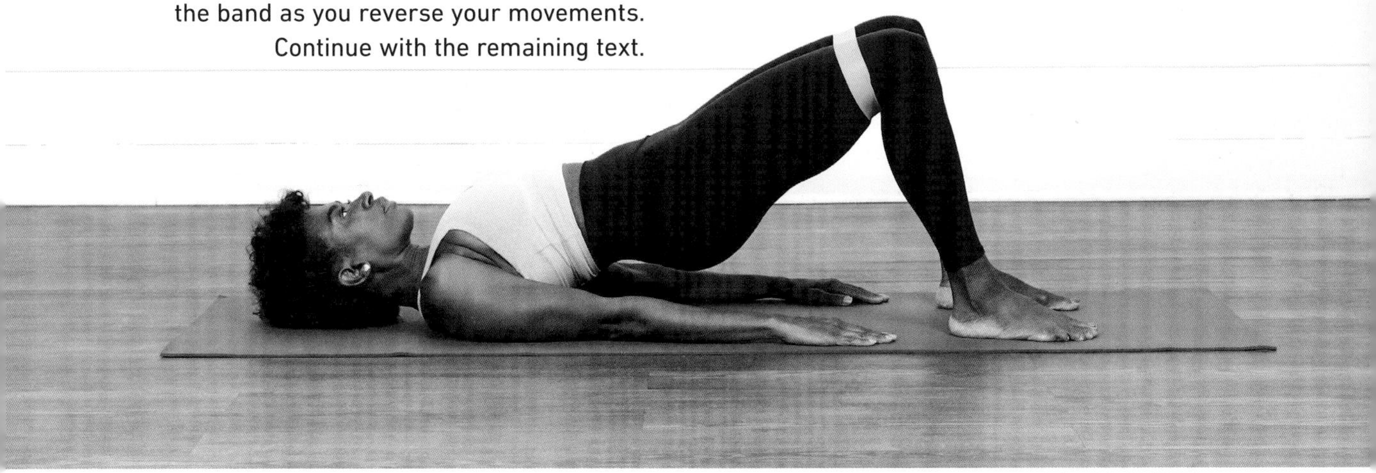

WITH A STABILITY BALL

In step 1, place your feet on a stability ball.

In step 2, press your feet into the ball as you raise and lower your glutes. Continue with the remaining text.

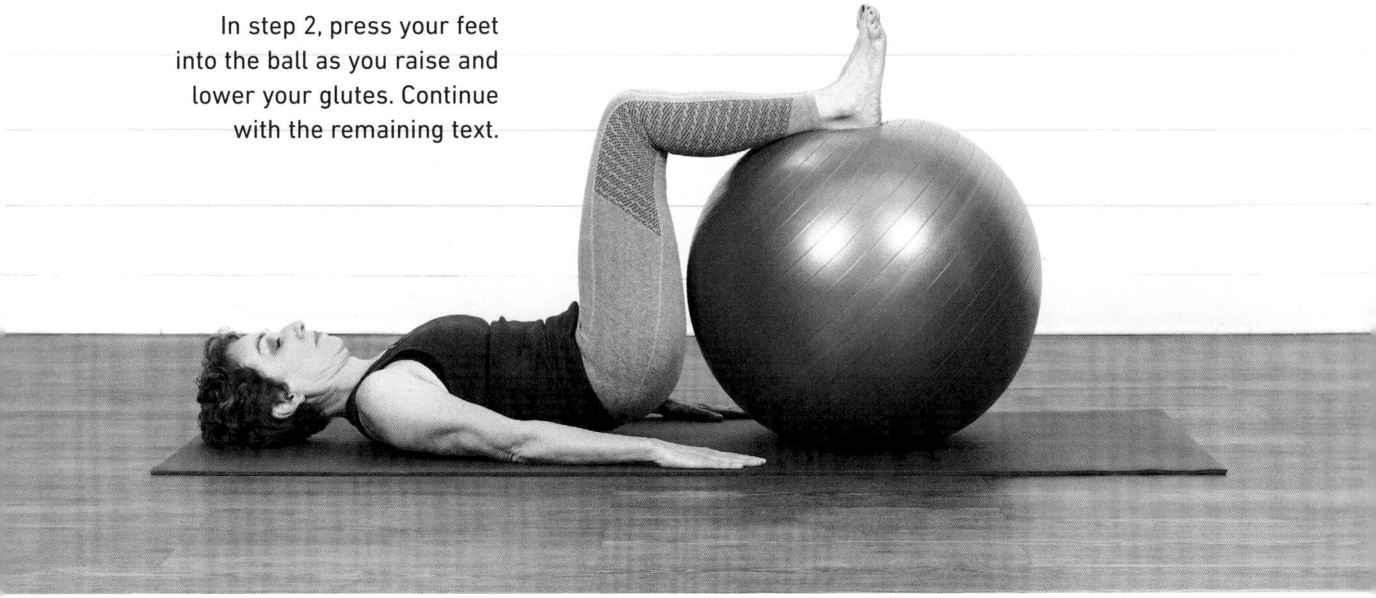

Clam

When you perform this exercise, you can strengthen your hip abductors and gluteus medius, which is responsible for stabilizing your pelvis. These movements can also help balance the muscular effort between your inner and outer thighs as well as your pelvic floor while increasing hip mobility. This exercise is often a part of a physical therapy regimen for knee injuries.

1 Lie on your left side with your head resting in your left hand. Place the fingertips of your right hand on the floor. Bend your knees to align your heels and glutes.

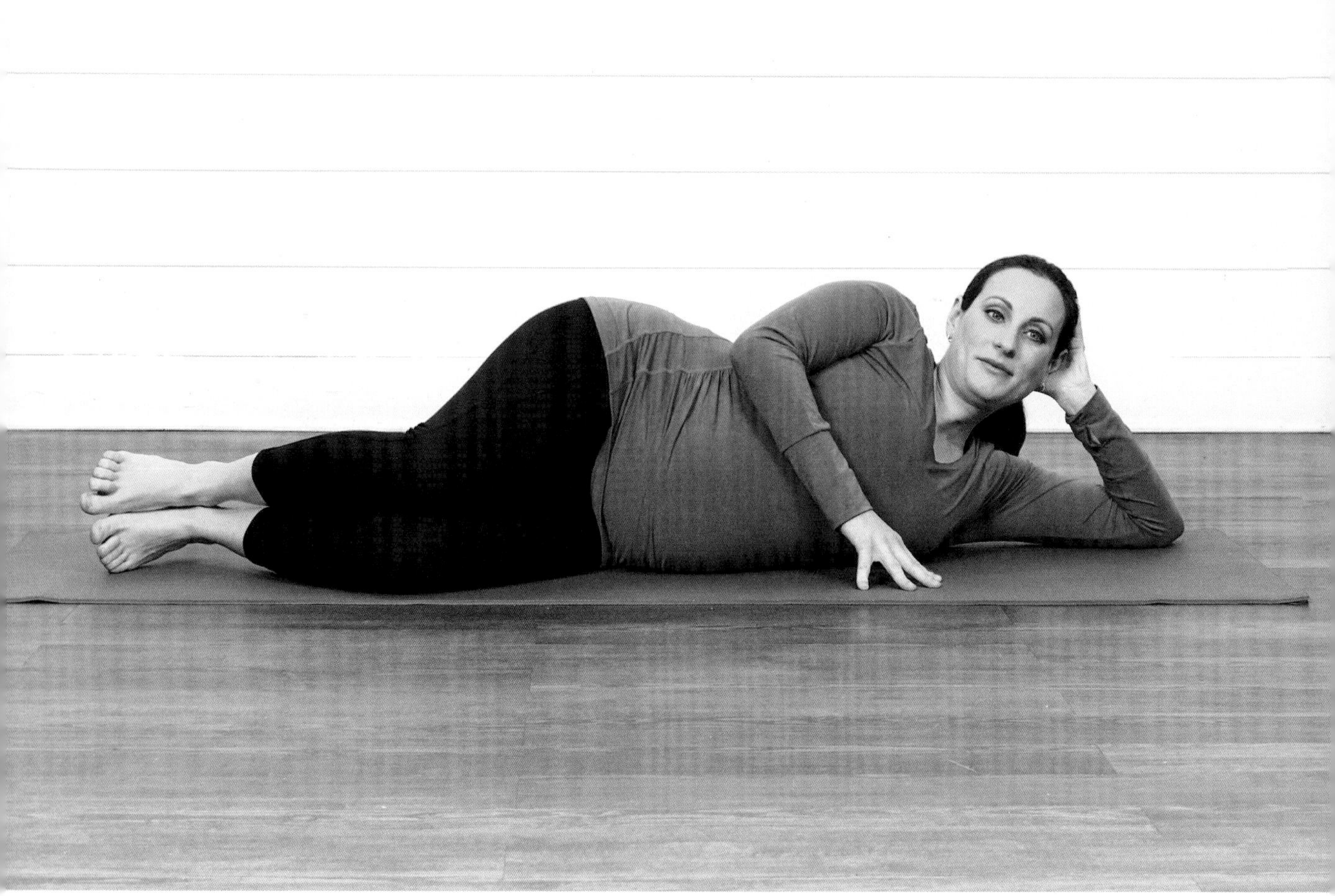

2 Lift your right leg off your left leg, keeping your feet together. Slowly reverse your movements to return to your starting position. Perform these steps 10 times. Repeat these steps on your right side.

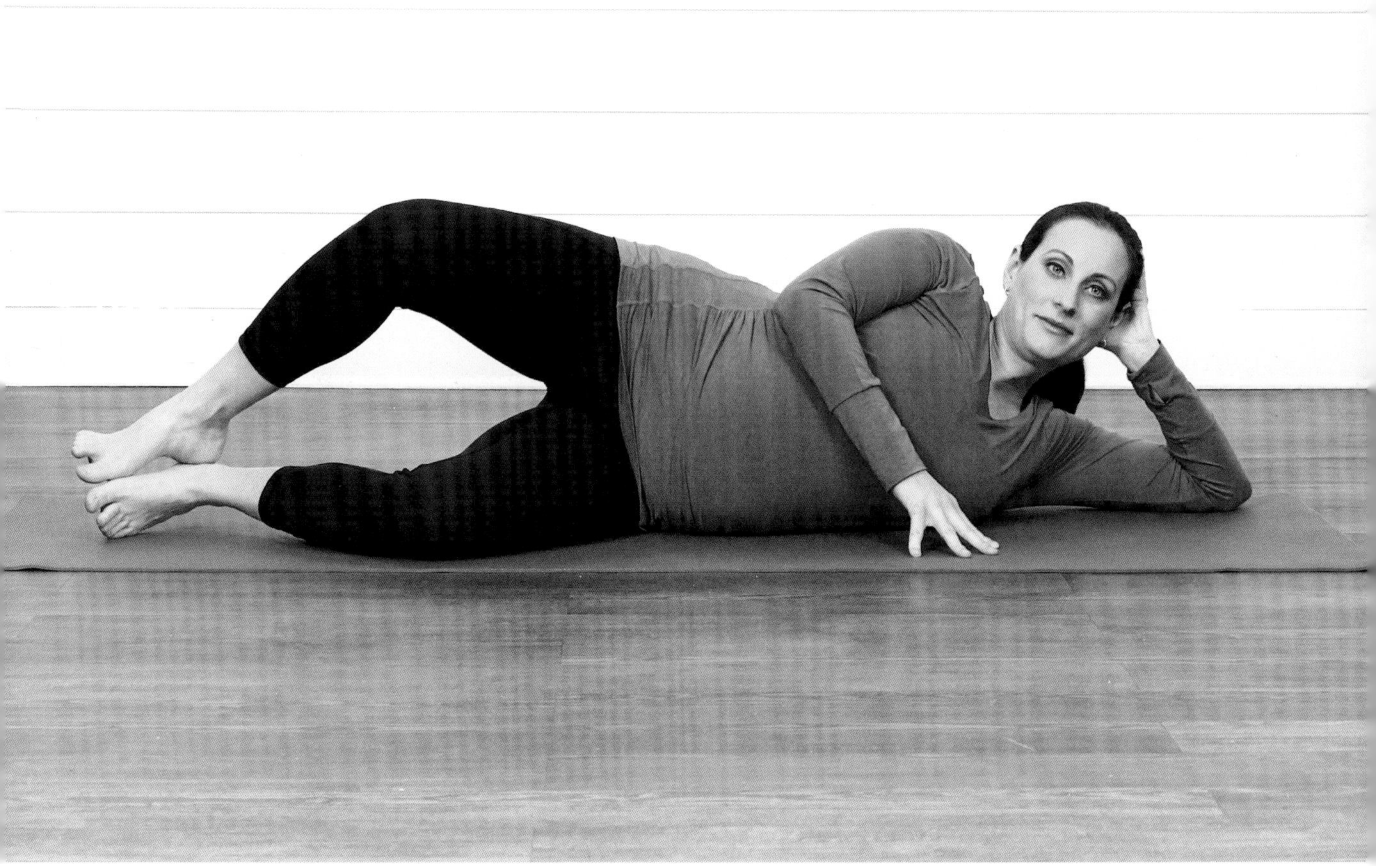

CLAM

VARIATIONS

Using the resistance of props can improve the quality of this exercise by helping recruit your stabilizing muscles, focusing your muscle control, and assisting with proper alignment. If you're unable to get down on the floor, the chair variation can prove effective.

WITH A LOOP BAND

In step 1, place a loop band around your legs just above your knees. Continue with the remaining text.

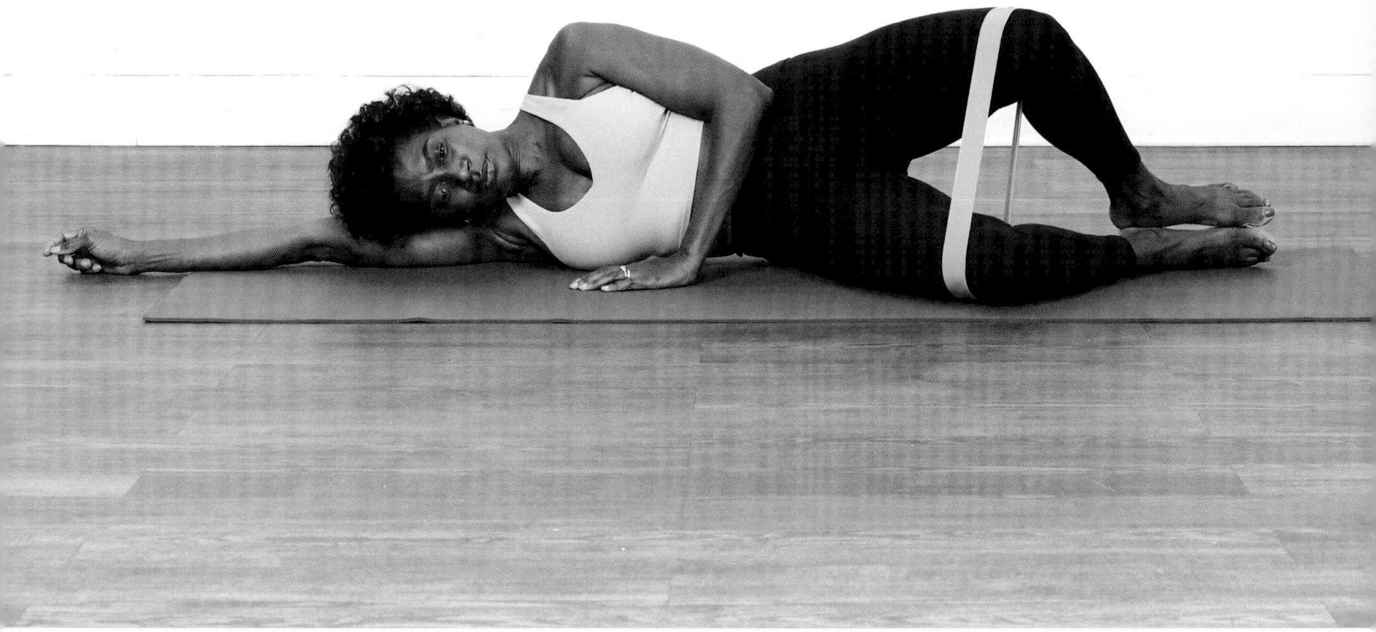

WITH THE MAGIC CIRCLE

In step 1, place your forearm flat on the floor. Place the pads of the Magic Circle between your legs just below your knees.

In step 2, squeeze and release the Magic Circle while lifting and lowering your leg. (If the Magic Circle is too tight, don't worry about trying to keep your feet together.) Continue with the remaining text.

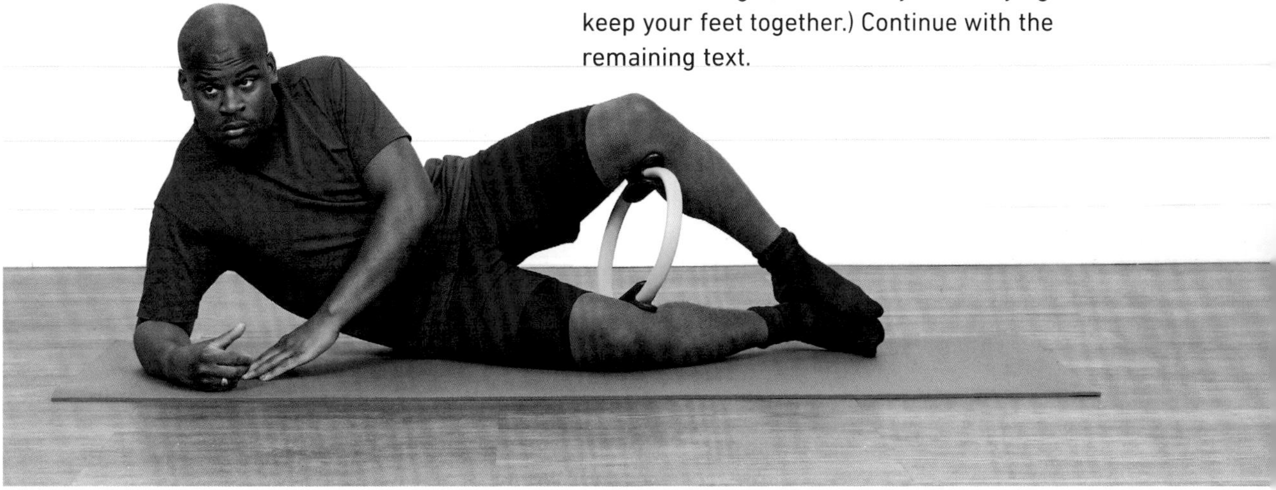

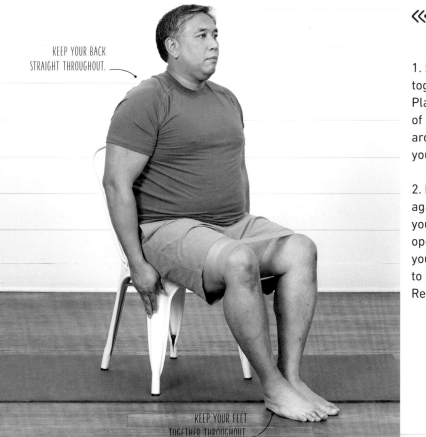

SITTING IN A CHAIR AND WITH A LOOP BAND

1. Sit in a chair with your feet together and flat on the floor. Place your hands on the sides of the chair. Place a loop band around your legs just above your knees.

2. Press your knees open against the band, engaging your gluteal muscles to open the band. Reverse your movements to return to your starting position. Repeat these steps 8 times.

Inner Thigh Lifts

As one of the most targeted inner thigh exercises in the Pilates mat repertoire, this lift can help strengthen your inner thighs by moving your leg toward your midline while requiring core engagement. Strong inner thighs are crucial for stability in your knee and hip joints.

1 Lie on your right side with your right elbow bent and your head resting in your right hand. Place the fingertips of your left hand on the floor. Bend your left knee and place your left foot behind your right knee.

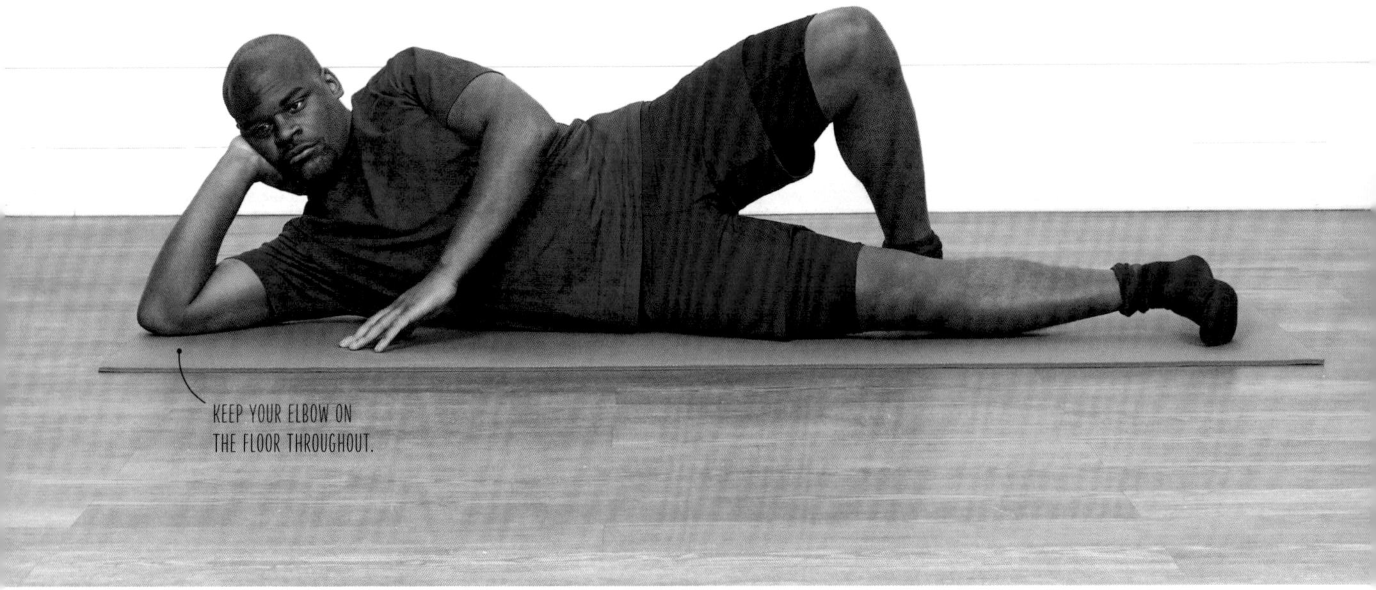

KEEP YOUR ELBOW ON THE FLOOR THROUGHOUT.

2 Slowly raise your right leg for 4 seconds. Perform this step 4 times. Repeat these steps on your left side.

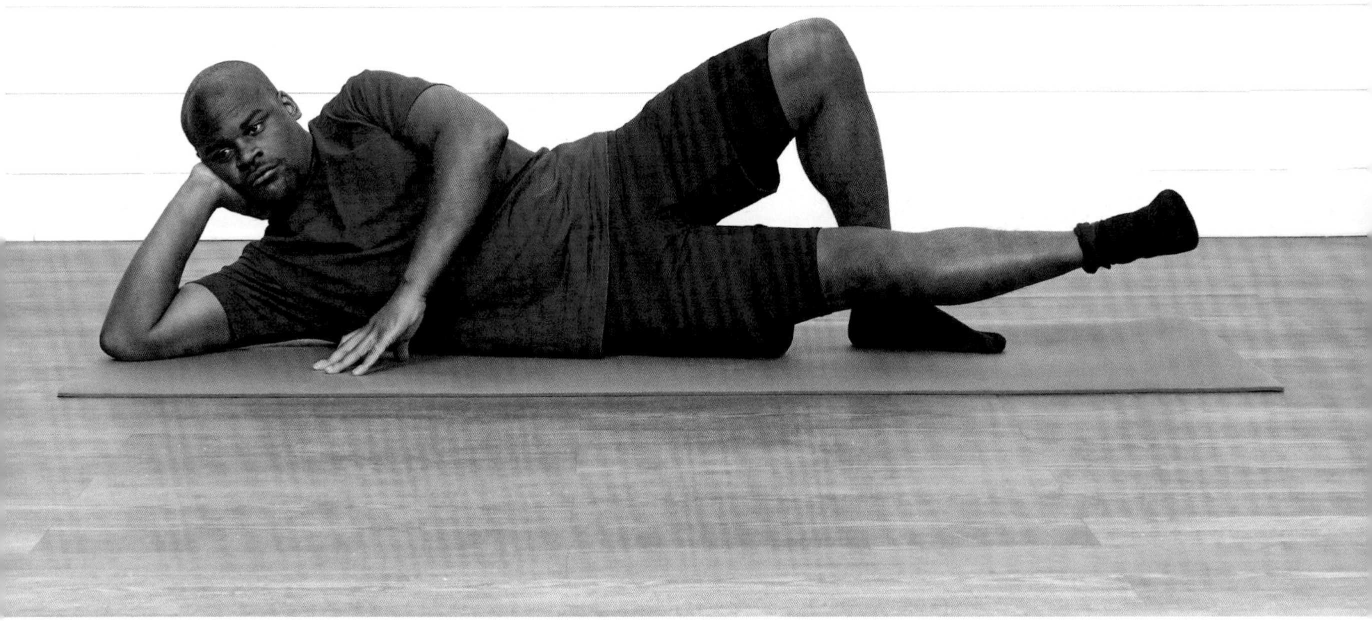

INNER THIGH LIFTS

VARIATIONS

Resistance can improve the quality of this exercise by helping recruit your stabilizing muscles, focusing muscle control, and assisting with proper alignment. Keeping your forearm flat on the floor can also help increase your range of motion.

WITH A SMALL PILATES BALL

1. Lie on your right side with your head resting in your right hand and your left hand flat on the floor. Place a small Pilates ball between your ankles.

2. Raise your legs 3 to 6 inches off the floor. Hold this position and squeeze the ball 10 times. Lower your legs to the floor. Repeat these steps on your left side.

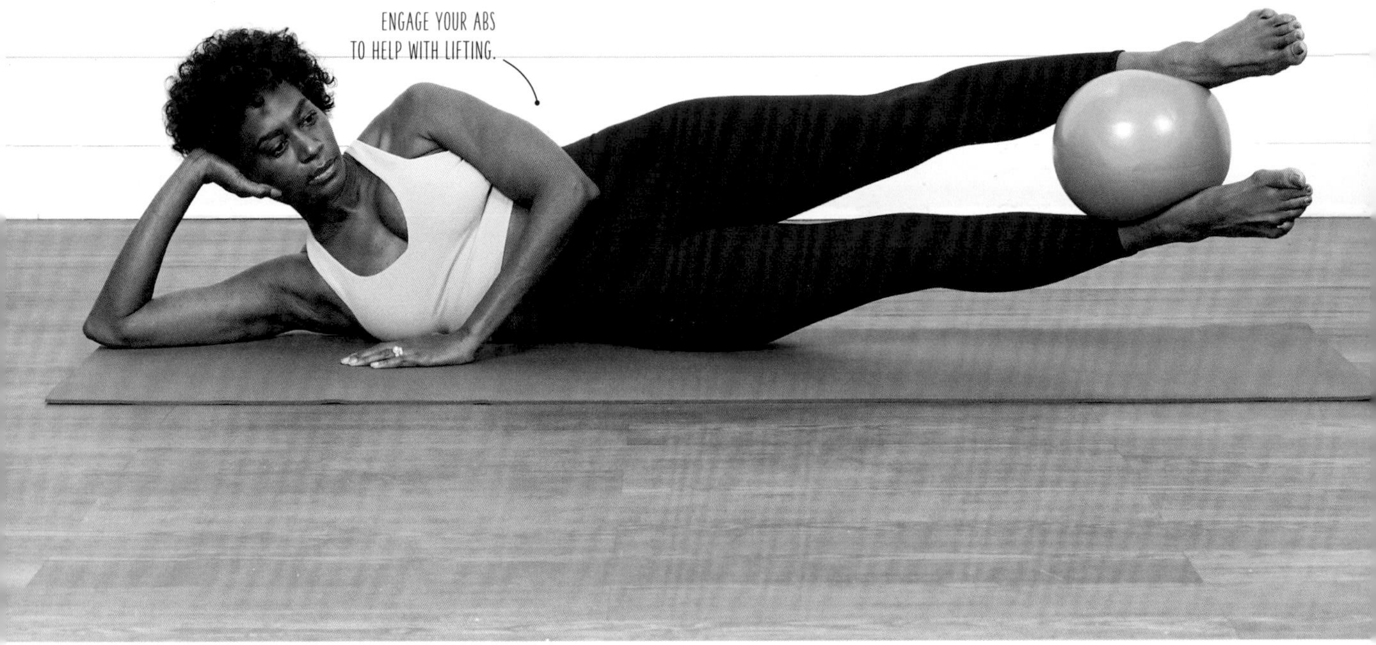
ENGAGE YOUR ABS
TO HELP WITH LIFTING.

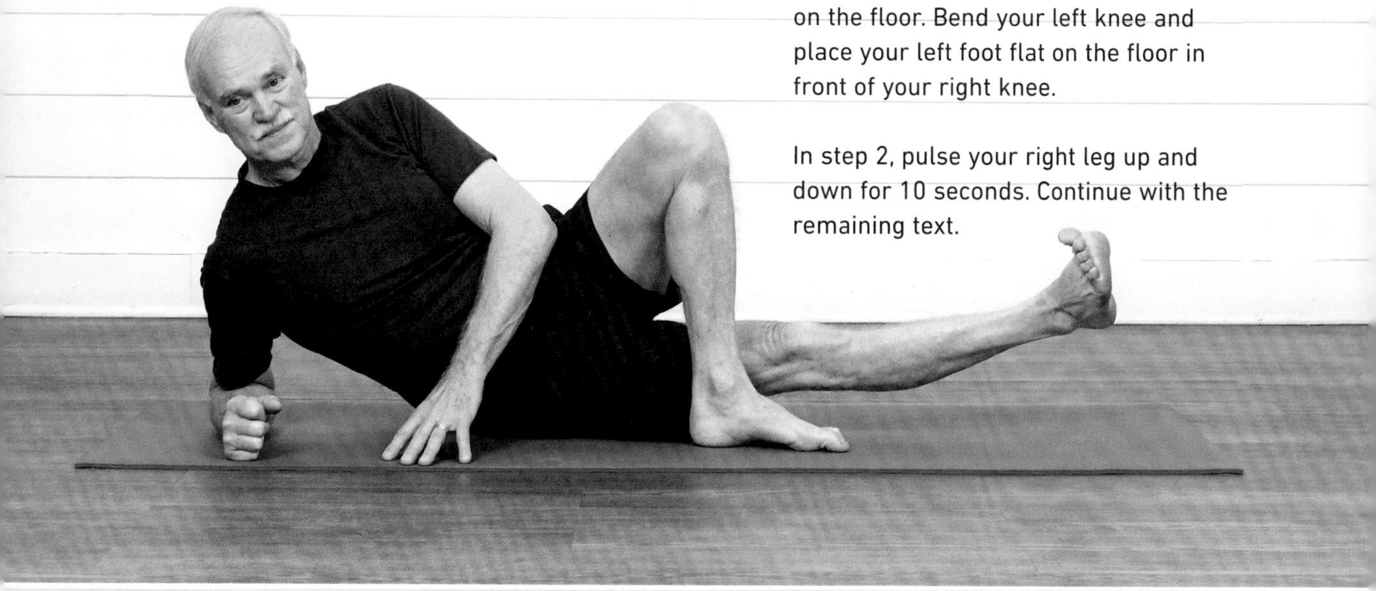

«« ON YOUR FOREARM

In step 1, place your right forearm flat on the floor. Bend your left knee and place your left foot flat on the floor in front of your right knee.

In step 2, pulse your right leg up and down for 10 seconds. Continue with the remaining text.

WITH THE MAGIC CIRCLE

1. Lie on your right side with your head resting in your right hand and your left hand flat on the floor. Place the Magic Circle between your ankles.

2. Press into the Magic Circle with both legs. Hold this position for 3 seconds. Repeat these steps on your left side.

ENGAGE YOUR ABS TO HELP WITH LIFTING.

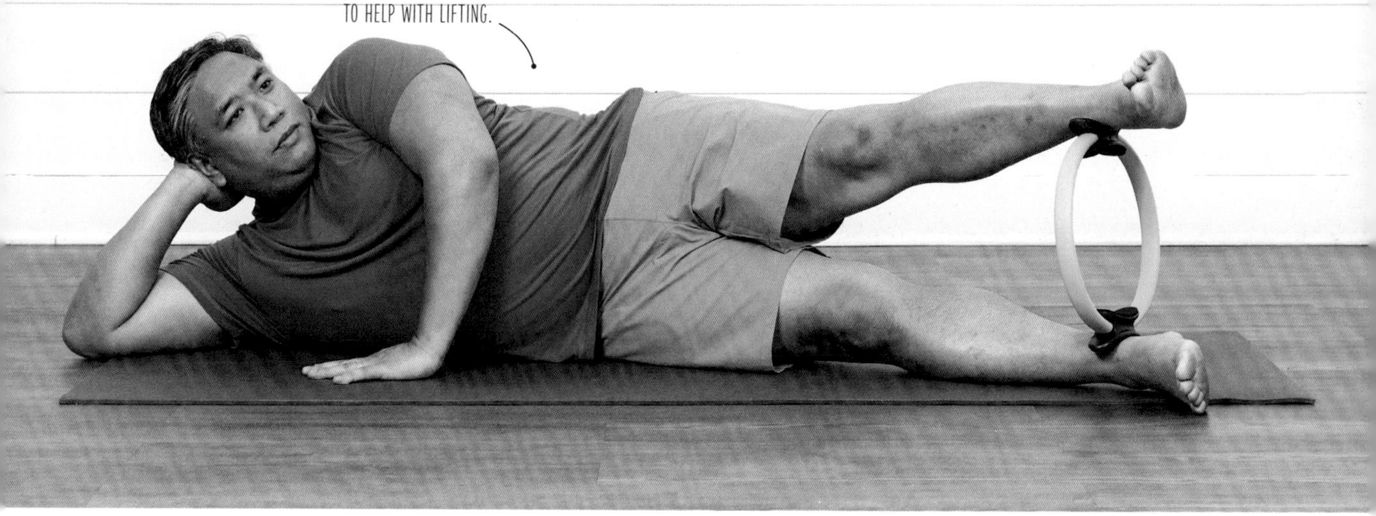

Side Kicks

Kicking movements can help develop core stability and strengthen your glutes, hips, abs, and back. This exercise works one leg at a time, which can help increase proprioception (the awareness of movement of your body) as well as reduce body and muscle imbalances. It can also release tight areas in your hips and thighs.

1 Lie on your right side with your left leg raised a few inches above your right leg. Angle your feet toward the front corner of the mat. Bend your right elbow and rest your head in your right hand. Place your left hand flat on the floor.

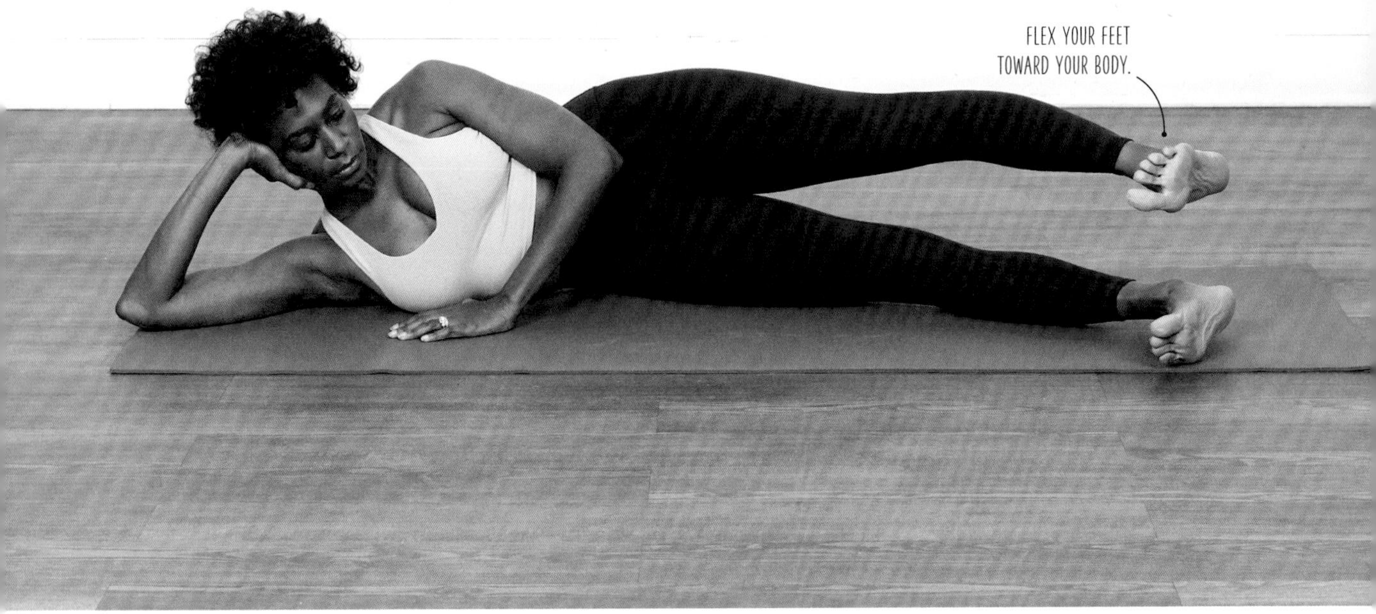
FLEX YOUR FEET TOWARD YOUR BODY.

2 Kick your left leg forward until perpendicular to your right leg.

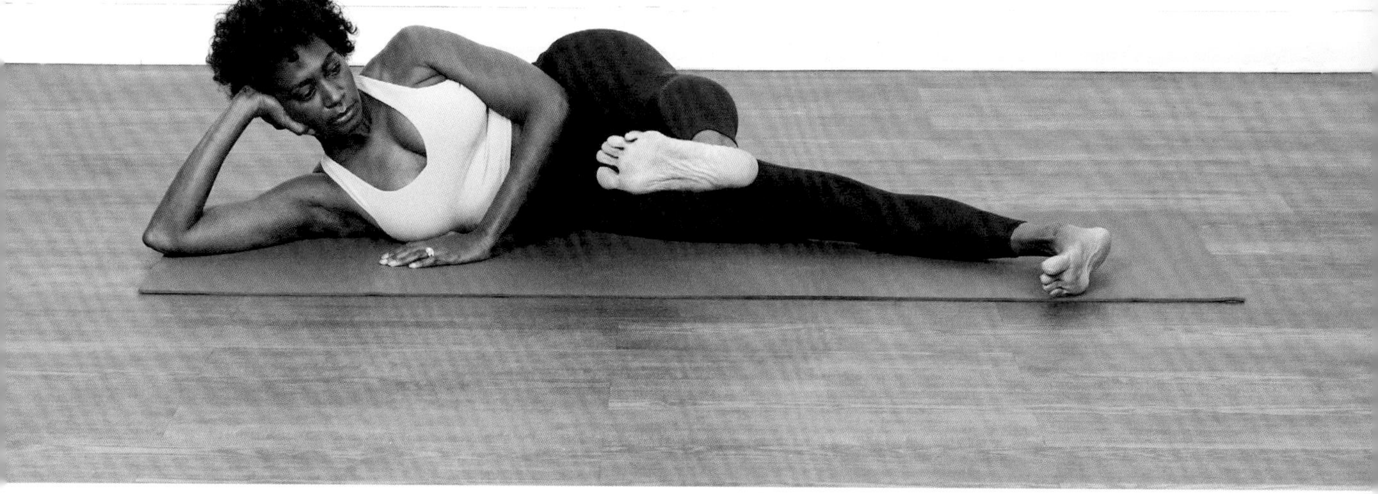

3 Kick your left leg backward as far as you can go. Perform the last two steps 6 times. Repeat these steps on your left side.

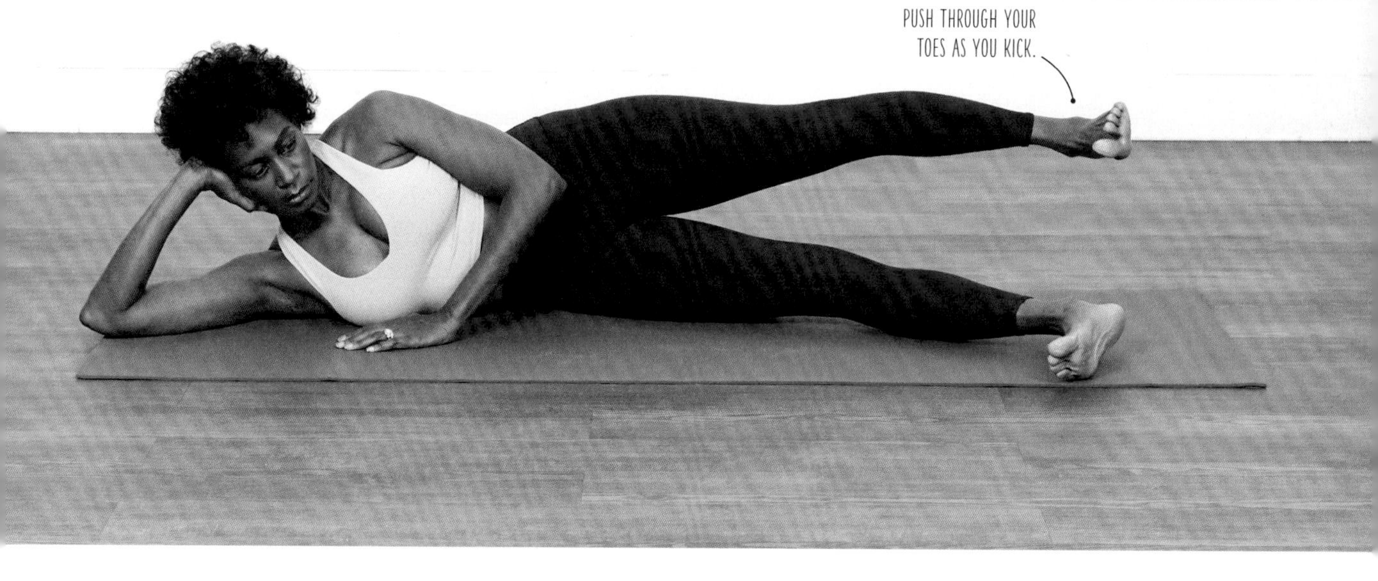
PUSH THROUGH YOUR
TOES AS YOU KICK.

SIDE KICKS

VARIATIONS

Coming up to your forearm and using a small Pilates ball can help increase your range of motion with this exercise as well as assist with proper alignment. Using a loop band adds resistance that can allow you to gain strength in a shorter amount of time.

WITH A LOOP BAND

In step 1, place a loop band around your legs just above your ankles. Continue with the remaining text.

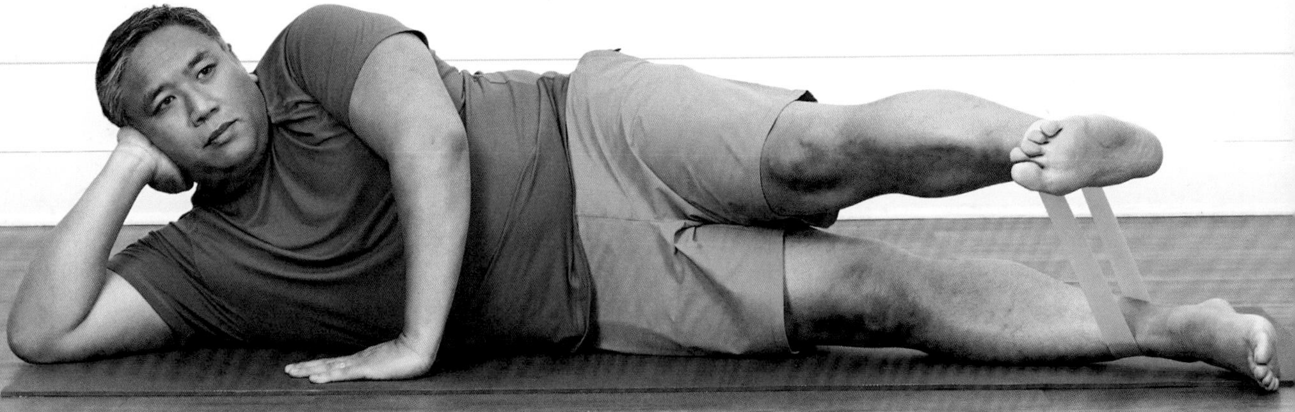

ON YOUR FOREARM

In step 1, place your right forearm flat on the floor and place the fingertips of your left hand on the floor. Continue with the remaining text.

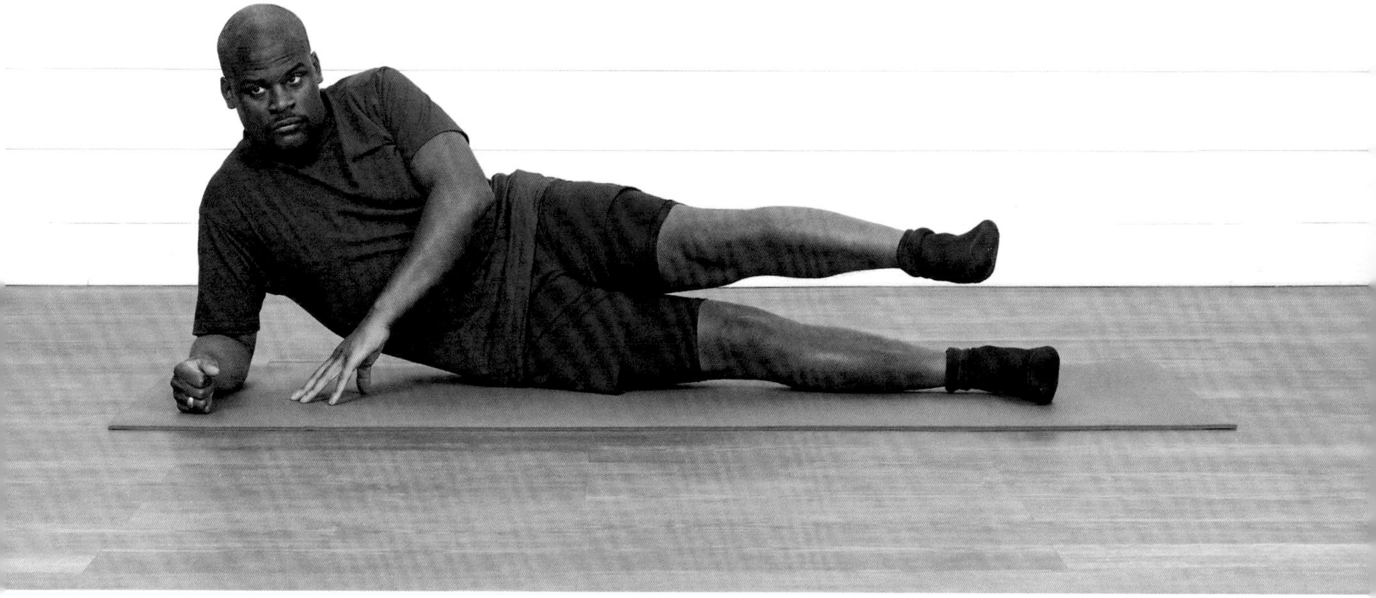

WITH A SMALL PILATES BALL

In step 1, place your right forearm flat on the floor. Place a small Pilates ball between your right hip and your ribs. Continue with the remaining text.

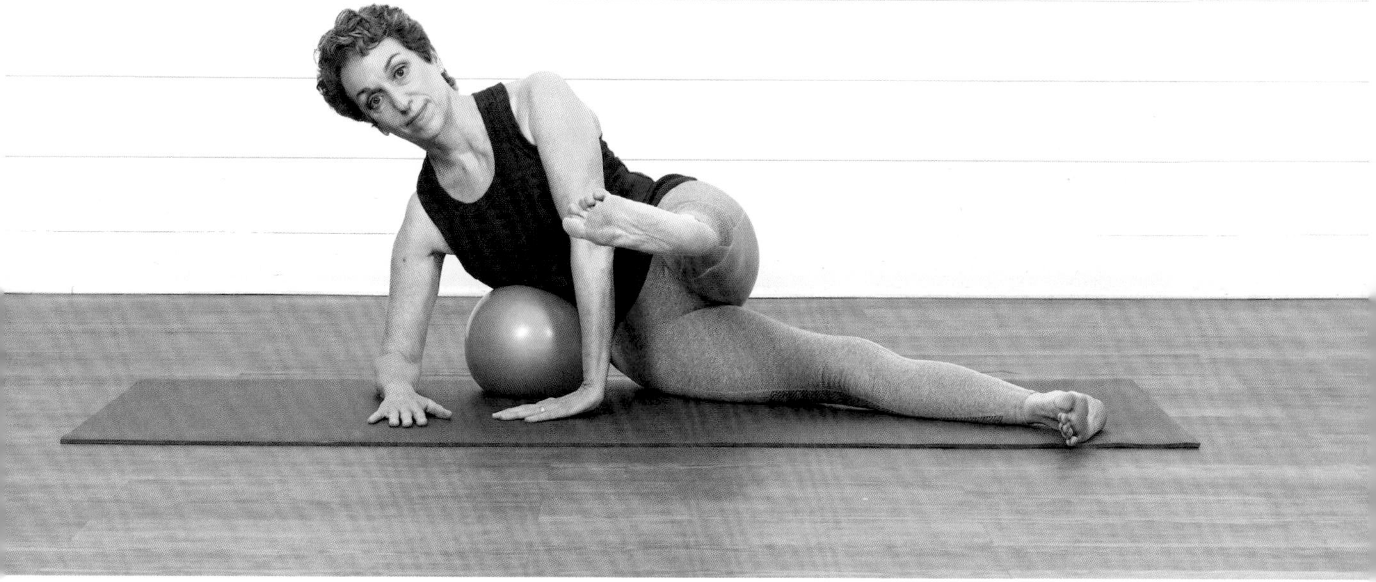

Single-Leg Kicks

Strengthen your hamstrings, upper back, triceps, shoulders, and abs with this exercise. Because of the unilateral movements, you can focus on the side you're working and maximize your range of motion during the exercise. You'll activate more muscle fibers because you're also working stabilizing muscles.

1 Lie on your stomach on the floor with your legs extended. Clasp your hands together and place your forearms flat on the floor. Press your glutes and inner thighs together and raise your chest off the floor.

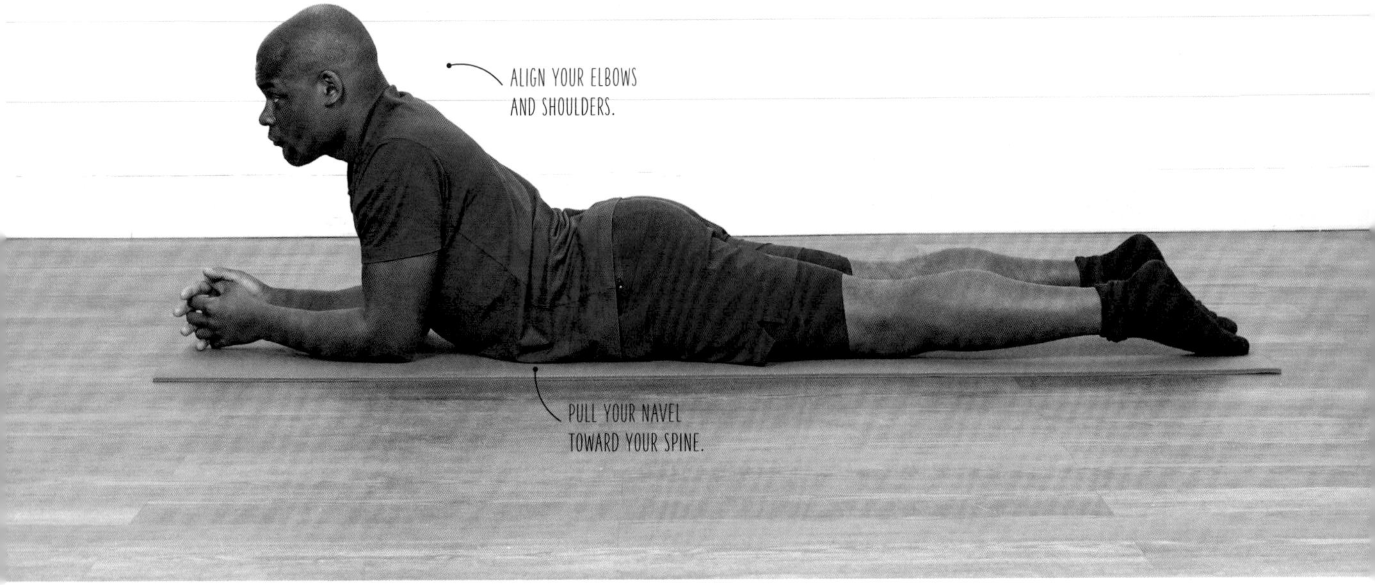
ALIGN YOUR ELBOWS AND SHOULDERS.
PULL YOUR NAVEL TOWARD YOUR SPINE.

2 Bend your left knee and pulse your left foot toward your glutes 2 times. Lower your left leg to the floor. Perform this step 2 times. Repeat these steps with your right leg.

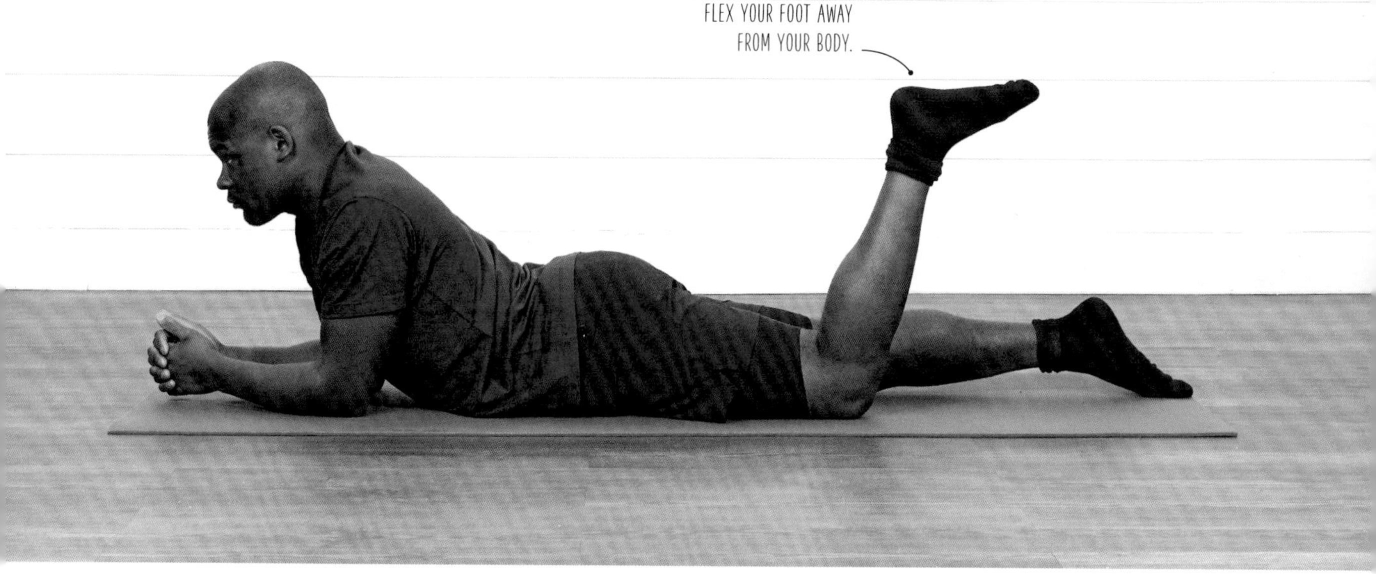
FLEX YOUR FOOT AWAY
FROM YOUR BODY.

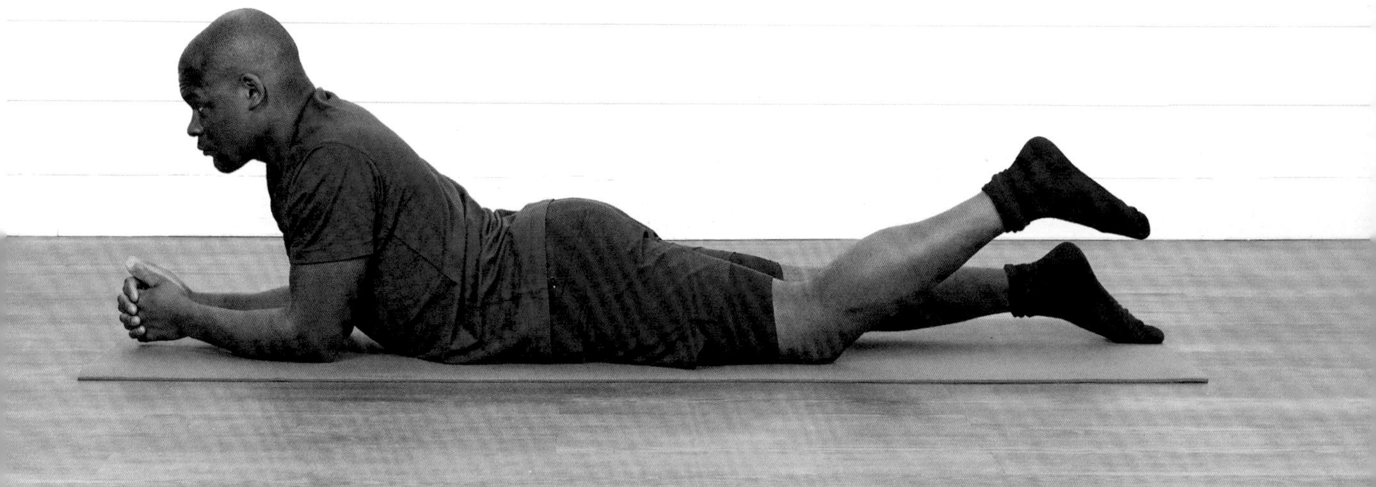

SINGLE-LEG KICKS

VARIATIONS

If you have a herniated disc or lower back pain, avoid performing the main exercise. Using a small Pilates ball or a stability ball might help you if you have lower back inflexibility by decreasing your range of motion for the movements and decreasing pressure on your lower back. The standing variation is a good option for pregnant people or those who have difficulty getting down to or up from the floor.

WITH A STABILITY BALL

1. Kneel in front of a stability ball. Place your forearms on the ball, rolling the ball slightly away, and lean your abs into the ball.

2. Bend your right knee and bring your right heel toward your buttocks. Reverse your movements to return to your starting position. Perform this step 2 times.

3. Bend your left knee and bring your left heel toward your buttocks. Reverse your movements to return to your starting position. Perform this step 2 times. Perform these steps 5 times.

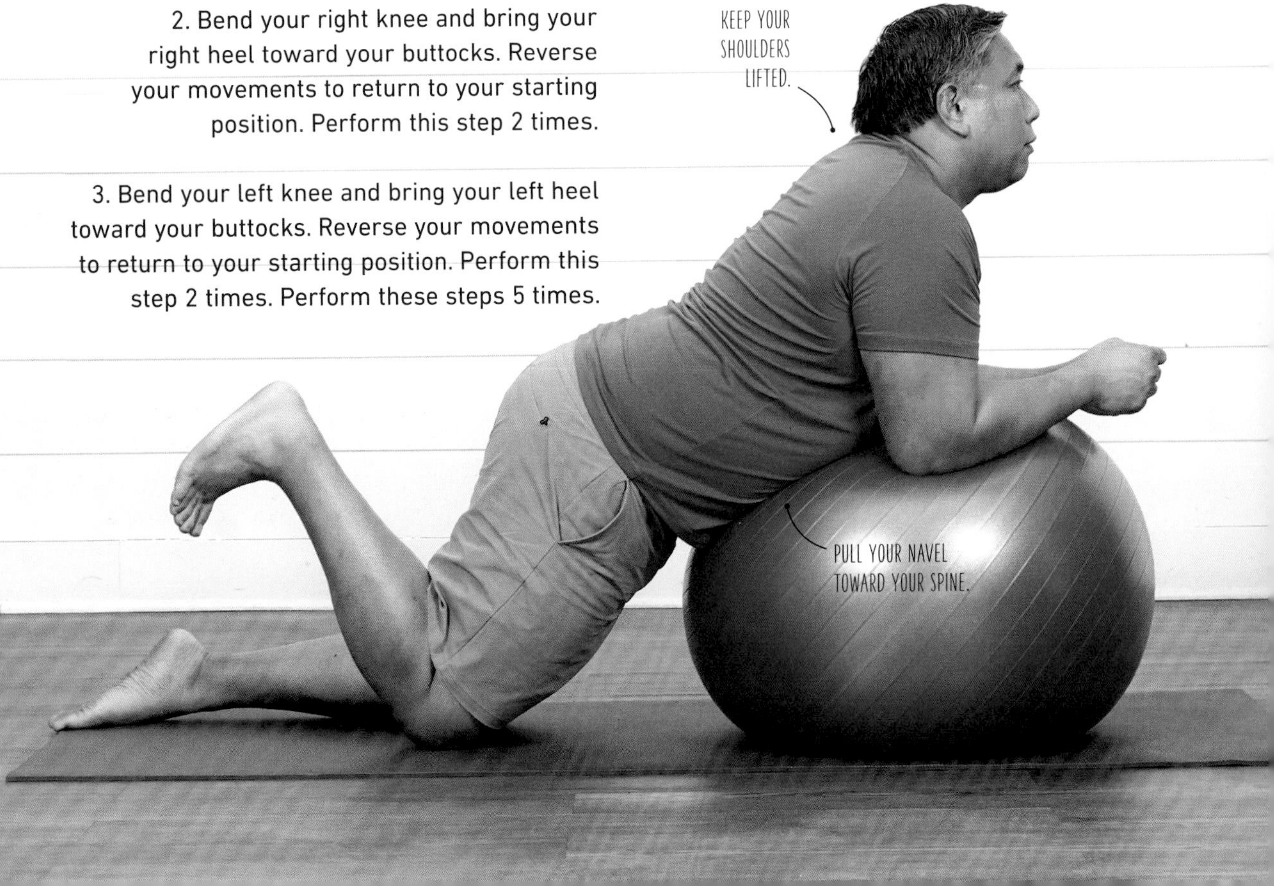
KEEP YOUR SHOULDERS LIFTED.
PULL YOUR NAVEL TOWARD YOUR SPINE.

WITH A SMALL PILATES BALL

In step 1, place a small Pilates ball under your body below your ribs. Continue with the remaining text.

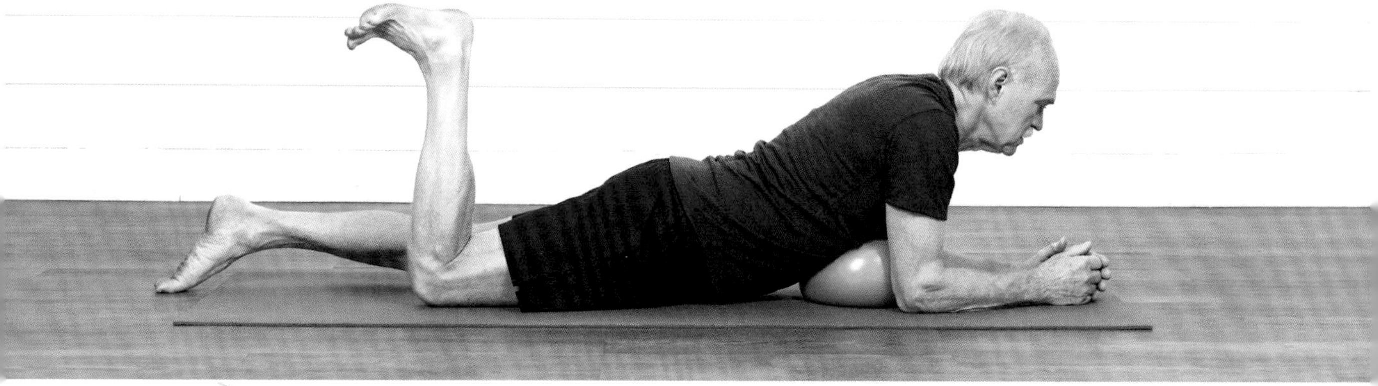

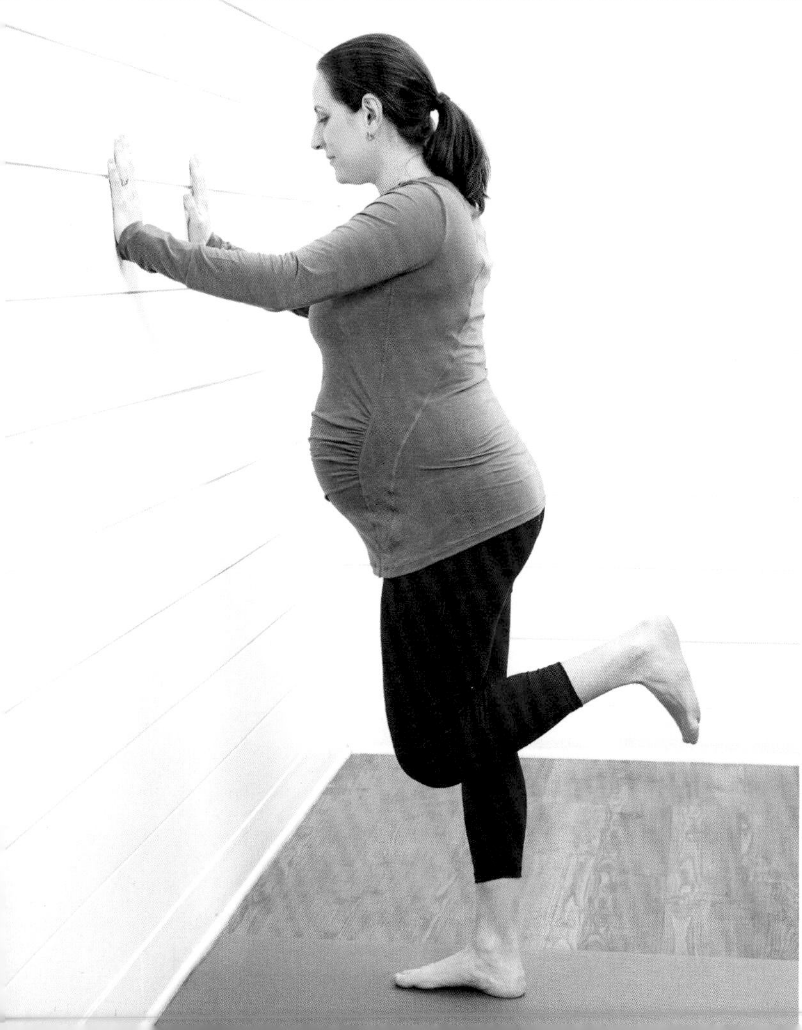

STANDING FACING A WALL

1. Stand an arm's length away from a wall with your legs shoulder width apart. Place your hands on the wall.

2. Bend your right knee and bring your right heel toward your buttocks. Reverse your movements to return to your starting position. Perform this step 2 times.

3. Bend your left knee and bring your left heel toward your buttocks. Reverse your movements to return to your starting position. Perform this step 2 times. Perform these steps 5 times.

ANDREW PETERSON

Shortly after birth, I was found alone. I was sent to a foster home, but I was later adopted. However, my birth mother drank alcohol during pregnancy, and because I have permanent brain damage from fetal alcohol syndrome, nothing in life has ever been easy for me.

In school, I tried my best. But I couldn't run, speak, or learn like other kids. Some laughed and called me names. Others walked by me like I didn't exist. All I wanted was to be included.

After a decade of physical therapy, including years of acrobatics and even tap dancing, I could actually move my arms and legs in a smooth motion. Finally, I was ready to move. I wasn't the fastest on the playground, but no one could run as far as me. I didn't slow down. I refused to stop. For the first time in my life, my disability didn't define me. But most people kept focusing on what I'd never be able to do. I showed them: I earned four varsity letters in high school cross-country.

At the same time, Special Olympics provided me with opportunities to train and become an athlete and leader. Several years later, I ran three personal bests and won three gold medals at the USA Games. I also gave hundreds of speeches to thousands of high school students about respect. One person *can* make a difference.

Then a new challenge emerged: marathons. Six days a week, I ran with runners faster than me. I became known more for my grit than my running form. And soon, I proved the skeptics wrong again. After running my fifth marathon in 2 hours and 57 minutes, I qualified for the prestigious Boston Marathon. I earned the name "No-Limits Andrew."

Life was great until my 12th marathon. For the first time, I experienced severe back pain while running. On mile 23 of my 13th marathon, I could run no farther. I had to stop. Since running with my father at age 8, I had never stopped. Until now. A week later, the X-ray didn't lie. Scoliosis. It went undiagnosed in my teens yet hadn't ever been a problem. My doctor knew better. Years of intense marathon training had left my hips and shoulders grossly misaligned. My muscles were no longer in sync. In fact, one leg was an inch longer than the other. Something that came so easy was now impossible. But would I be able to run again?

After three months of intense physical therapy, I felt new. Then I discovered Pilates and all its benefits. With exercises that focused on my postural alignment, core strength, and muscular balance, I regained much of my former self. Within three months, I ran another marathon. Decent time. And best of all, absolutely no discomfort.

To maintain my health today, I meticulously follow my Pilates routine twice a day. The results are clear. My body continues to feel great, with no hint of back pain. Rather than my body controlling me and my performance, I control it—thanks to Pilates.

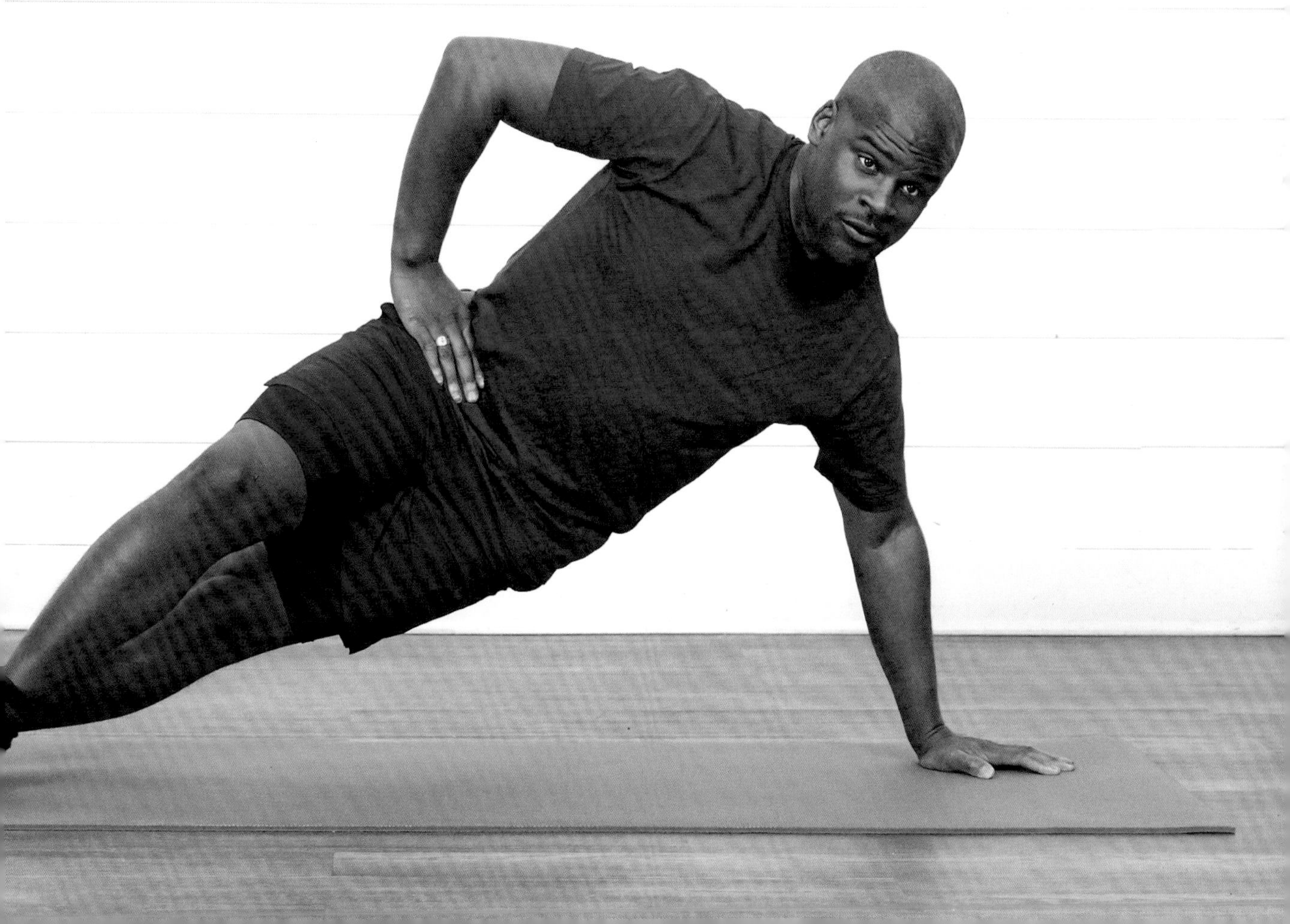

Heel Beats

This exercise can strengthen your lower back, your gluteal muscles, and the backs of your legs while encouraging core control. It can also strengthen the inner thighs while requiring core engagement. These movements can help with the mind-body connection and your overall coordination.

1 Lie on your stomach on the floor. Fold your arms on top of each other and rest your forehead on your top forearm.

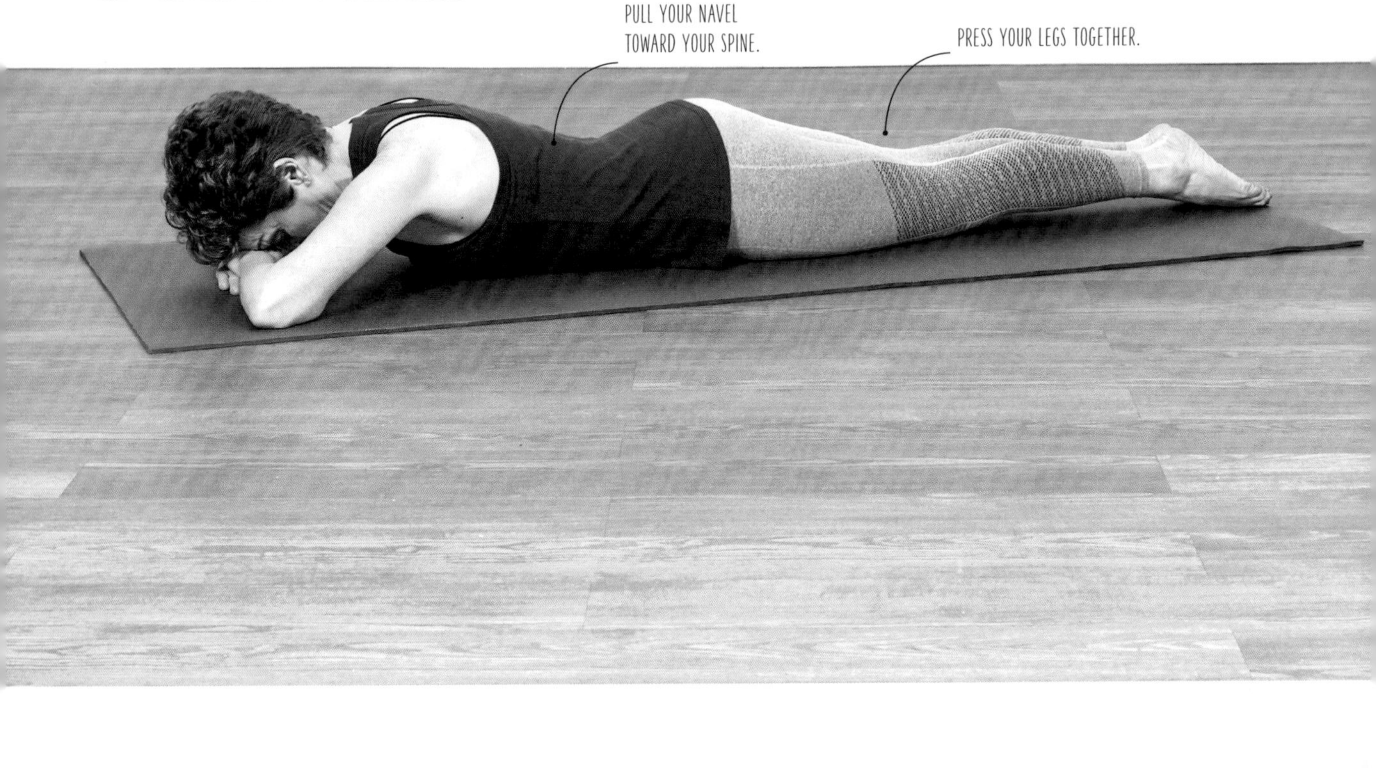

PULL YOUR NAVEL TOWARD YOUR SPINE.
PRESS YOUR LEGS TOGETHER.

2 Press your glutes together and raise your legs off the floor.

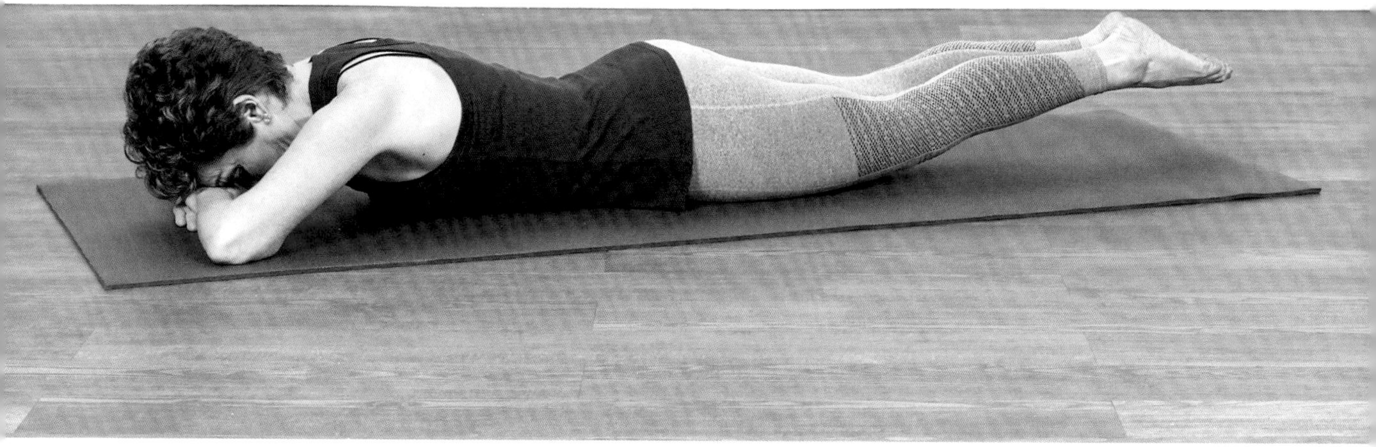

3 Extend your legs to your sides and hold this position for 10 seconds. Reverse your movements to return to your position in step 2. Perform the last two steps 3 times.

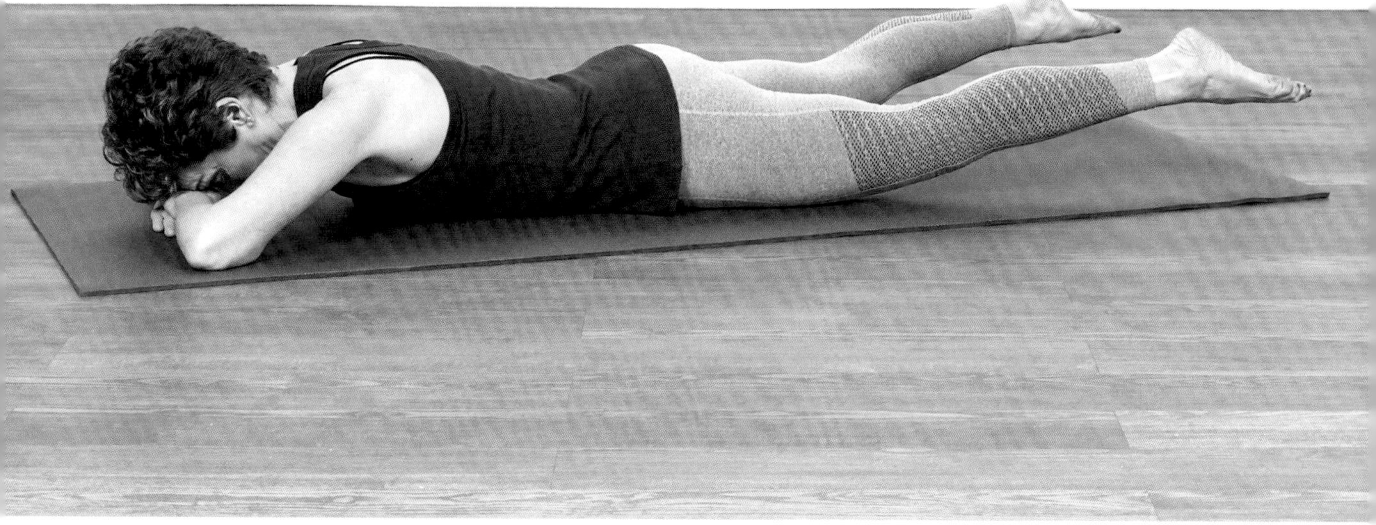

HEEL BEATS

VARIATIONS

Using a small Pilates ball or lying on your back decreases the range of motion needed for this exercise and decreases the pressure on your lower back. The seated variation is a good option for pregnant people or those who have difficulty getting down to or up from the floor.

ON YOUR BACK

1. Lie on your back on the floor and extend your legs toward the ceiling, keeping your legs together. Relax your arms by your sides.

2. Point your toes toward your sides and turn your legs to allow your heels to touch. Tap the insides of your heels together for a count of 10. Perform this step 3 times.

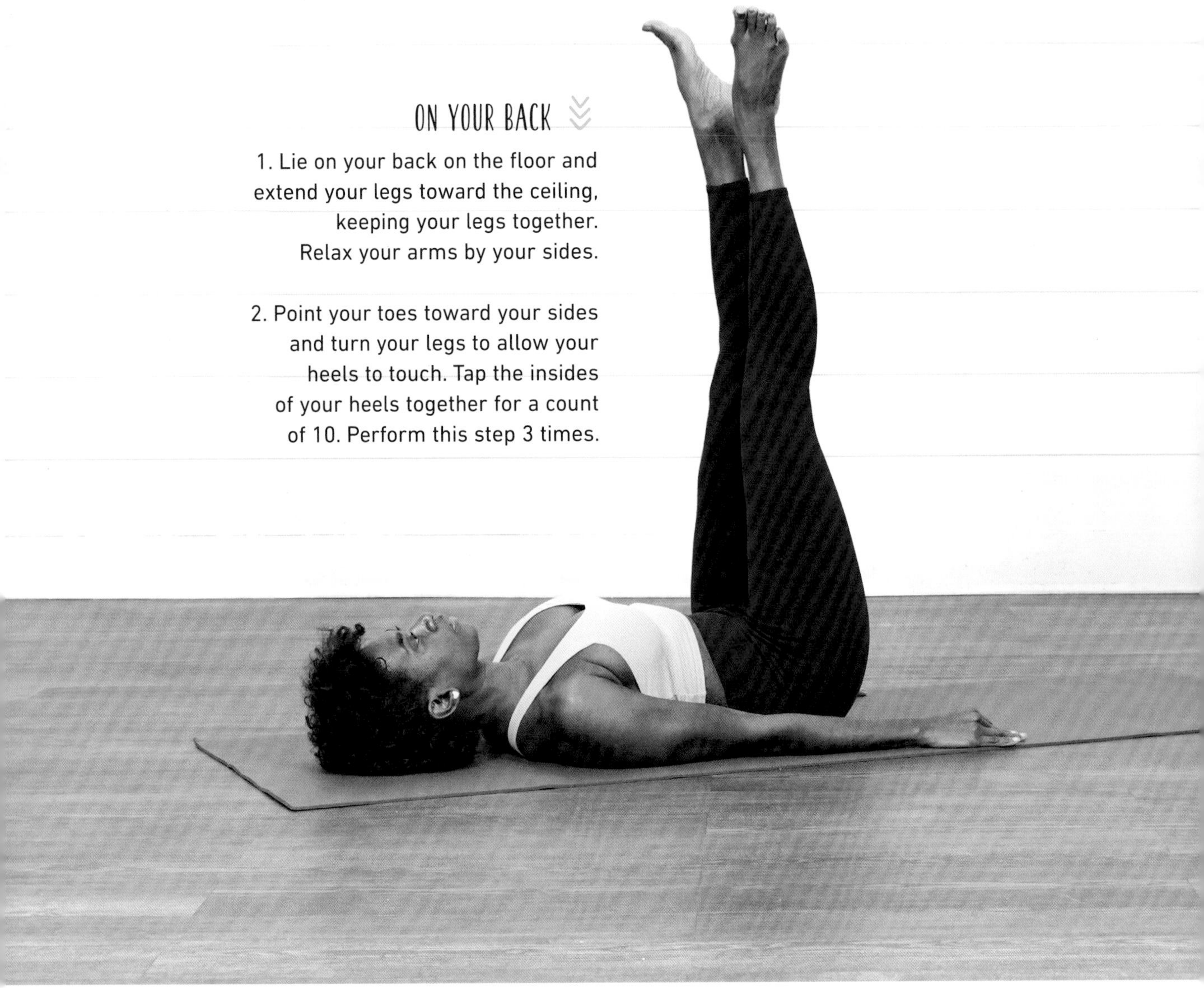

WITH A FOLDED TOWEL

In step 1, place a folded towel under your chest at your breastbone.

In step 3, return to your starting position in step 1. Continue with the remaining text.

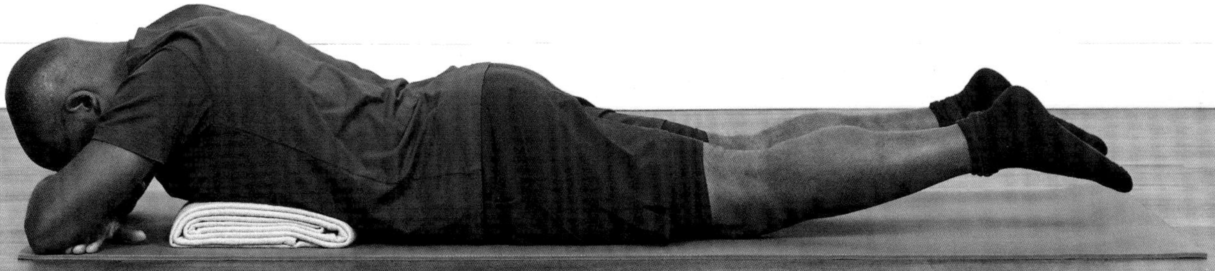

SITTING IN A CHAIR

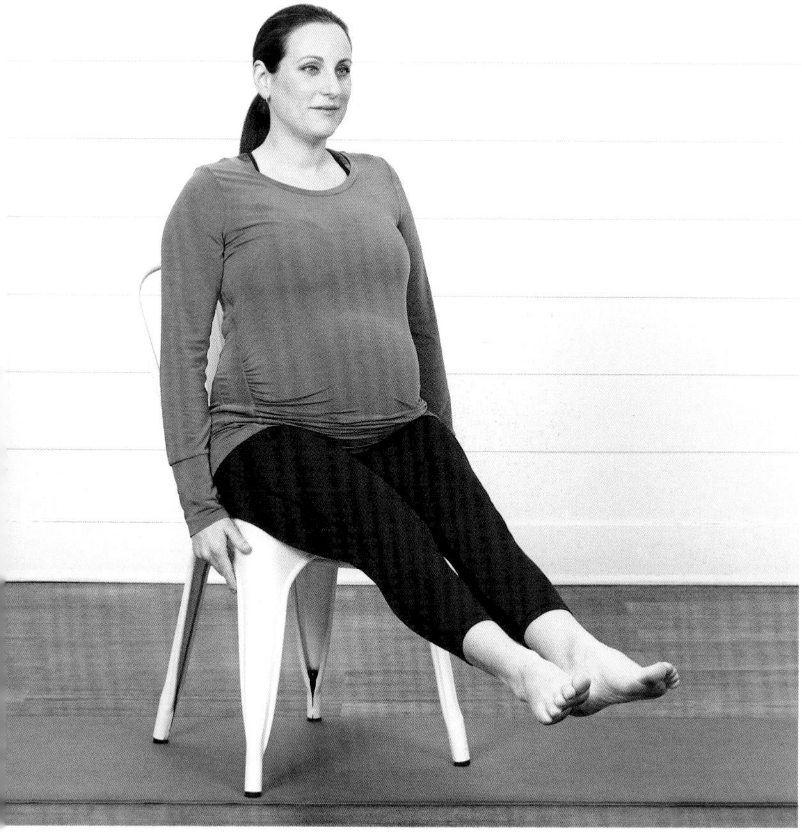

1. Sit in a chair with your feet flat on the floor and your legs together. Place your hands on the sides of the chair.

2. Raise your legs until parallel with the floor or as high as you feel comfortable. Point your toes toward your sides and turn your legs to allow your heels to touch. Tap the insides of your heels together for 10 seconds. Lower your legs to the floor. Perform this step 3 times.

Leg Circles

Rotating your legs can strengthen your glutes, hip muscles, and core. This exercise can also improve pelvic stability—the pelvic muscles are strong and able to prevent excessive movement from destabilizing the balance of joints. Pelvic stability helps stabilize your spine and prevents injury.

1 Lie on your right side on the floor with your legs stacked. Extend your right arm toward the top of the mat and rest your head on your right biceps. Place your left hand flat on the floor.

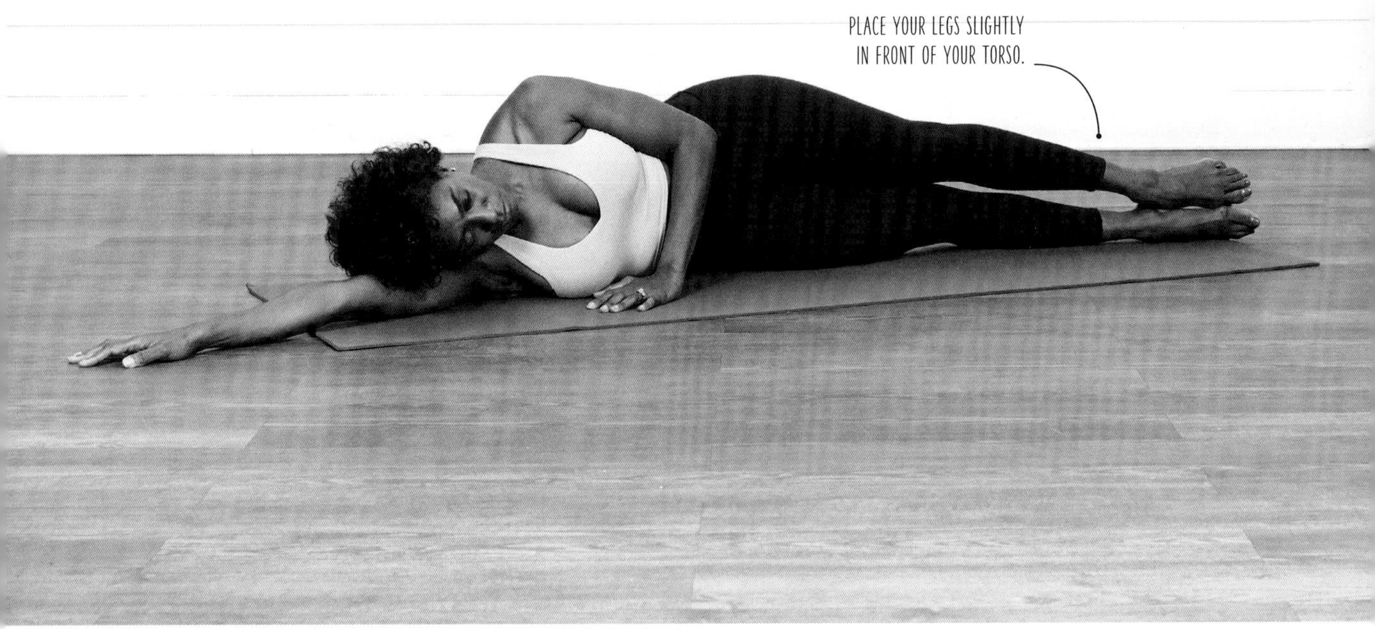

PLACE YOUR LEGS SLIGHTLY IN FRONT OF YOUR TORSO.

2 Raise your left leg and trace clockwise circles a little larger than a basketball. Perform this step 5 times. Return your left leg to atop your right leg.

3 Raise your left leg and trace counterclockwise circles a little larger than a basketball. Perform this step 5 times. Return your left leg to atop your right leg. Repeat these steps on your left side.

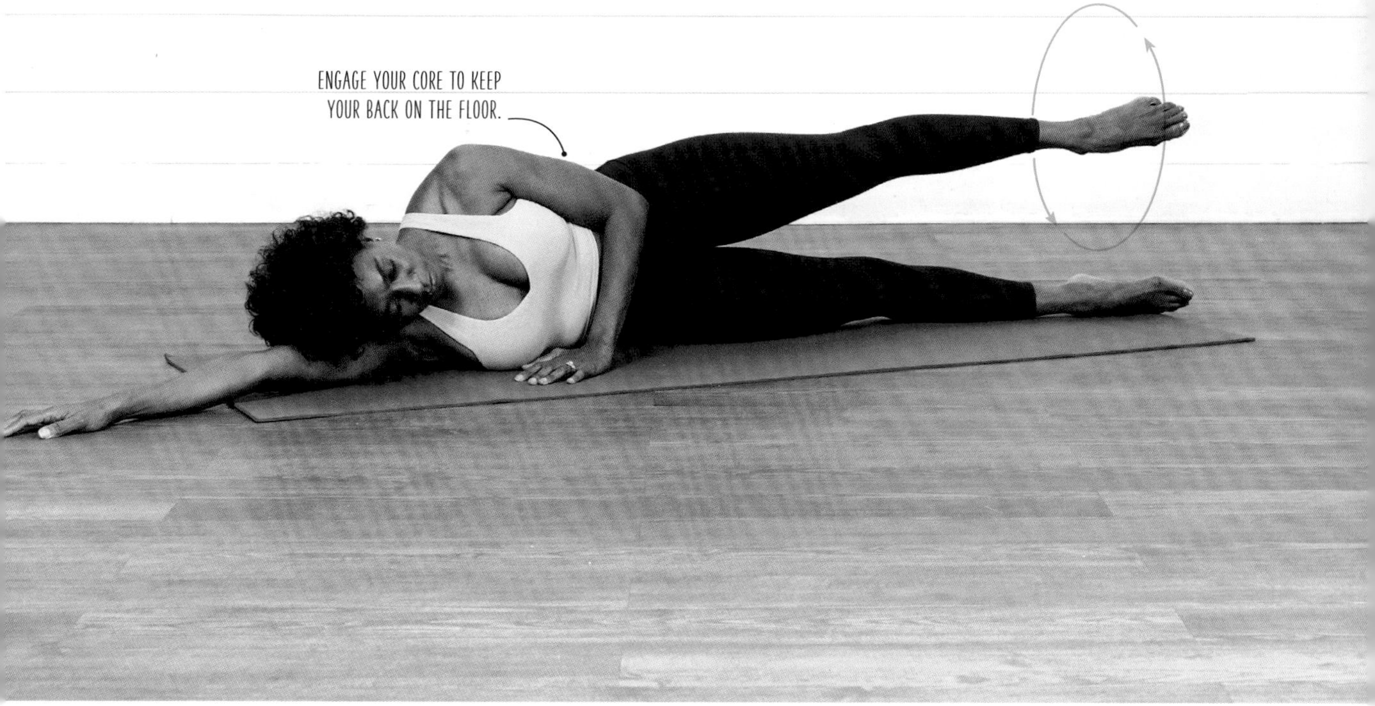
ENGAGE YOUR CORE TO KEEP YOUR BACK ON THE FLOOR.

LEG CIRCLES

VARIATIONS

If you can't straighten your leg because you lack flexibility in your hamstrings, the bent knee or the seated variation can help you perform this exercise. Using a resistance band can also assist in keeping your pelvic region stable.

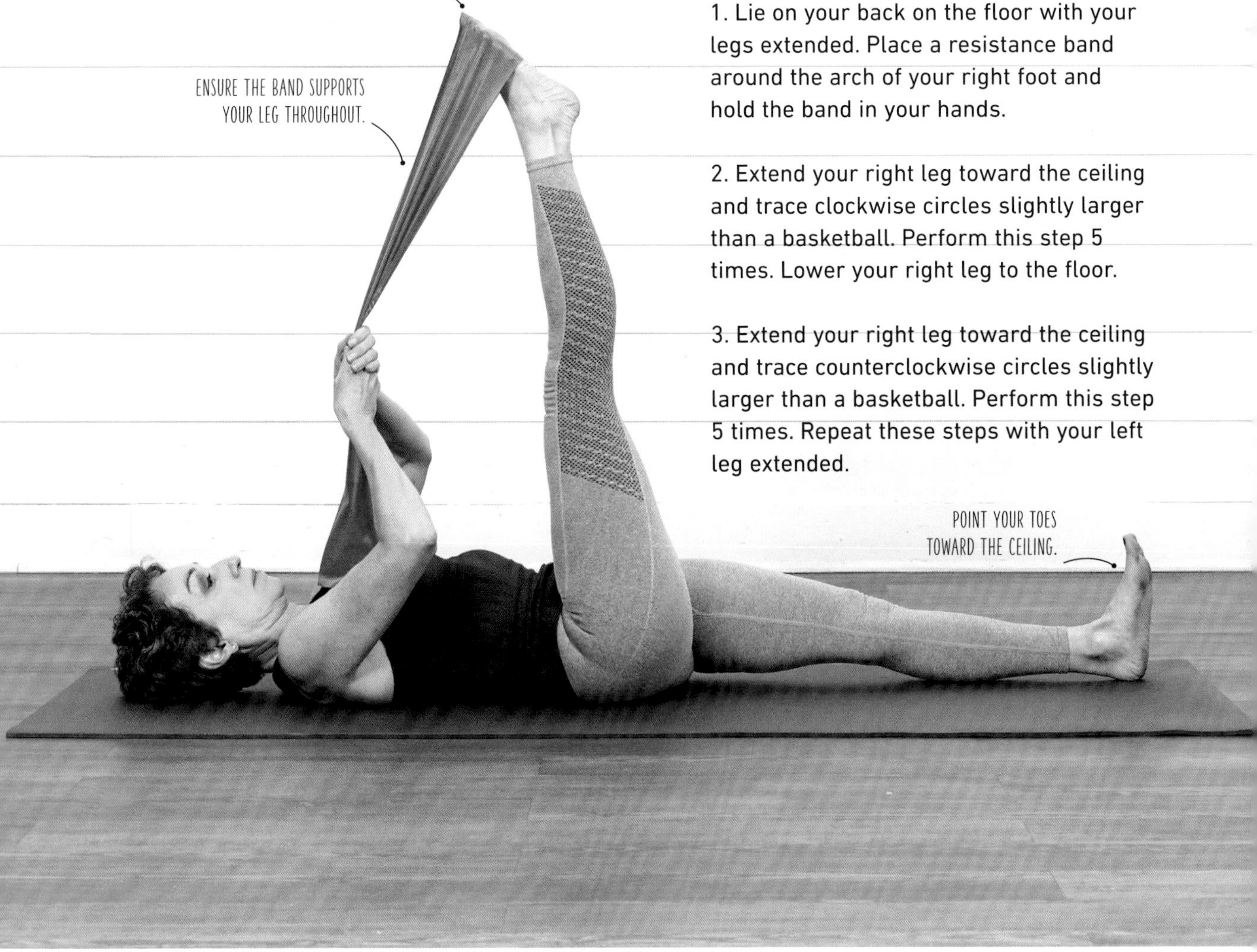

FLEX YOUR FOOT TOWARD YOUR BODY.
ENSURE THE BAND SUPPORTS YOUR LEG THROUGHOUT.
POINT YOUR TOES TOWARD THE CEILING.

WITH A RESISTANCE BAND

1. Lie on your back on the floor with your legs extended. Place a resistance band around the arch of your right foot and hold the band in your hands.

2. Extend your right leg toward the ceiling and trace clockwise circles slightly larger than a basketball. Perform this step 5 times. Lower your right leg to the floor.

3. Extend your right leg toward the ceiling and trace counterclockwise circles slightly larger than a basketball. Perform this step 5 times. Repeat these steps with your left leg extended.

WITH BENT KNEES

In step 2, bend your left knee. Continue with the remaining text.

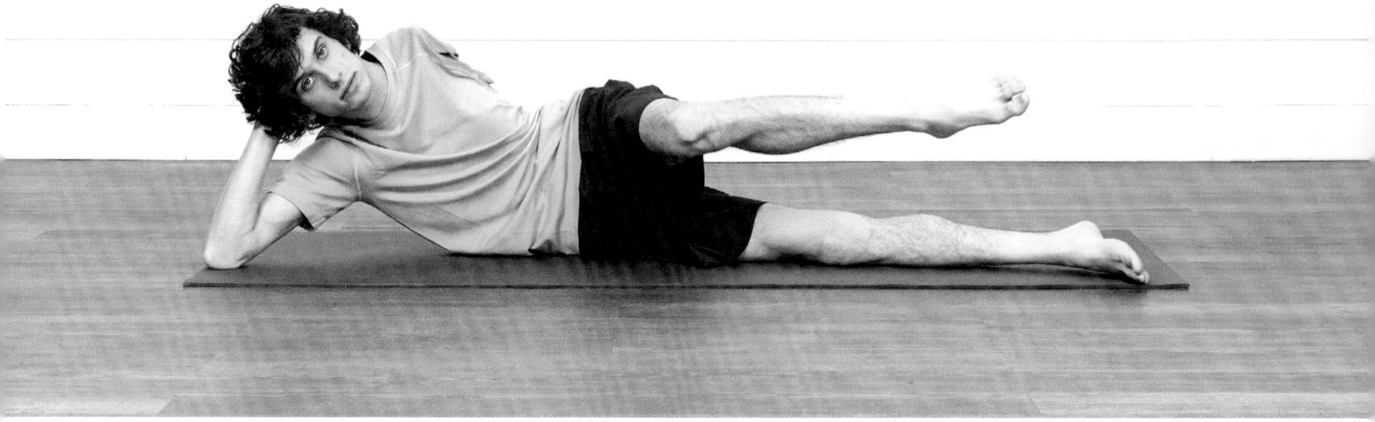

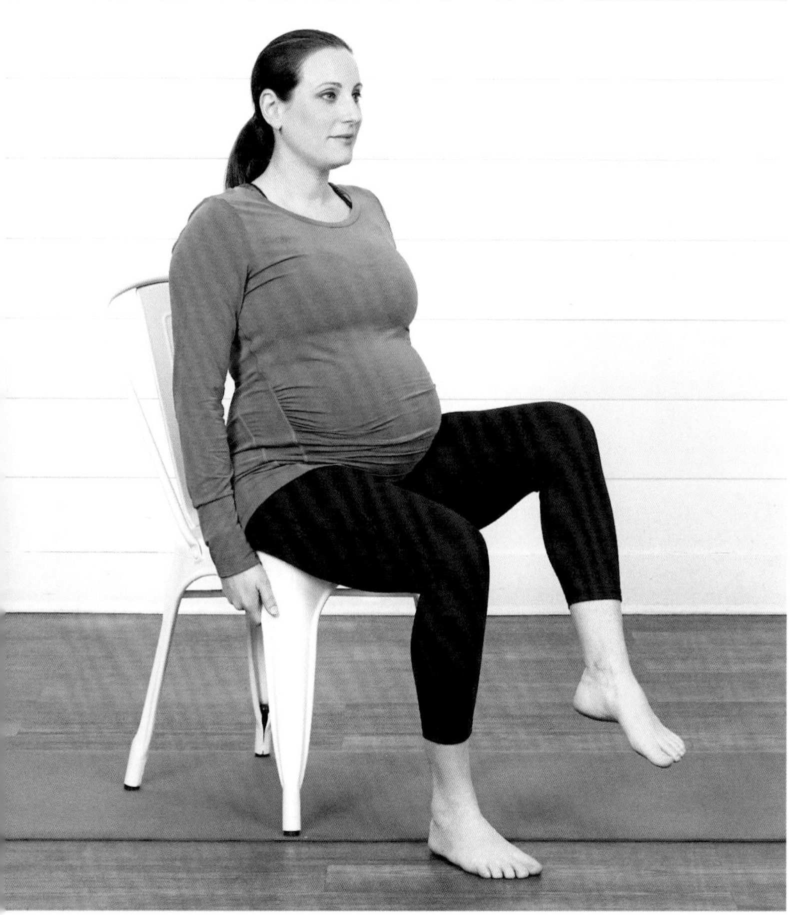

SITTING IN A CHAIR

1. Sit in a chair with your feet flat on the floor. Place your hands on the sides of the chair.

2. Raise your left foot off the floor, keeping your left knee bent, and trace clockwise circles the size of a basketball with your left knee 5 times.

3. Reverse your movements to trace counterclockwise circles the size of a basketball with your right knee 5 times. Lower your right leg to the floor. Repeat these steps with your left leg raised and your left knee bent.

Double Straight-Leg Stretches

This exercise challenges your abdominal muscles (especially those hard-to-target lower abdominal muscles) and stabilizes your torso. Executing these movements works your hip flexors, quadriceps, and gluteal muscles. You can also strengthen your deep core stabilizers, which might protect your lower back from injury.

1 Lie on your back on the floor with your hands behind your head. Extend your legs toward the ceiling to form a 90-degree angle with your body. Raise your head and shoulders off the floor.

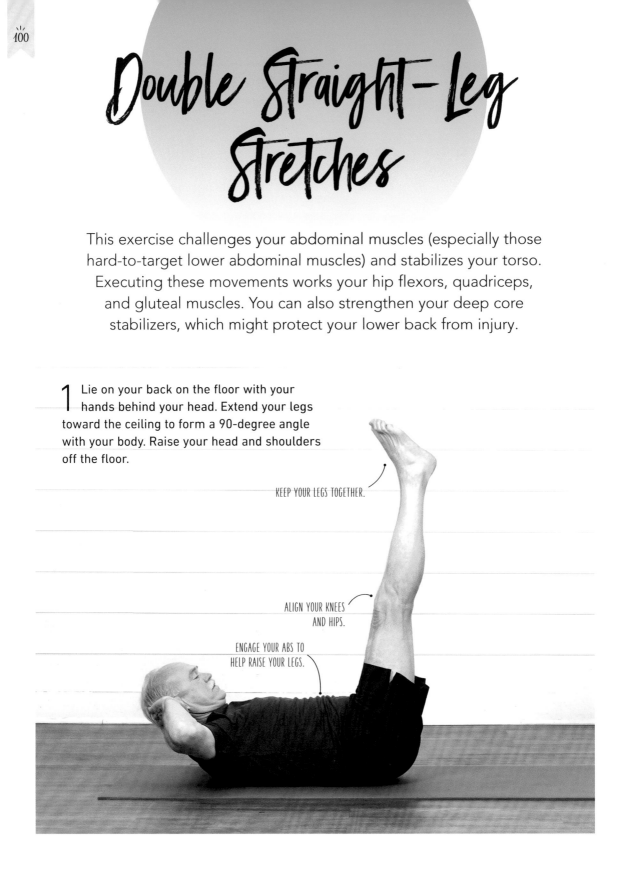

KEEP YOUR LEGS TOGETHER.
ALIGN YOUR KNEES AND HIPS.
ENGAGE YOUR ABS TO HELP RAISE YOUR LEGS.

2 Press your inner thighs and glutes together as you lower your legs toward the floor until they form a 45-degree angle with your body. Press your inner thighs and glutes together as you reverse your movements to return to your starting position. Perform these steps 6 times.

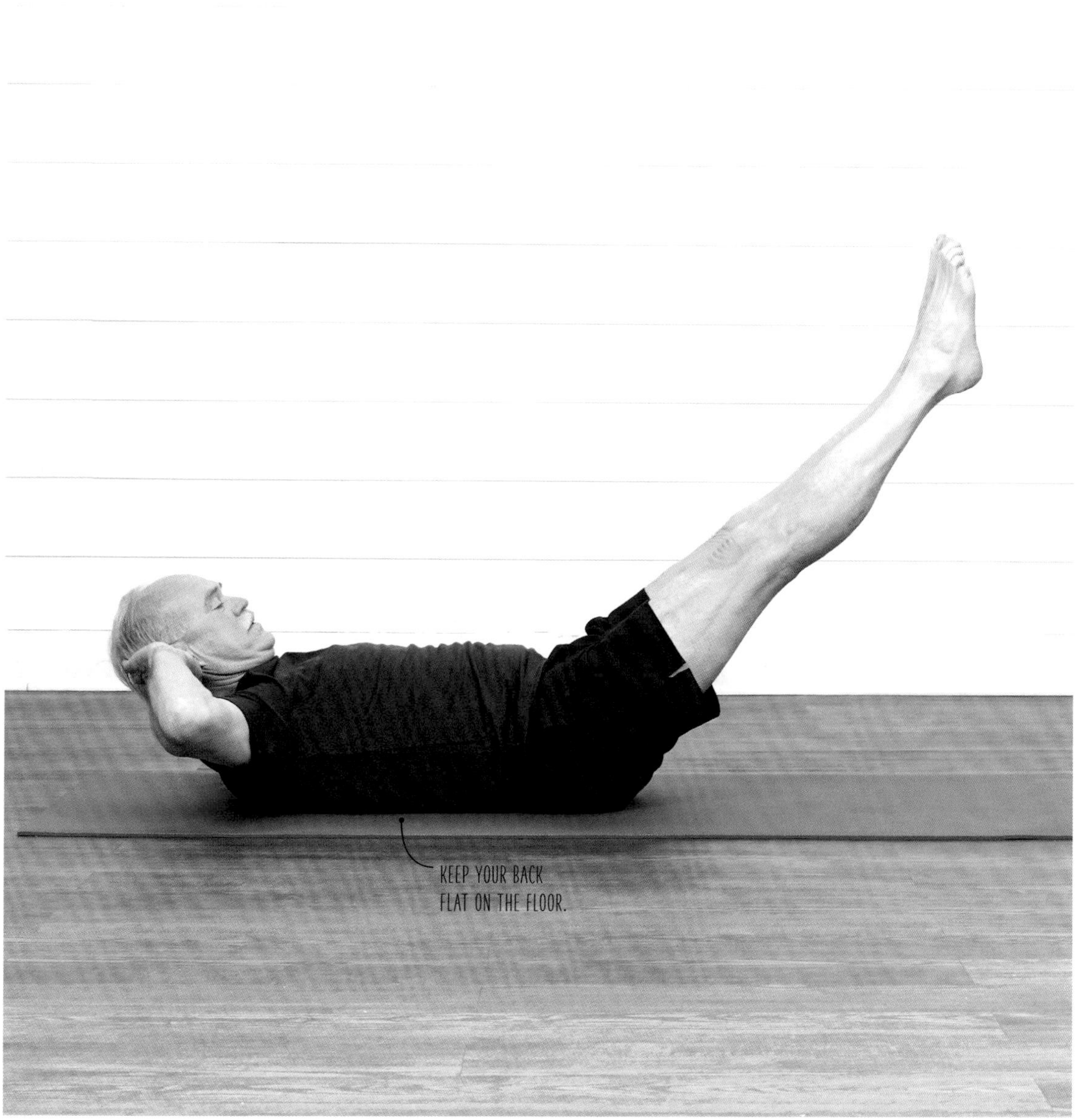
KEEP YOUR BACK
FLAT ON THE FLOOR.

DOUBLE STRAIGHT-LEG STRETCHES

VARIATIONS

When your neck and shoulders aren't properly supported in an exercise, they do too much work. If you feel a strain when lifting your head off the floor, keeping your head down can provide relief. Using resistance bands can also help support the weight of your legs and take pressure off your lower back.

WITH YOUR HEAD DOWN

In step 1, keep your head and shoulders on the floor. Continue with the remaining text.

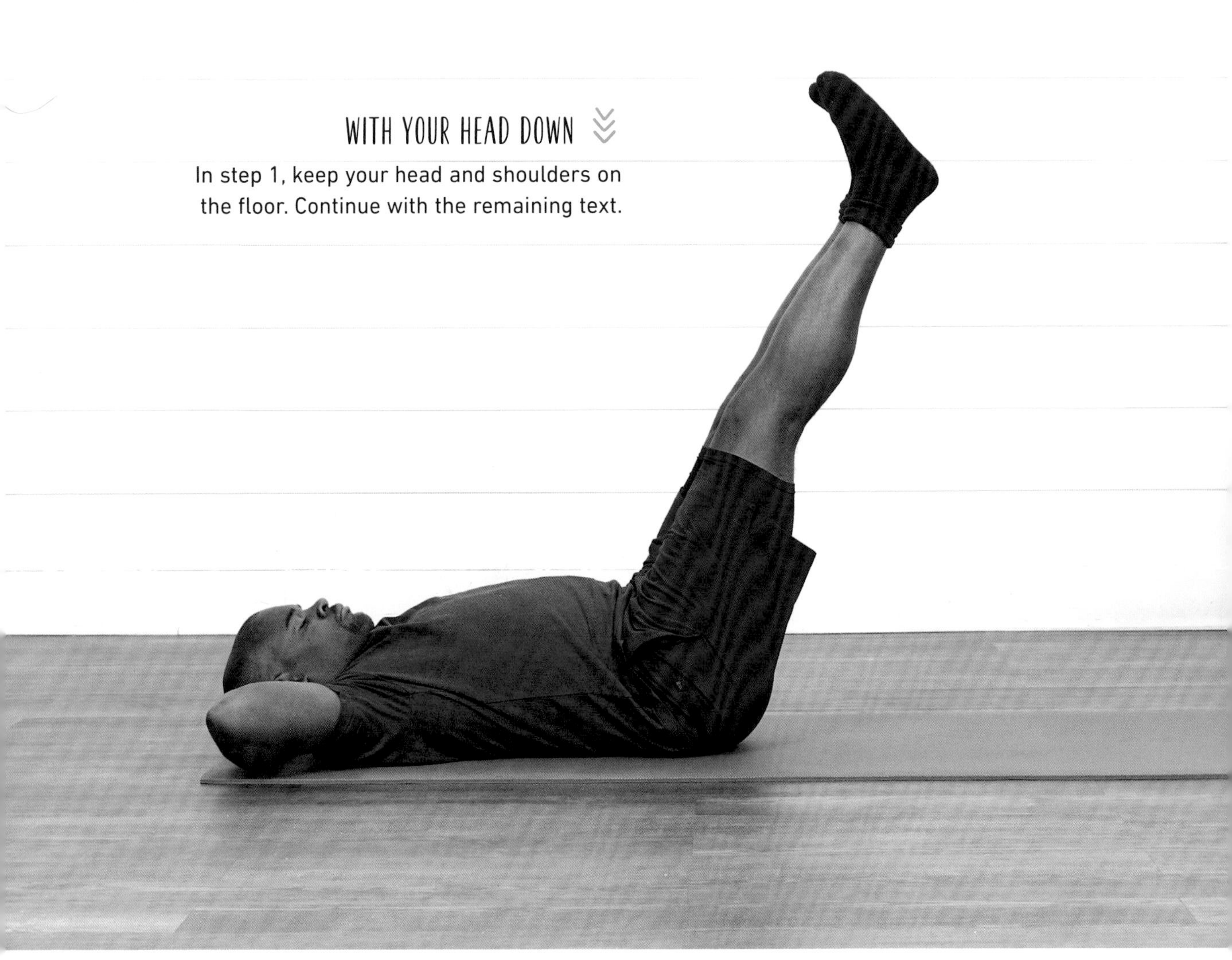

WITH YOUR HEAD DOWN AND KNEES BENT

In step 1, keep your head and shoulders on the floor.

In step 2, bend your knees to form a 90-degree angle with the floor. (You can lower your legs separately or together.) Continue with the remaining text.

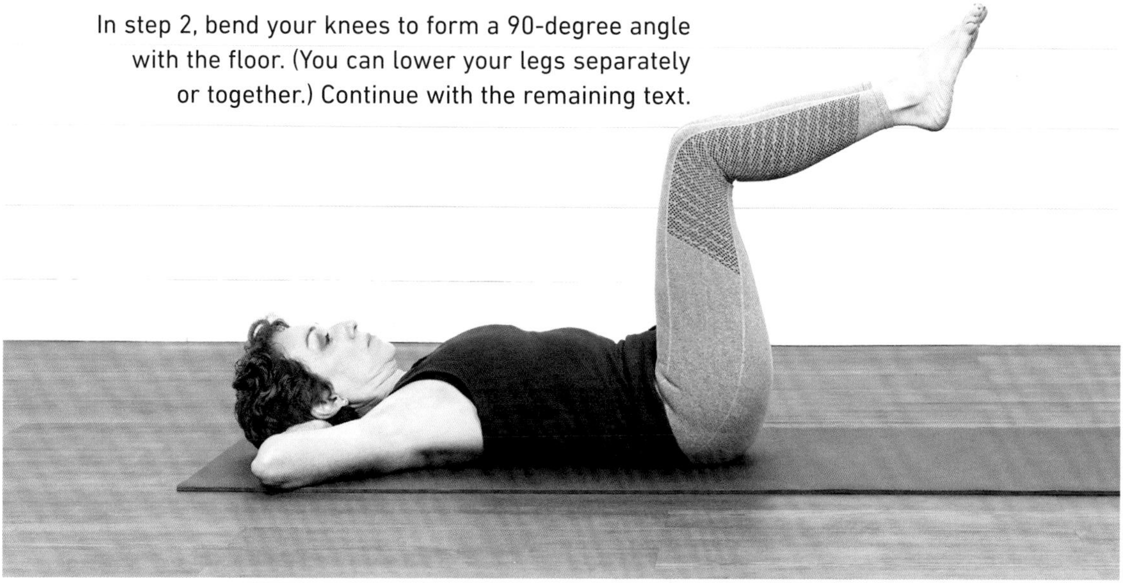

WITH A LOOP BAND

In step 1, place a loop band around your ankles. Keep your head and shoulders on the floor throughout.

In step 2, widen your feet slightly. Continue with the remaining text.

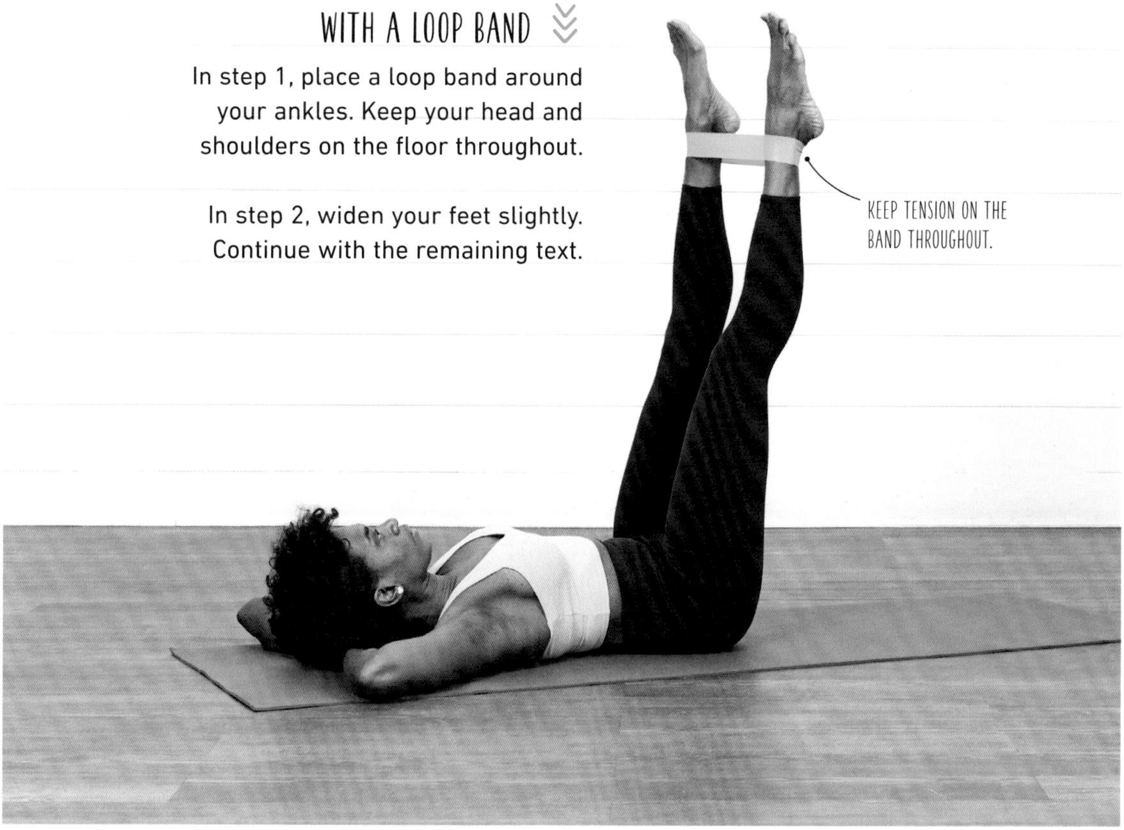

KEEP TENSION ON THE BAND THROUGHOUT.

Hip Flexor Lunges

Tight hips make it harder for your pelvis to rotate properly, which can cause your lower back to overcompensate and might put you at a higher risk for injury. Performing this exercise can help lengthen the hip flexor muscles, providing better flexibility and increased range of motion.

1 Stand with your feet together and your arms relaxed at your sides.

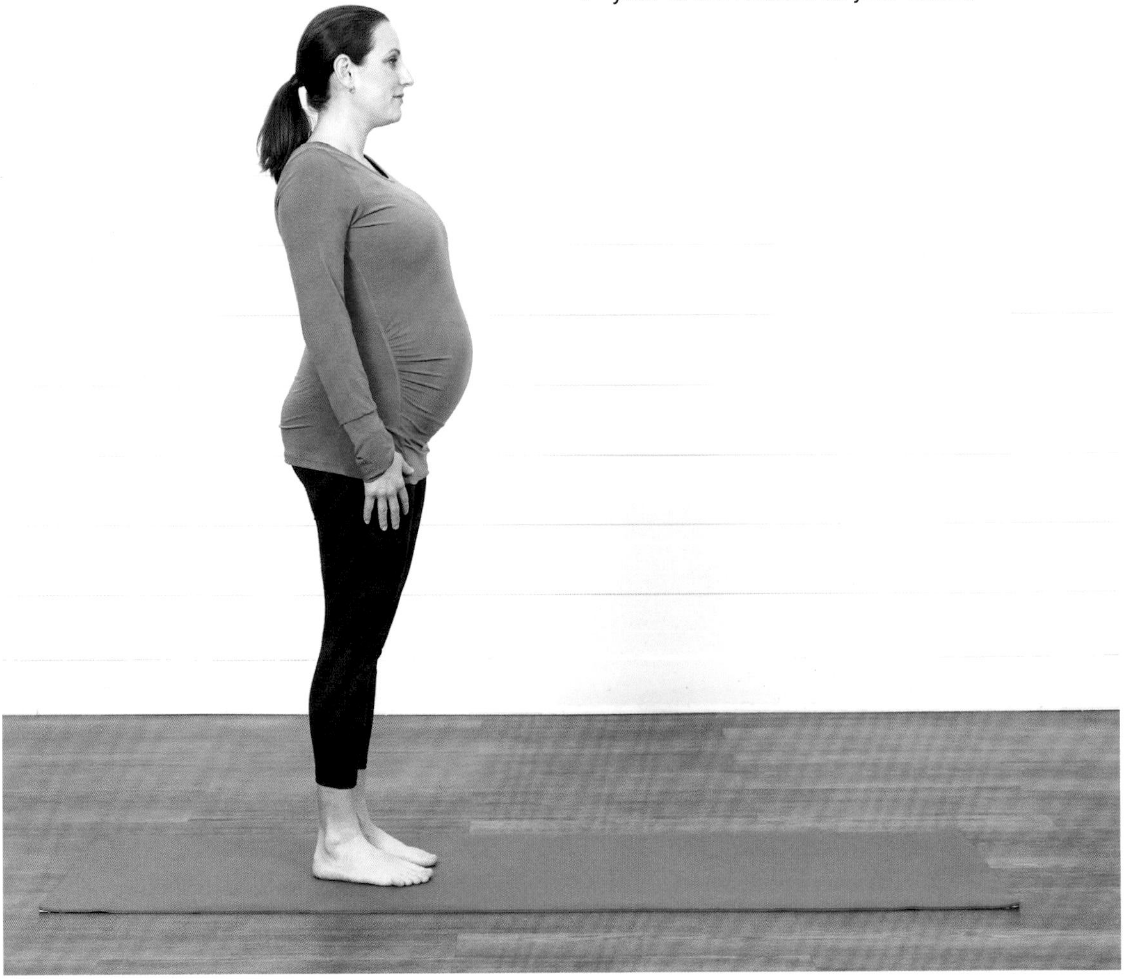

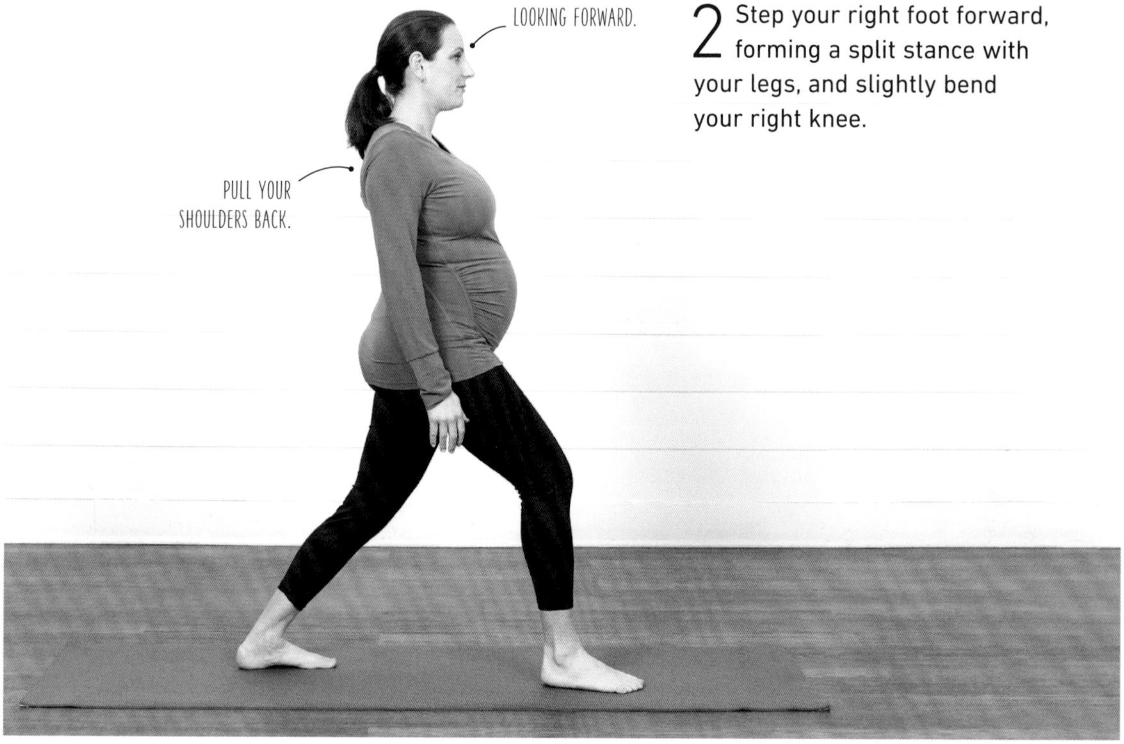
KEEP YOUR GAZE
LOOKING FORWARD.
PULL YOUR
SHOULDERS BACK.

2 Step your right foot forward, forming a split stance with your legs, and slightly bend your right knee.

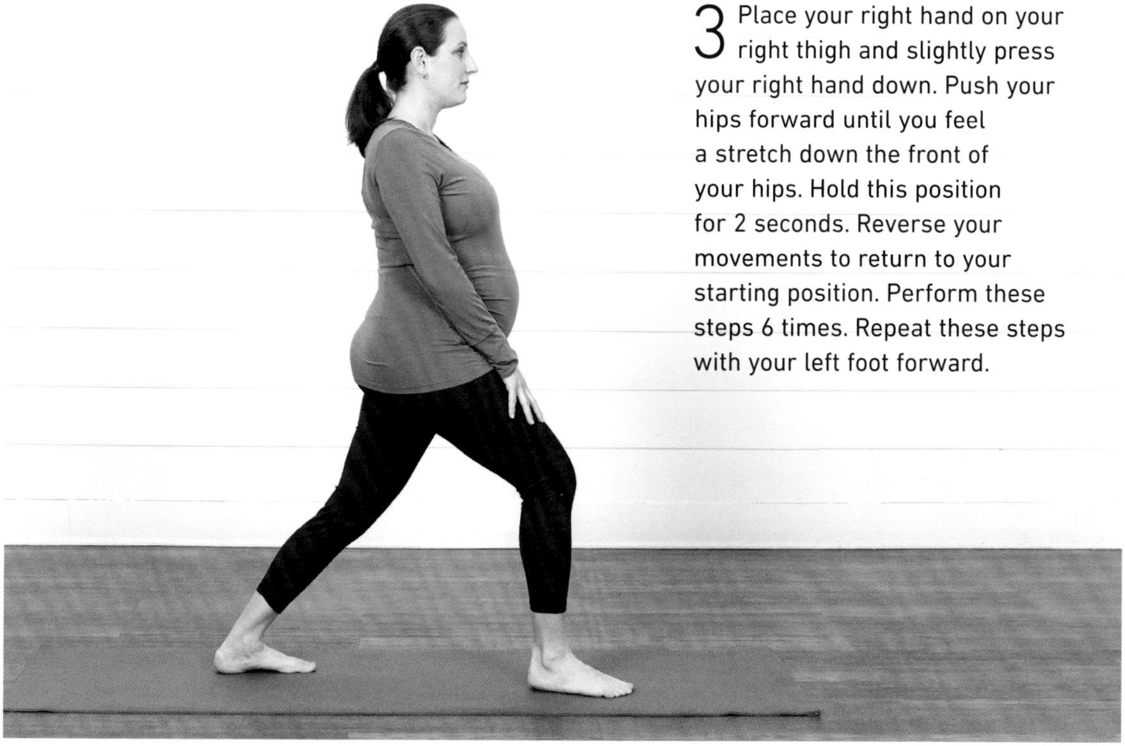

3 Place your right hand on your right thigh and slightly press your right hand down. Push your hips forward until you feel a stretch down the front of your hips. Hold this position for 2 seconds. Reverse your movements to return to your starting position. Perform these steps 6 times. Repeat these steps with your left foot forward.

HIP FLEXOR LUNGES

VARIATIONS

If you have difficulty balancing or standing, using a chair or kneeling on the floor can help with this exercise. Adding the stability ball in the kneeling position can also offer assistance and help create a greater mind-body connection.

KNEELING >>>

1. Kneel on the floor and rest your hands on your hips.

2. Step your right foot forward to form a 90-degree angle with your right leg.

3. Lean your body forward until you feel a stretch in your hips. Hold this position for 2 seconds. Reverse your movements to return to your starting position. Perform these steps 6 times. Repeat these steps with your left leg forward.

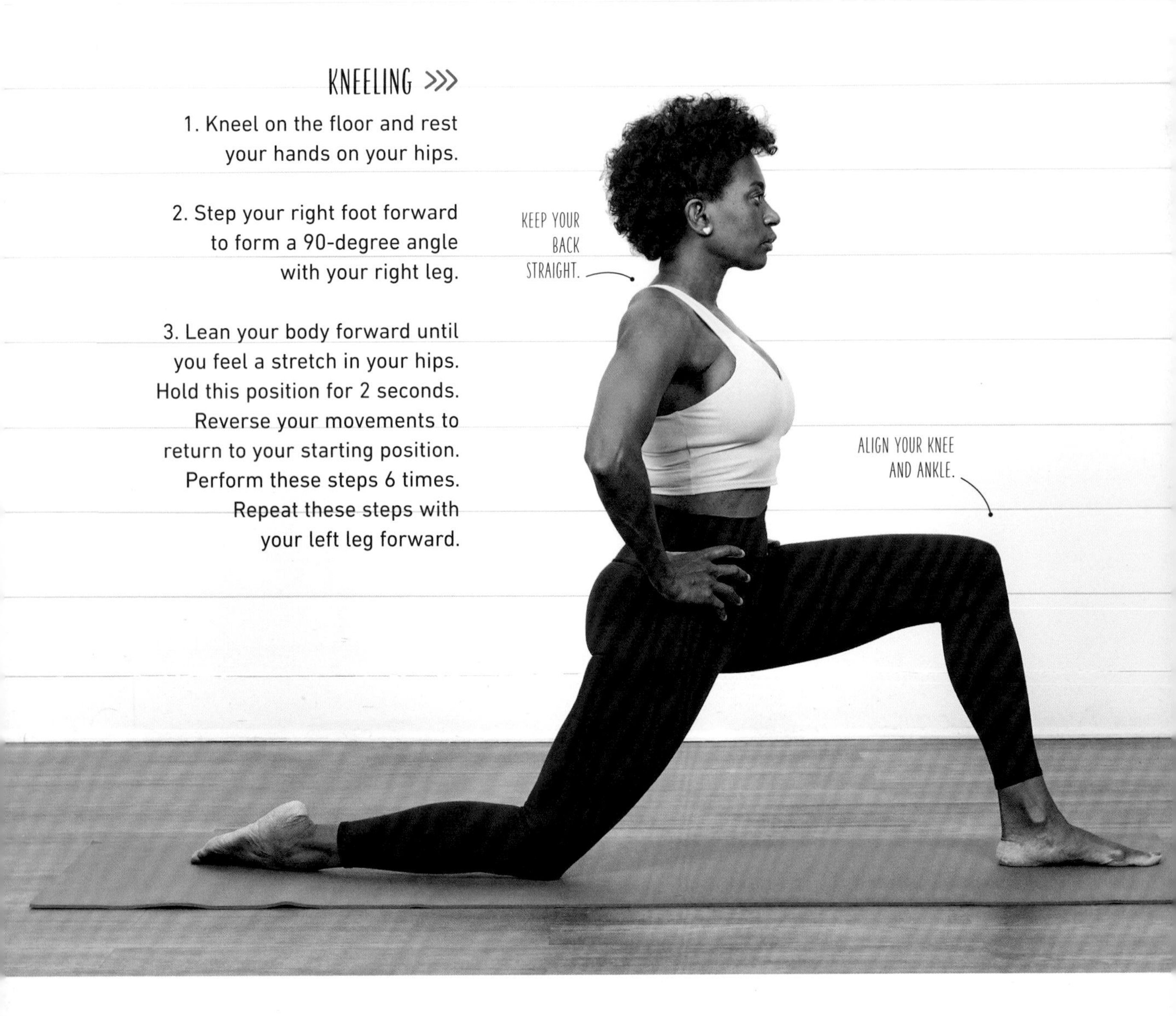

KEEP YOUR BACK STRAIGHT.
ALIGN YOUR KNEE AND ANKLE.

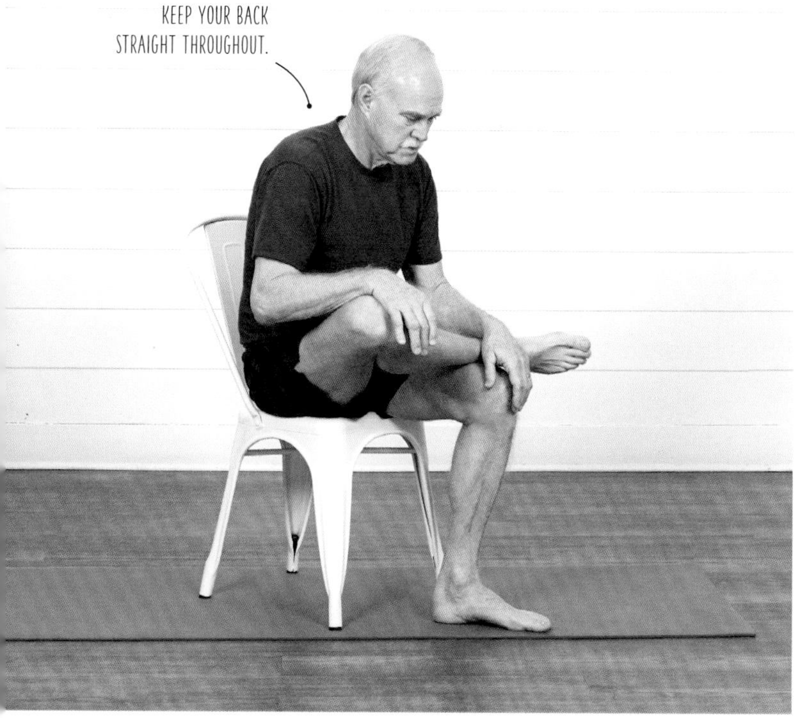

⋘ SITTING IN A CHAIR

1. Sit in a chair with your right ankle on top of your left knee and your left foot flat on the floor. Rest your hands on your knees.

2. Gently lean your body forward and reach through the top of your head until you feel a stretch in your hips. Hold this position for 5 seconds. Reverse your movements to return to your starting position. Perform these steps 6 times. Repeat these steps with your left ankle on top of your right knee.

WITH A STABILITY BALL ⋙

1. Kneel on the floor behind a stability ball. Place your right hand on the ball and relax your left arm at your side.

2. Step your left foot forward to form a 90-degree angle with your right leg.

3. Roll the ball forward until you feel a stretch. Hold this position for 2 seconds. Reverse your movements to return to your starting position. Perform these steps 6 times. Repeat these steps with your right foot forward.

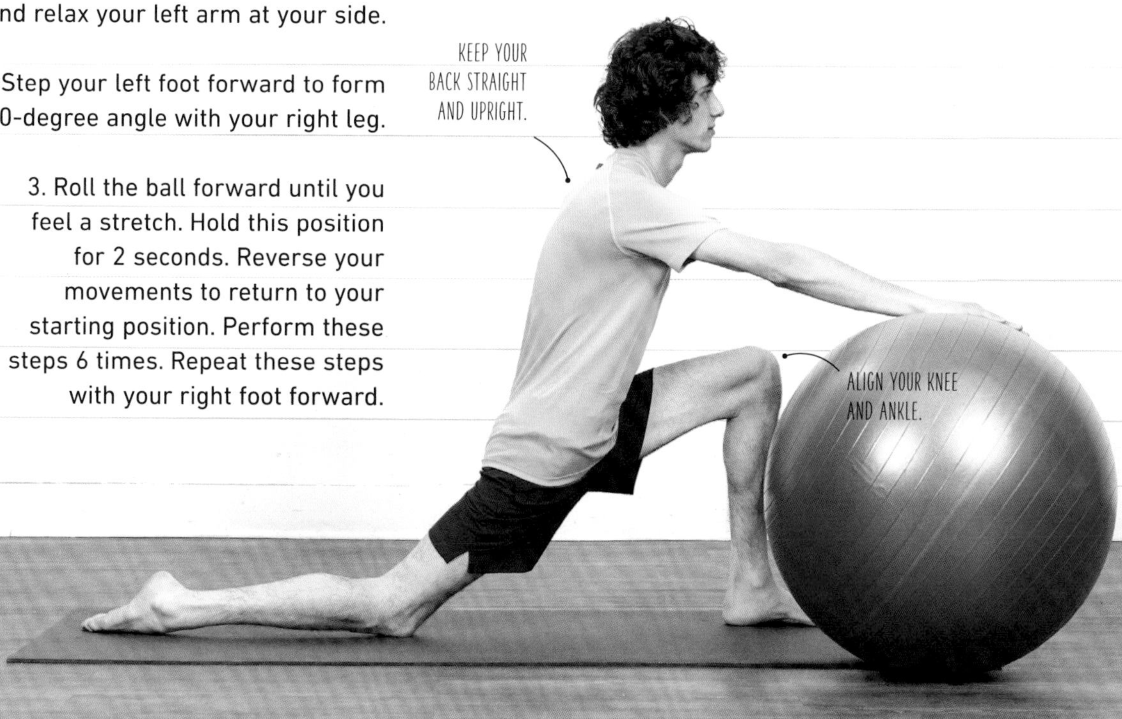
KEEP YOUR
BACK STRAIGHT
AND UPRIGHT.
ALIGN YOUR KNEE
AND ANKLE.

Forearm V-Lifts

Strengthening your abs, hip flexors, and quadriceps while building core stability is what this exercise can do for you. Core stability refers to keeping your spine from moving during physical activity, such as walking and running. Your core muscles protect your spine from excessive loads and transfer force from your lower body to your upper body and vice versa. Having a strong, stable core helps prevent injuries.

1 Sit on the floor with your knees bent and your legs shoulder width apart. Lean backward and place your forearms flat on the floor. Balance your feet on the tips of your toes.

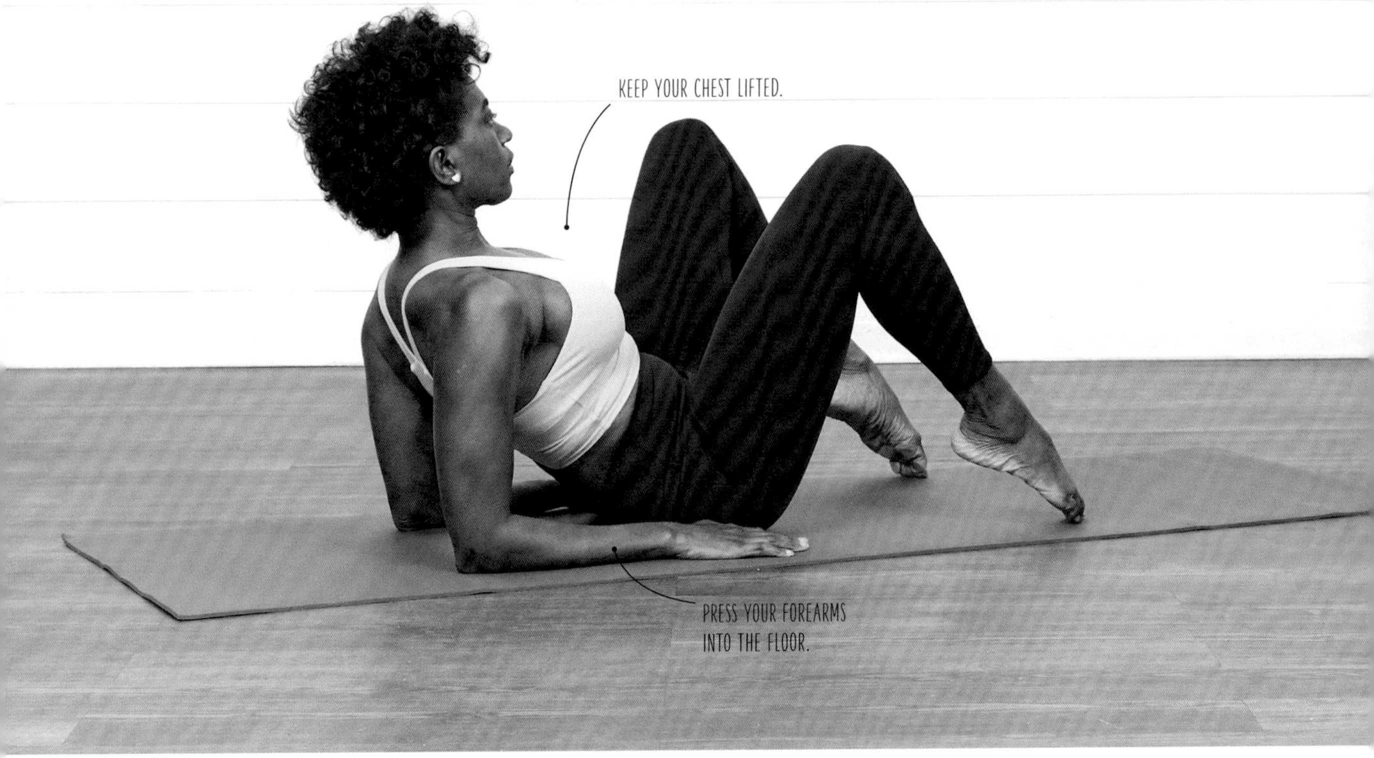

KEEP YOUR CHEST LIFTED.
PRESS YOUR FOREARMS INTO THE FLOOR.

2 Extend your legs toward the ceiling and separate your legs to form a V. Hold this position for 2 seconds. Reverse your movements to return to your starting position. Perform these steps 6 times.

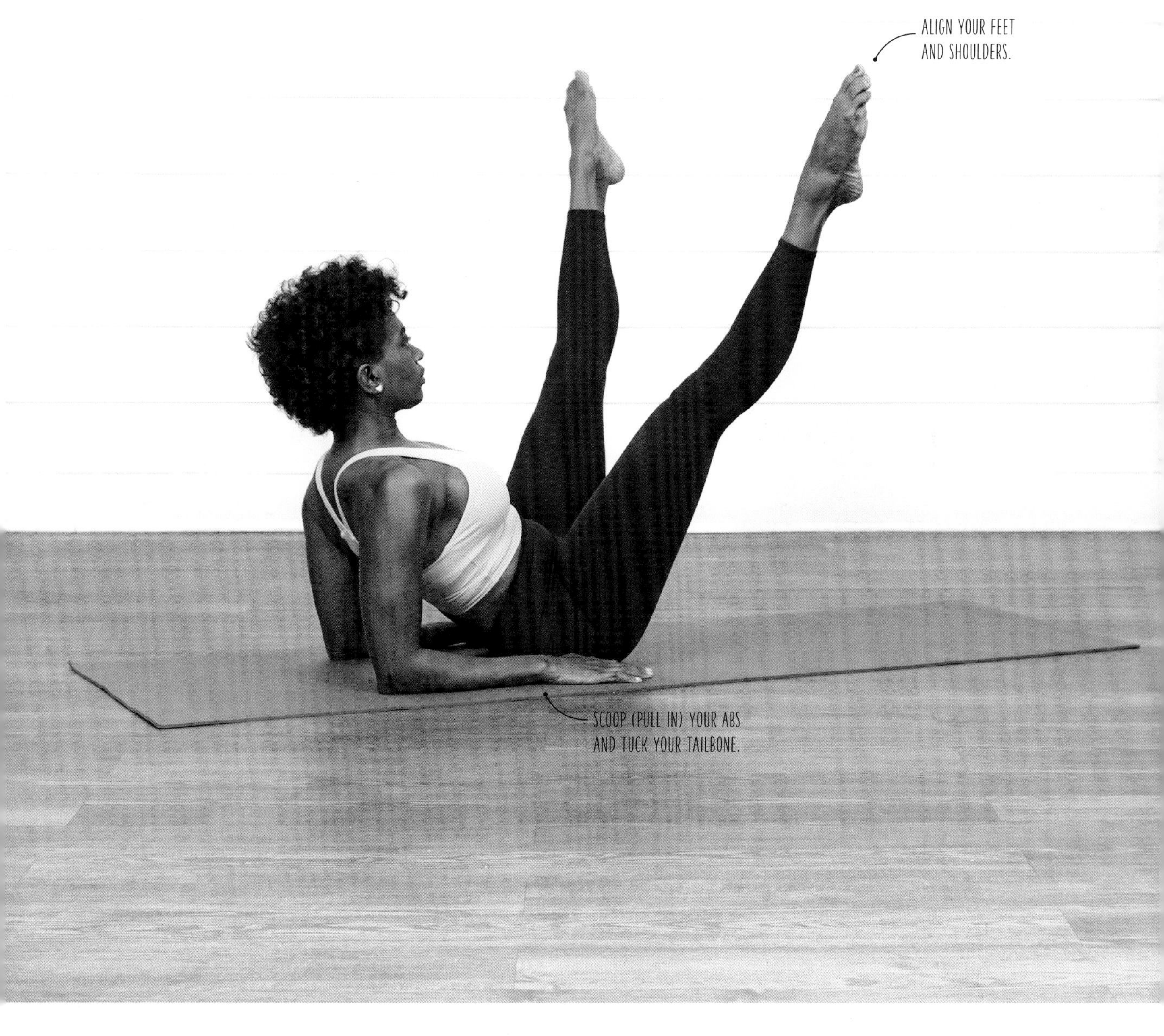

ALIGN YOUR FEET AND SHOULDERS.
SCOOP (PULL IN) YOUR ABS AND TUCK YOUR TAILBONE.

FOREARM V-LIFTS

VARIATIONS

If you lack core strength or core stability, placing a small Pilates ball under your back and/or lifting one leg at a time can reduce the stress on your lower back. Pregnant people or those who have difficulty getting down to or up from the floor might find the chair variation more accessible and just as beneficial.

ONE LEG AT A TIME >>>

In step 1, place your feet flat on the floor.

In step 2, extend one leg at a time. (You can either complete 6 reps with one leg, alternate legs within one rep, or use any method you prefer.) Continue with the remaining text.

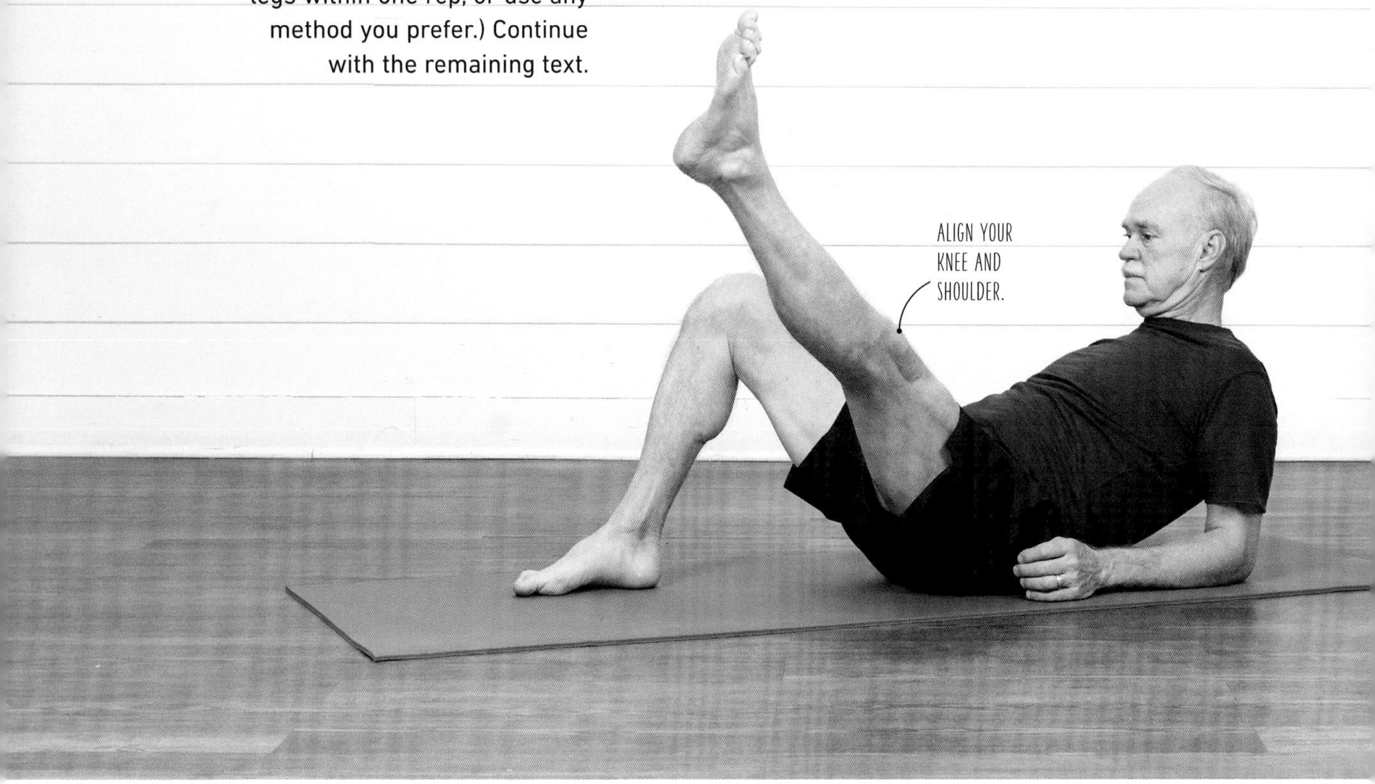
ALIGN YOUR KNEE AND SHOULDER.

WITH A SMALL PILATES BALL >>>

In step 1, place a small Pilates ball at your lower back and lean back on the ball. Keep your feet flat on the floor. Continue with the remaining text.

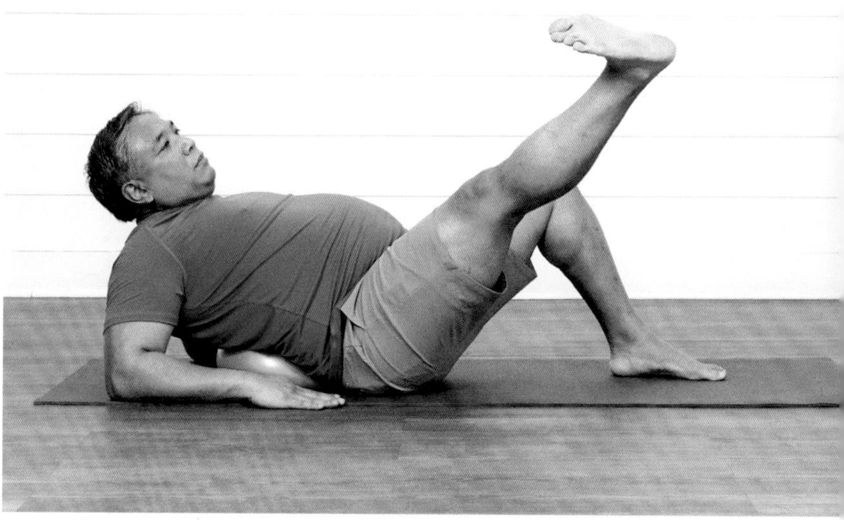

<<< SITTING IN A CHAIR

1. Sit in a chair with your feet shoulder width apart. Place your hands on the sides of the chair.

2. Raise your legs until parallel with the floor or as high as you feel comfortable. Hold this position for 2 seconds. Reverse your movements to return to your starting position. Perform these steps 8 times.

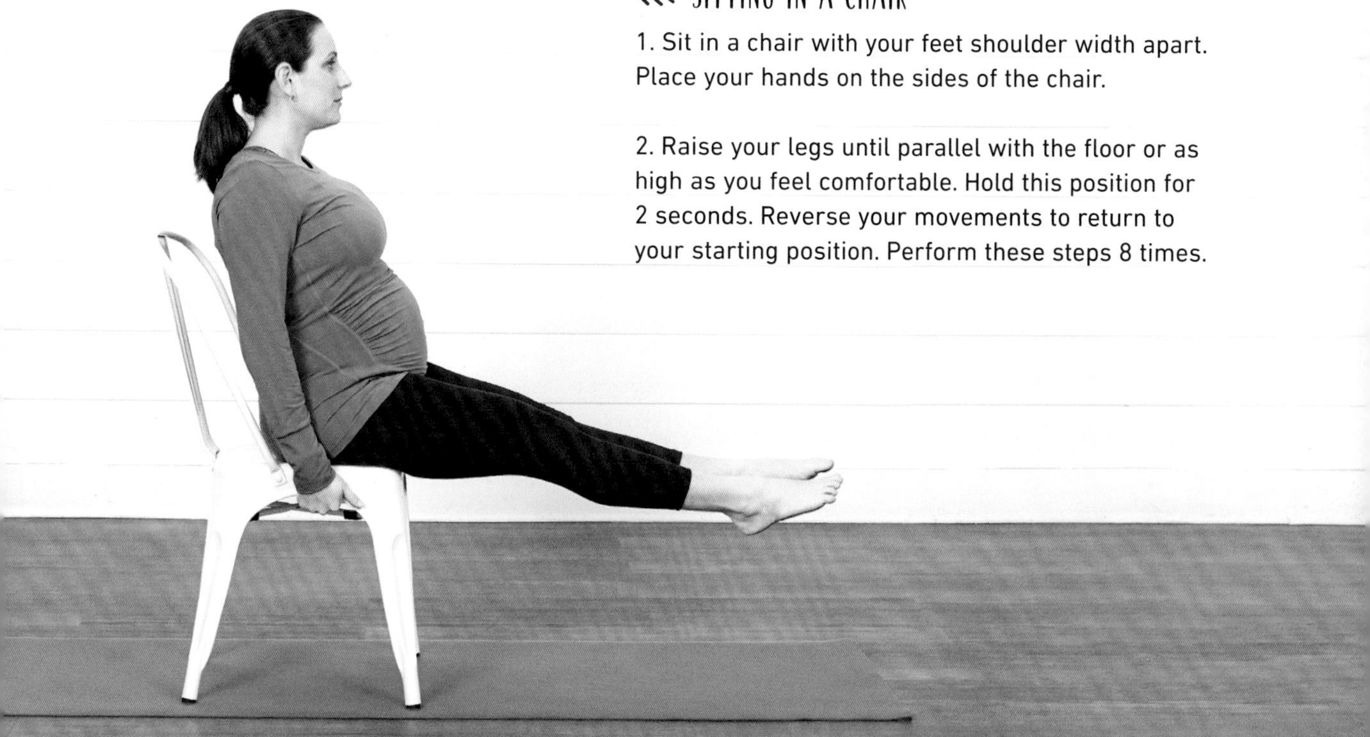

Hamstring Lunge Stretches

Lengthening your hamstrings and increasing your flexibility and range of motion are benefits of this exercise. Having tight hamstrings reduces pelvis mobility, which can put pressure on your lower back. Keeping your hamstrings flexible can help you avoid lower back pain, improve your posture, and prevent injury.

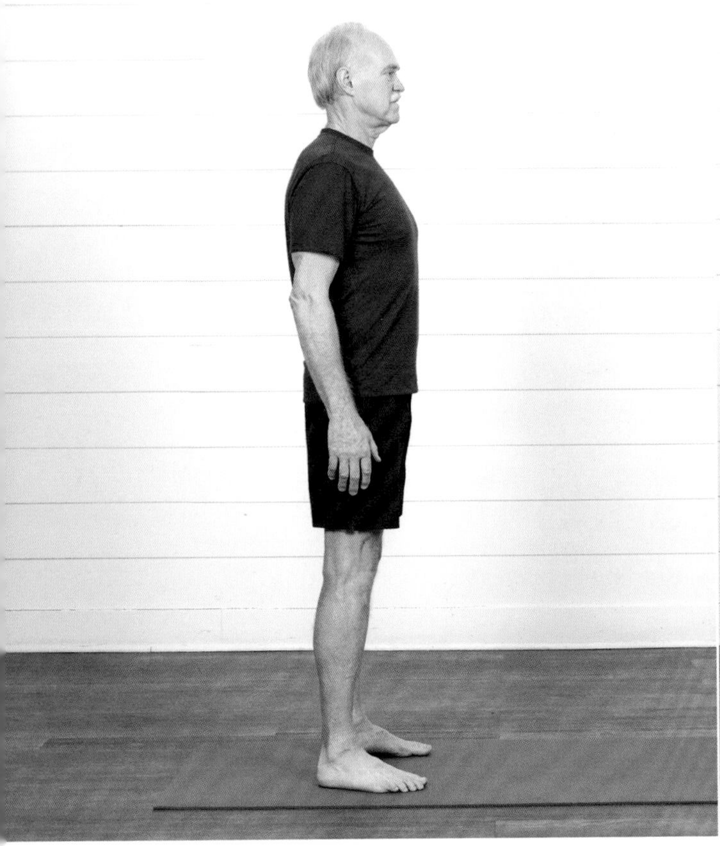

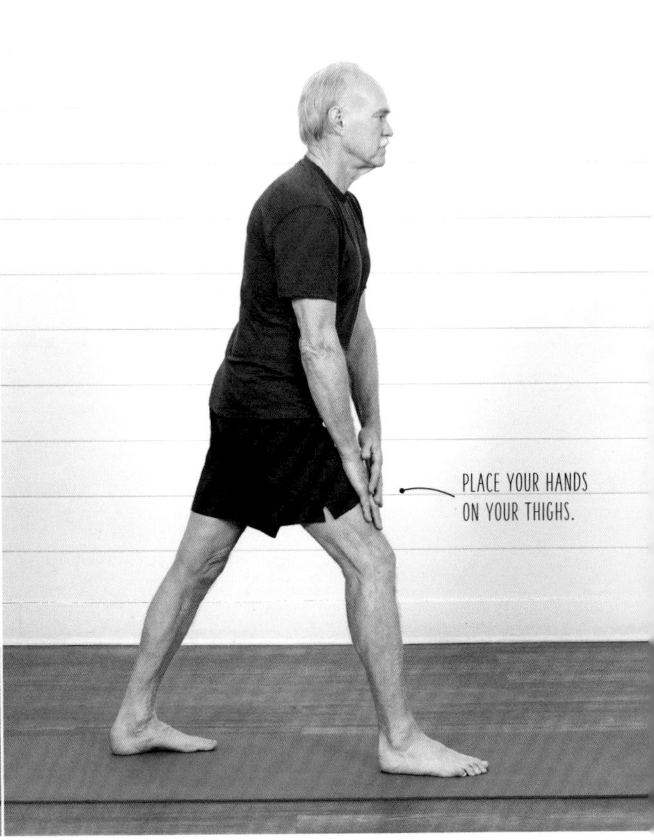
PLACE YOUR HANDS ON YOUR THIGHS.

1 Stand with your legs shoulder width apart and your arms relaxed at your sides.

2 Step your right foot forward to form a split stance, keeping your feet flat on the floor.

3 Gently lean forward and press your hands into your right thigh. Hold this position for 20 to 30 seconds. Reverse your movements to return to your position in step 2. Perform the last two steps 3 times. Repeat these steps with your left foot forward.

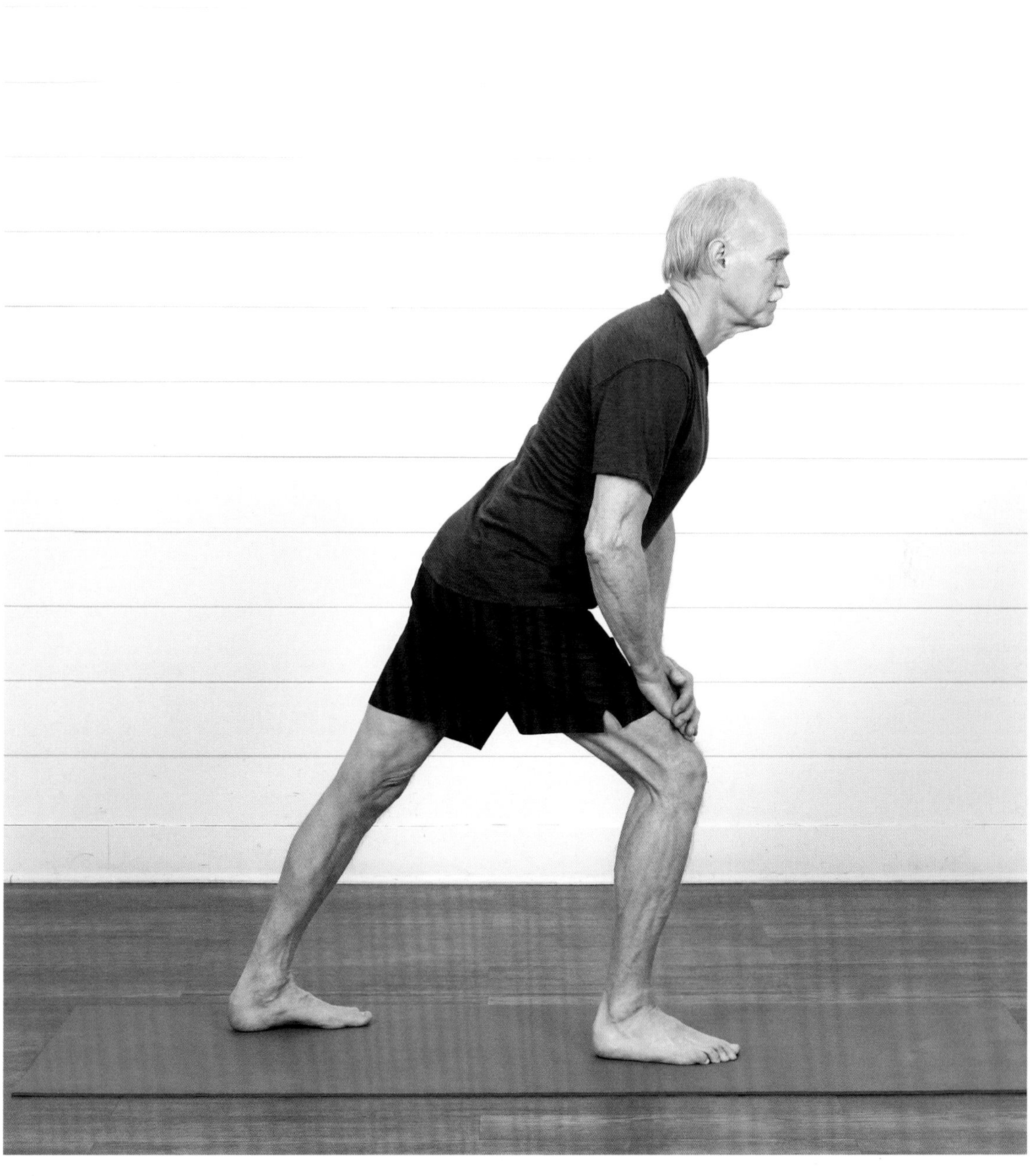

HAMSTRING LUNGE STRETCHES

VARIATIONS

If you suffer from lower back pain, you might benefit from hamstring stretching exercises that are done while lying on your back. These modifications are the least stressful on your lower back. If you have difficulty getting down to the floor, the seated version is quite effective.

ON THE FLOOR

1. Lie on your back on the floor. Wrap a towel around the back of your right thigh and hold the ends of the towel in your hands. (You can also slightly bend your right knee.)

2. Extend your right leg toward the ceiling until you feel a stretch in the back of your right thigh. Hold this position for 10 seconds to begin. Gradually work up to 30 seconds. Reverse your movements to return to your starting position. Repeat these steps with your left leg.

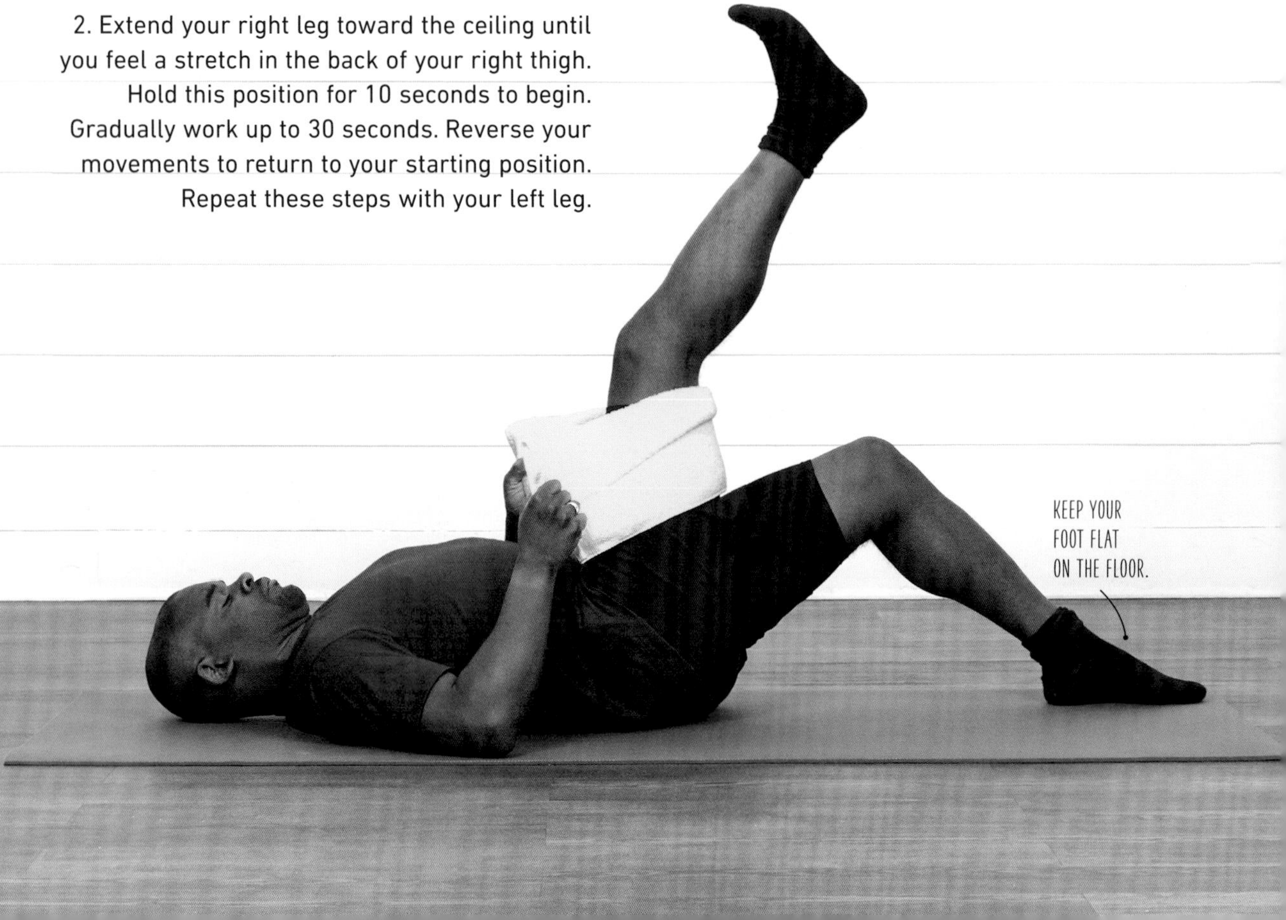
KEEP YOUR FOOT FLAT ON THE FLOOR.

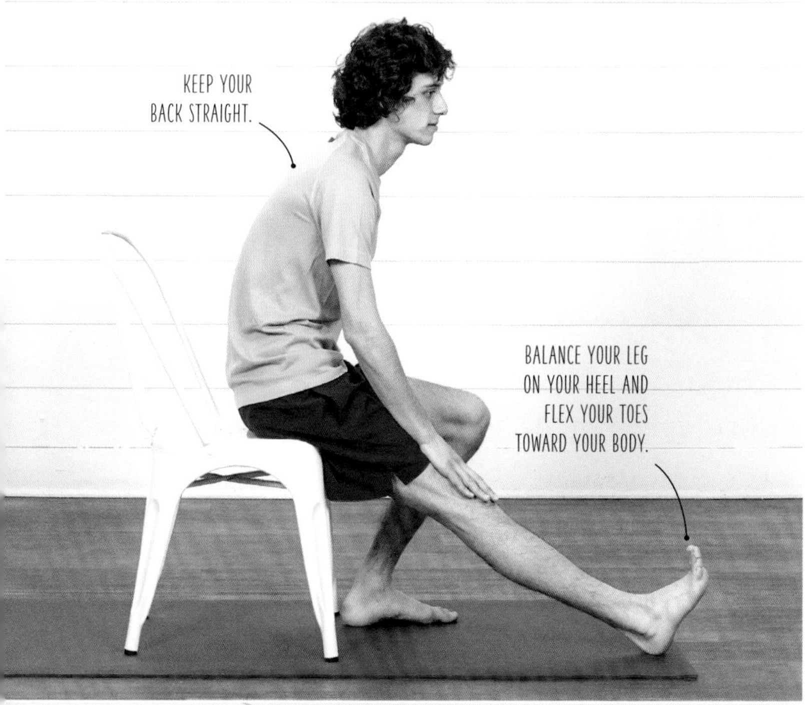

KEEP YOUR
BACK STRAIGHT.
BALANCE YOUR LEG
ON YOUR HEEL AND
FLEX YOUR TOES
TOWARD YOUR BODY.

<<< SITTING IN A CHAIR

1. Sit on the front edge of a chair with your right leg extended and your left foot flat on the floor. Place your right hand on your right knee and place your left hand on the side of the chair.

2. Bend at your waist to fold forward over your right leg. Hold this position for 10 to 20 seconds. Reverse your movements to return to your starting position. Perform these steps 3 times. Repeat these steps with your left leg.

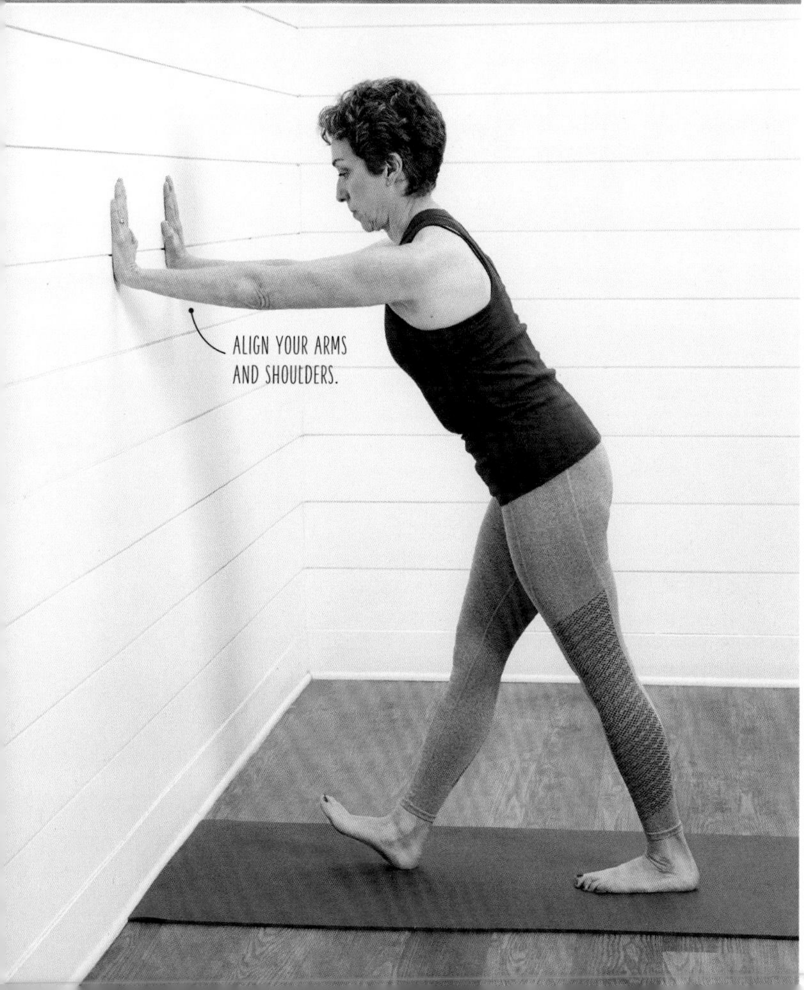

ALIGN YOUR ARMS
AND SHOULDERS.

<<< WITH A WALL

1. Stand facing 2 feet away from a wall. Extend your arms to place your hands flat on the wall.

2. Extend your right leg forward, balancing your right leg on your right heel and flexing your right toes toward the ceiling.

3. Bend at your waist to fold forward over your right leg. Hold this position for 10 to 20 seconds. Reverse your movements to return to your position in step 2. Perform the last two steps 3 times. Repeat these steps with your left leg.

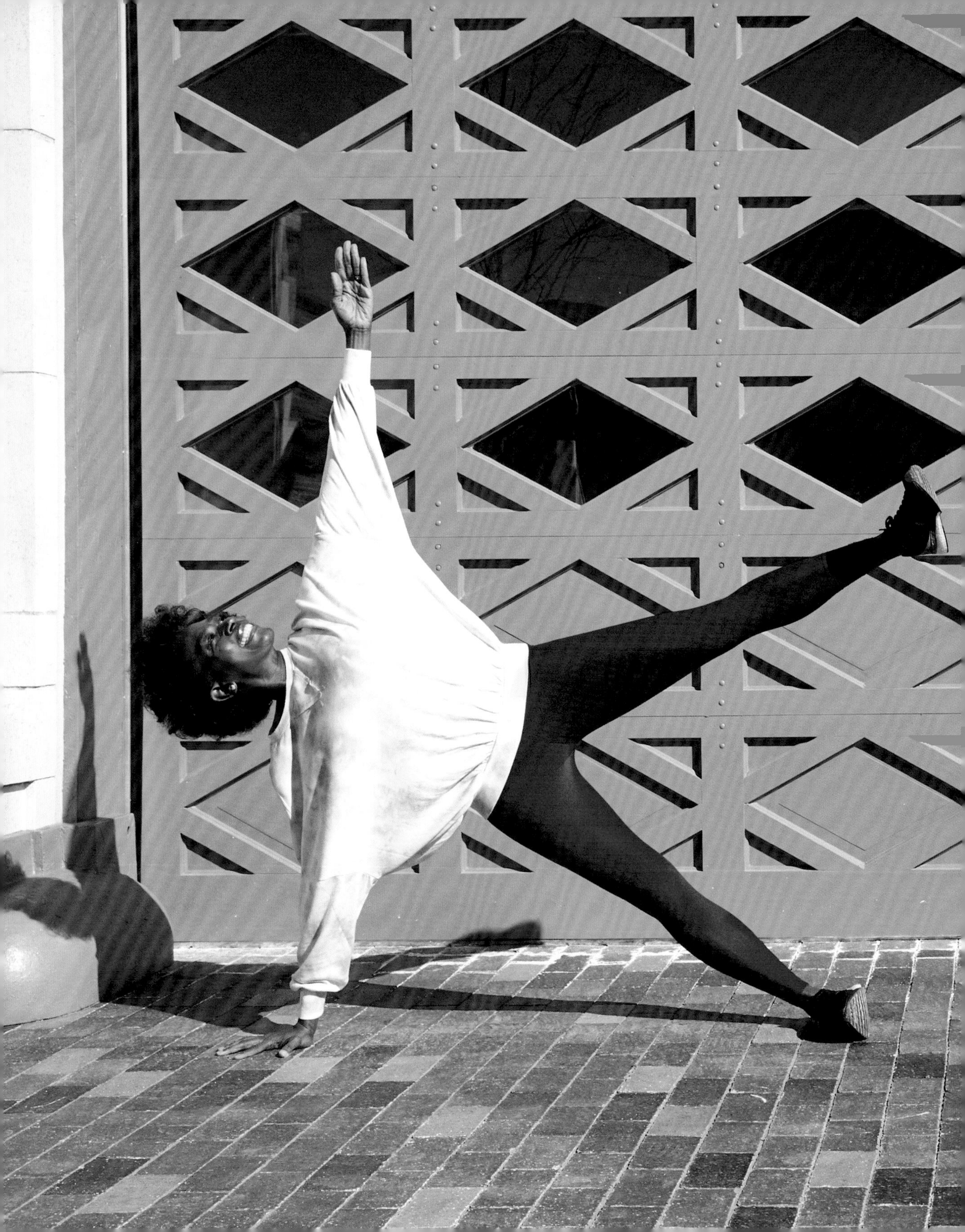

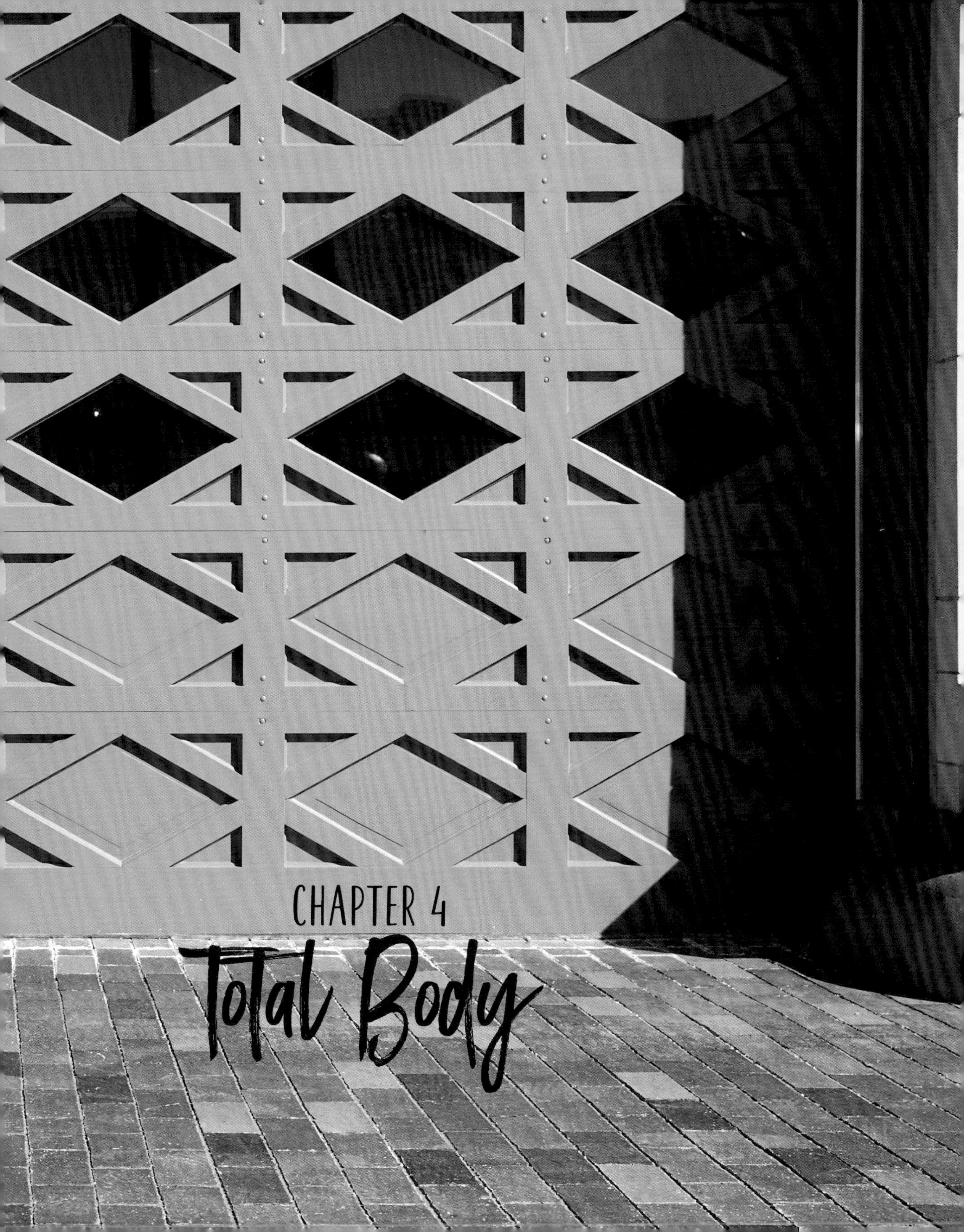

CHAPTER 4

Total Body

Teaser Prep

Executing these movements engages your abs, spinal extensors, quadriceps, and hip flexors. This exercise can help improve your balance, spinal mobility, and core strength. The main purpose of Teaser Prep is to build the strength required to perform Teaser. But Teaser Prep can also act as a modification for Teaser.

1 Lie on your back on the floor. Bend your knees to form a 45-degree angle with your legs and keep your feet flat on the floor. Extend your arms toward the ceiling.

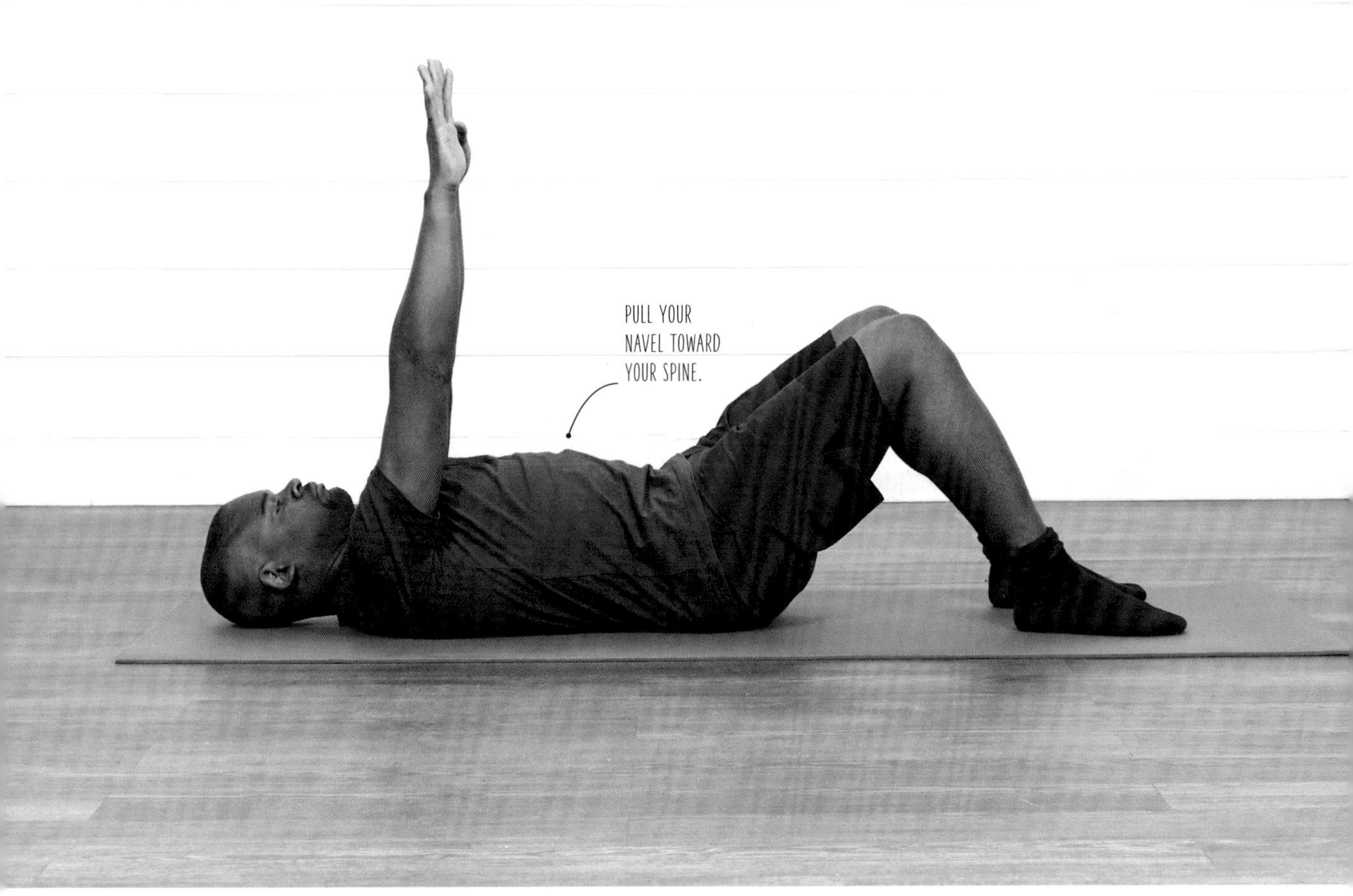
PULL YOUR NAVEL TOWARD YOUR SPINE.

2 Roll through your spine one vertebra at a time to raise your head and upper back off the floor. Lower your arms until parallel with your upper legs. Hold this position for 3 seconds. Reverse your movements to return to your starting position. Perform these steps 3 times.

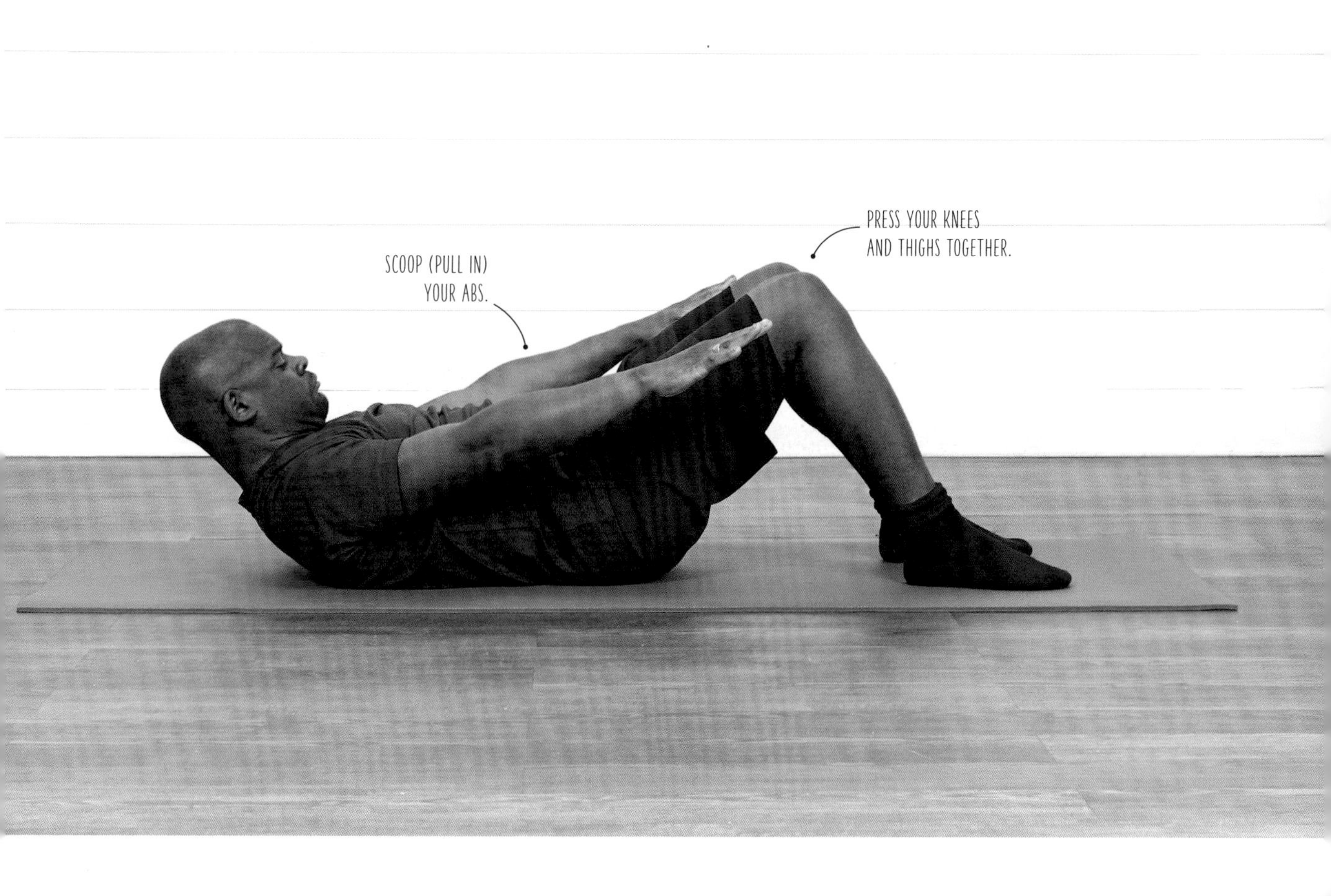
SCOOP (PULL IN) YOUR ABS.
PRESS YOUR KNEES AND THIGHS TOGETHER.

TEASER PREP

VARIATIONS

Supporting the weight of your legs without the assistance of your arms is an arduous task, requiring full-body activation. To perform this classic Pilates exercise, proper conditioning and prepping are important to prevent overuse of the hip flexors and lower back injuries. These modifications should help.

WITH A STABILITY BALL AND ONE LEG EXTENDED

In step 1, place a stability ball at your feet.

In step 2, raise your right leg and place it on top of the ball. Continue with the remaining text. Perform these steps with your left leg raised.

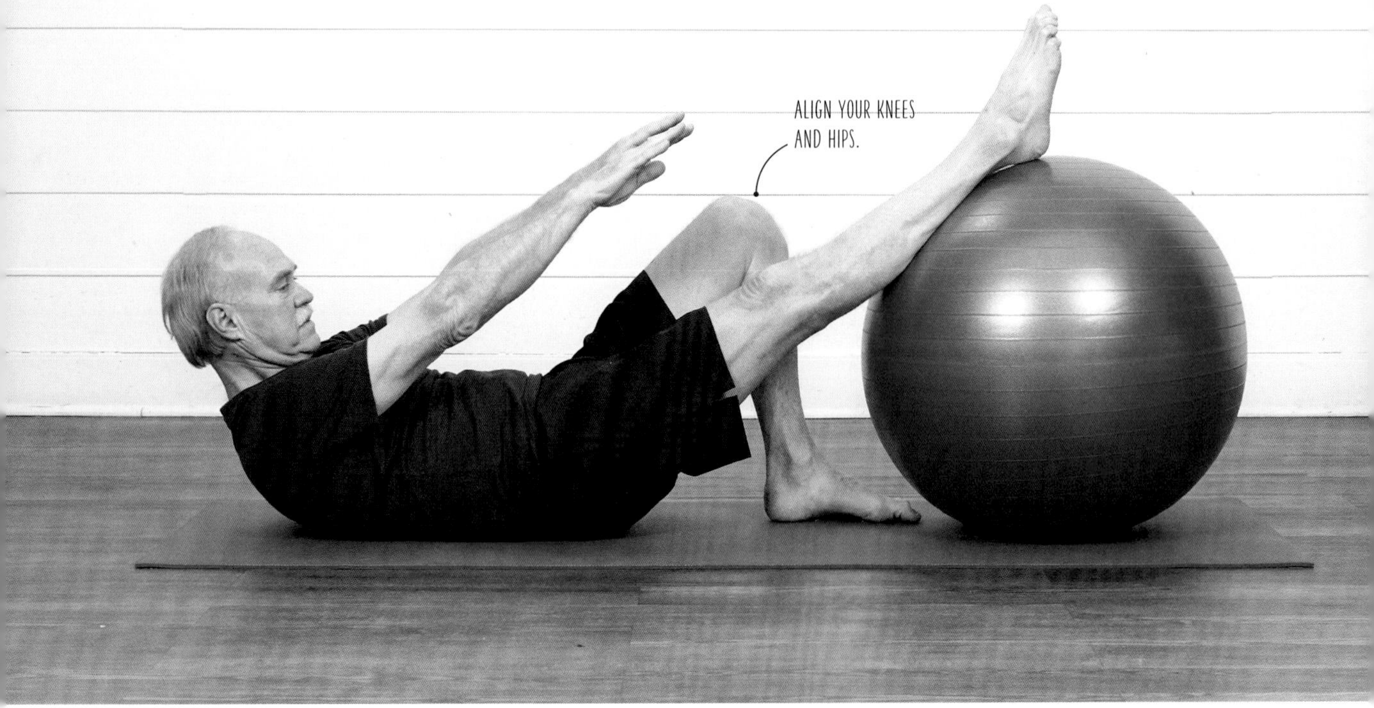
ALIGN YOUR KNEES AND HIPS.

WITH A STABILITY BALL

In step 1, place your lower legs on top of a stability ball, keeping your legs straight. Continue with the remaining text.

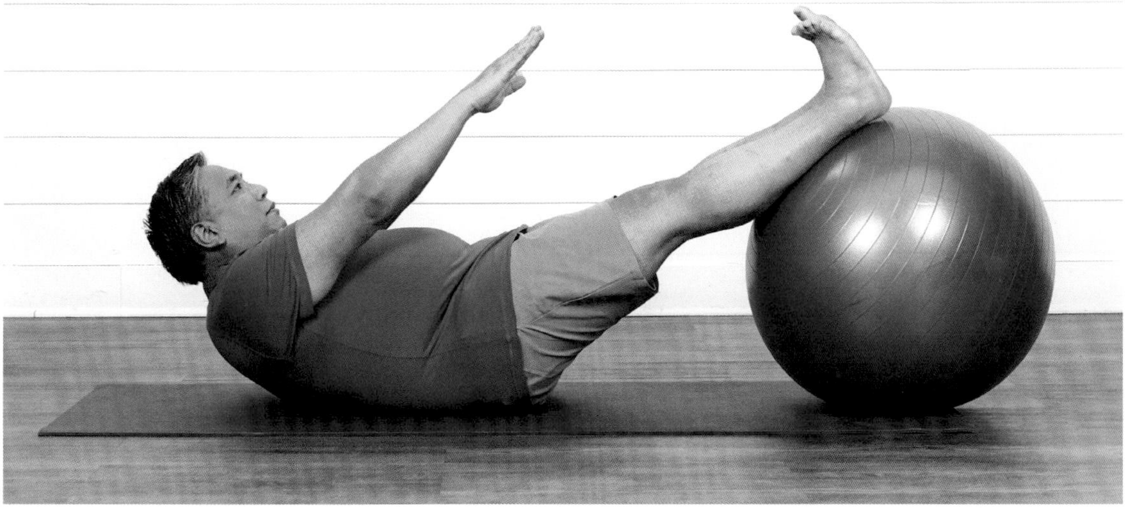

WITH A SMALL PILATES BALL

In step 1, place a small Pilates ball between your knees.

In step 2, squeeze the ball when you raise and lower your arms. Continue with the remaining text.

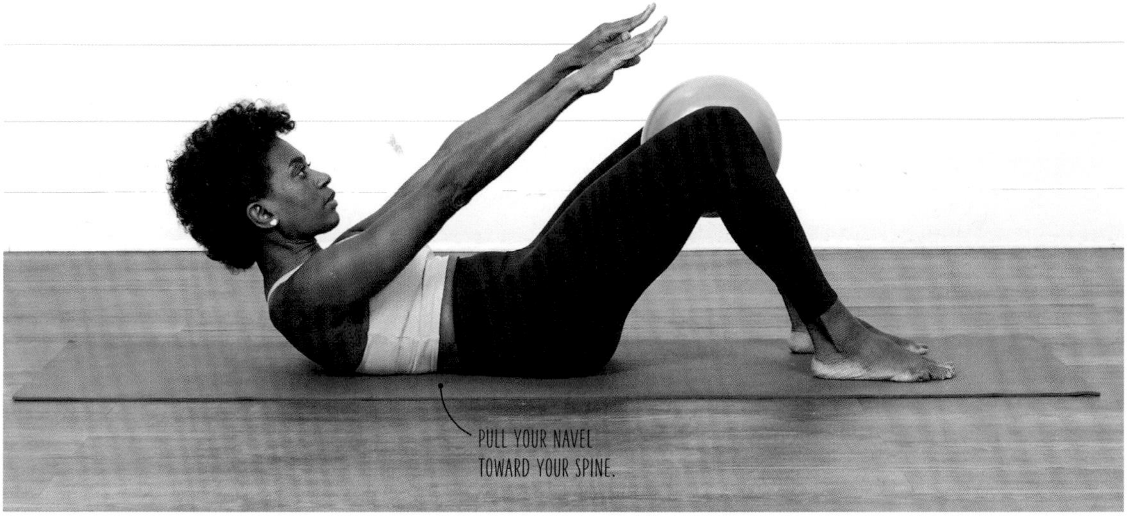
PULL YOUR NAVEL
TOWARD YOUR SPINE.

Teaser

This exercise engages your abs, spinal extensors, quadriceps, and hip flexors. These movements are much more effective than traditional crunches at targeting your external obliques and rectus abdominis. Plus, it's wonderful for balance and flexibility as well as developing spinal mobility and core strength.

1 Lie on your back on the floor with your legs extended. Extend your arms toward the ceiling, keeping your head and shoulders flat on the floor.

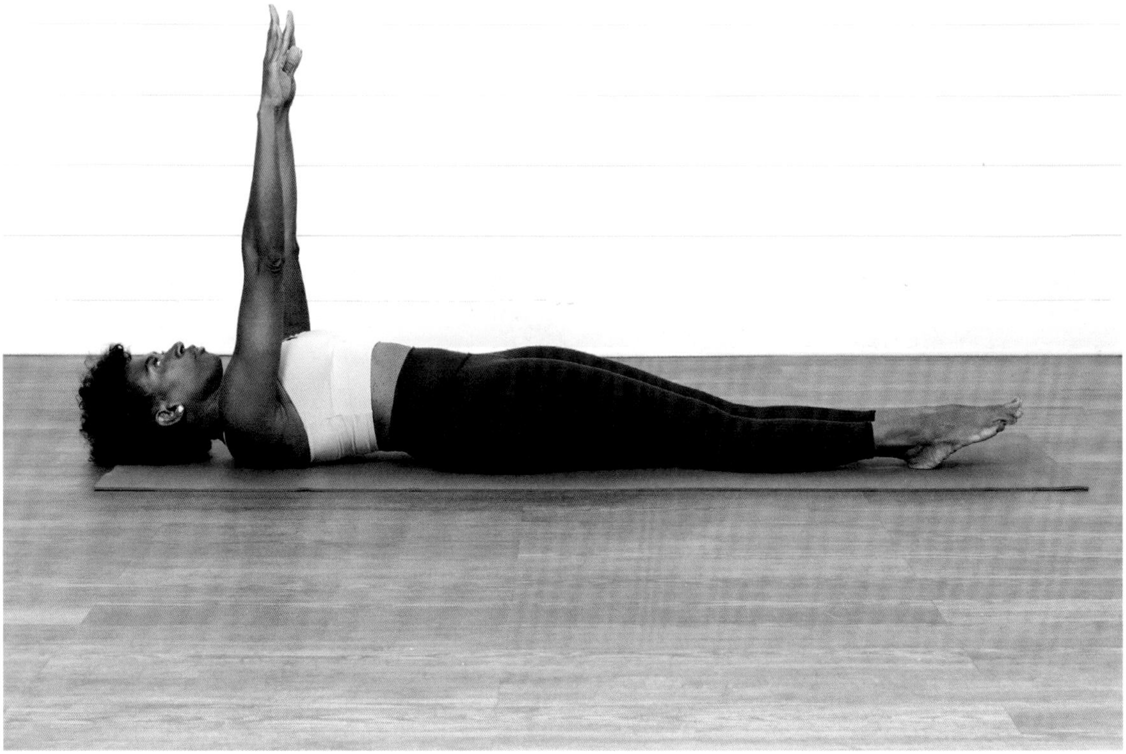

2 Raise your legs until they're parallel with your arms. Raise your head and shoulders off the floor and lower your chin toward your chest.

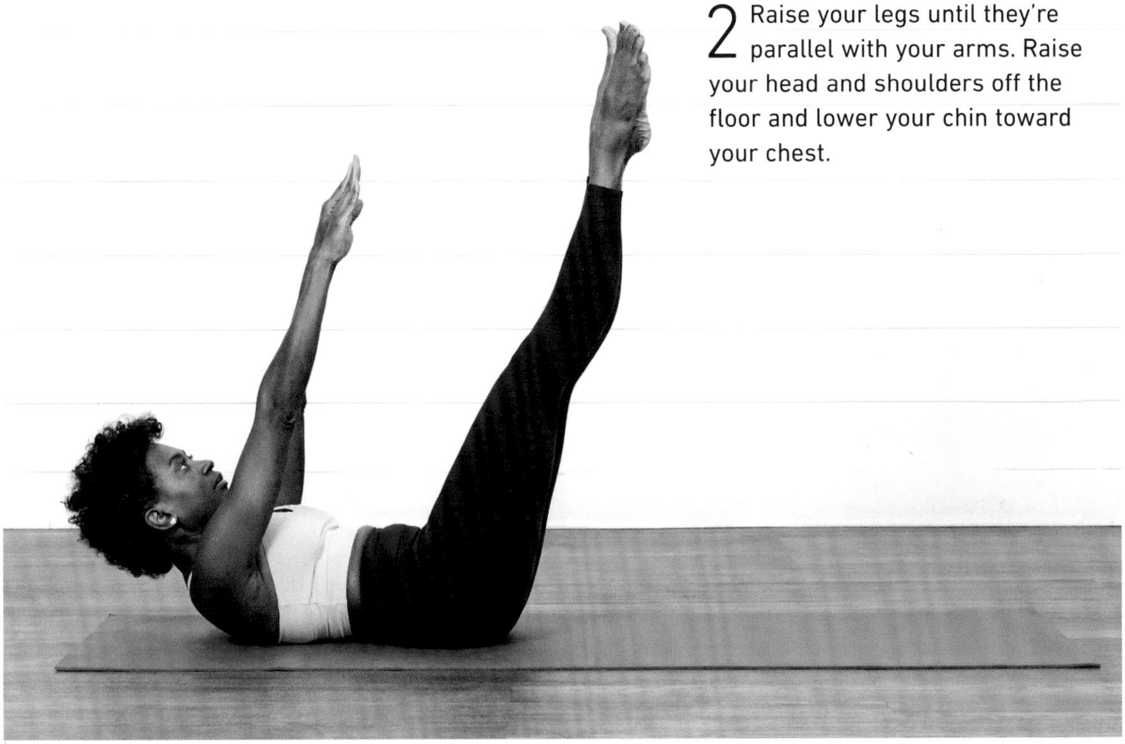

3 Raise your upper body off the floor to form a V with your body. Reverse your movements to return to your starting position. Perform these steps 3 times.

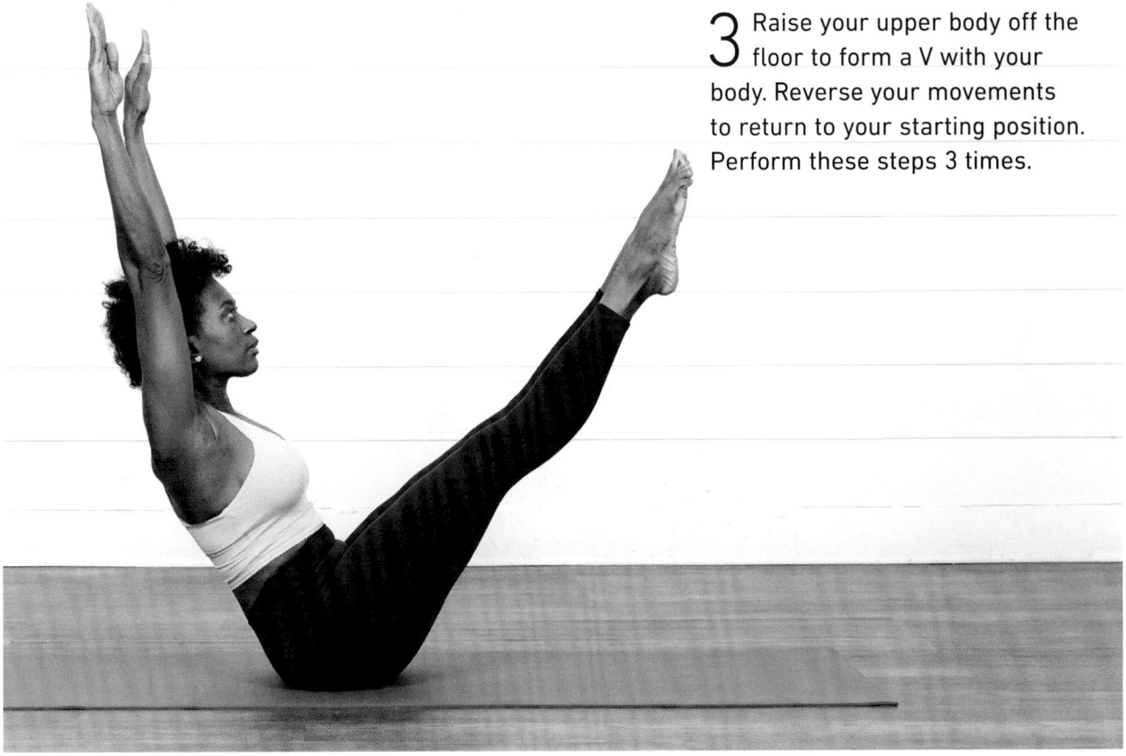

TEASER

VARIATIONS

Teaser is an exercise with many fitness components that can be challenging to master alone. Putting all those difficult components together makes for an even more challenging endeavor. If you have tight hamstrings, lack core strength, or have issues with hip flexor mobility, these variations can help you perform this exercise with a little more ease.

WITH A SMALL PILATES BALL

1. Sit on the floor with your legs extended. Place a small Pilates ball at your lower back. Lower your upper body backward until your forearms and hands are flat on the floor.

2. Raise your legs to form a V with your body. Hold this position for 3 seconds. Reverse your movements to lower your legs to the floor. Perform these two steps 6 times.

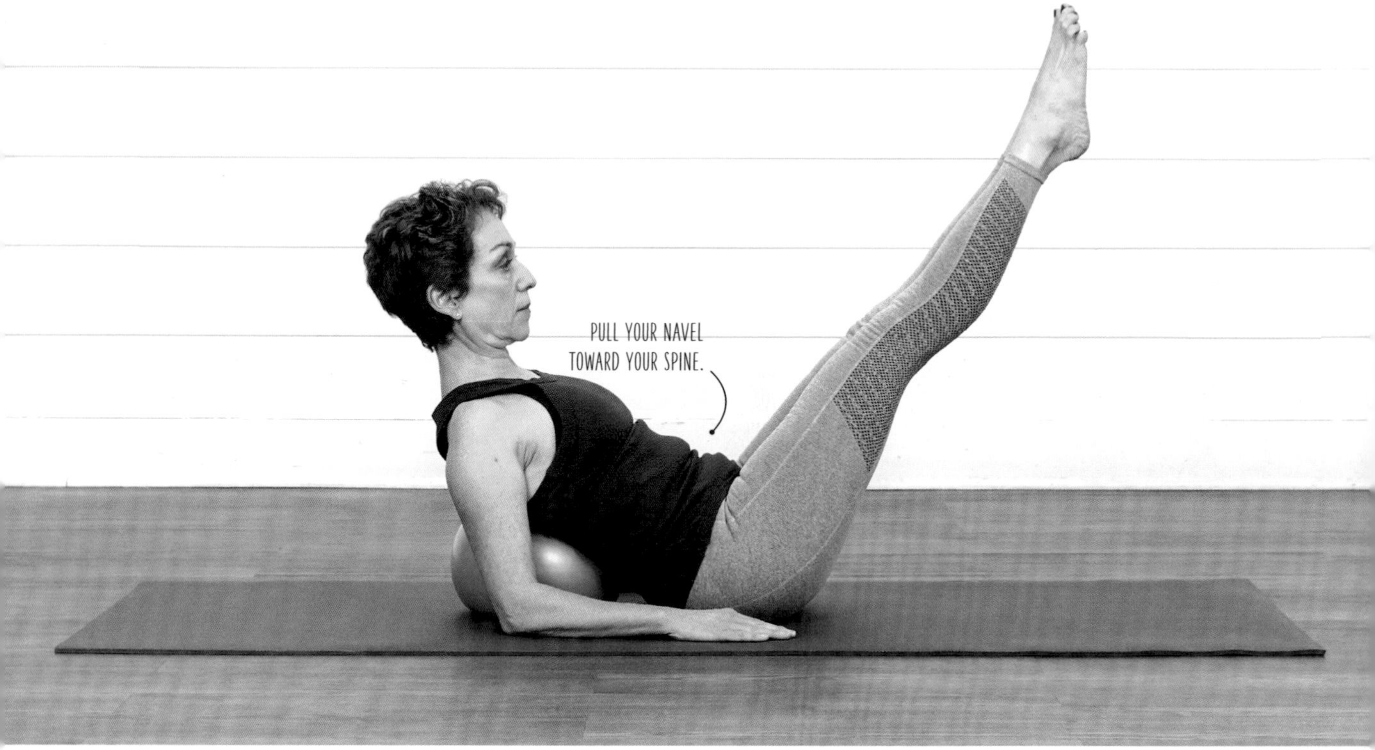
PULL YOUR NAVEL TOWARD YOUR SPINE.

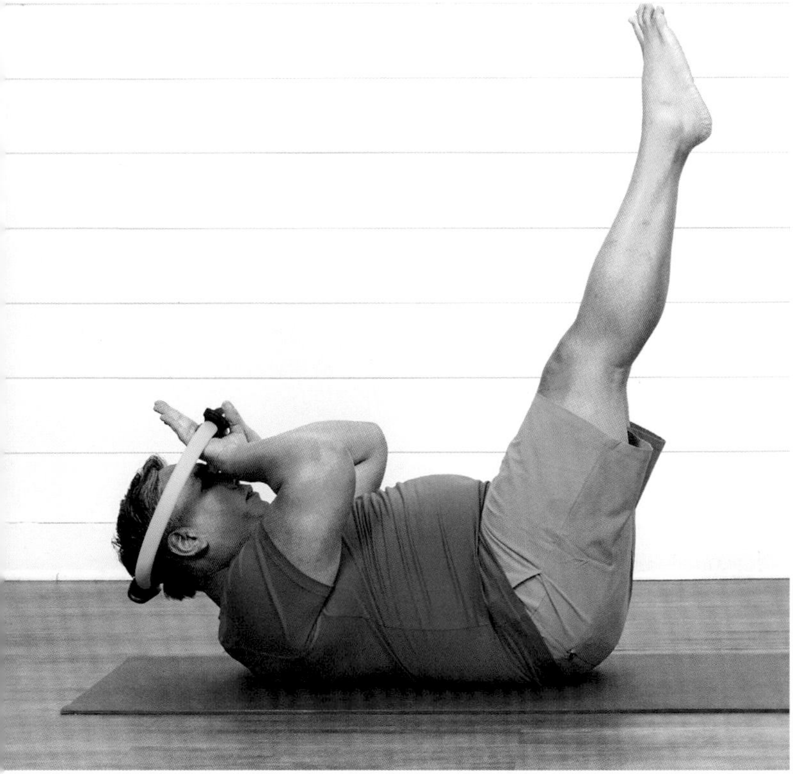

<<< WITH THE MAGIC CIRCLE

1. Lie on your back on the floor with your legs extended toward the ceiling. Place the Magic Circle under your head, with one pad at the base of your skull and your hands on the inside, holding the other pad.

2. Pull your navel toward your spine as you raise your head and shoulders off the floor. Hold this position for 3 seconds. Reverse your movements to return to your starting position. Perform these steps 6 times.

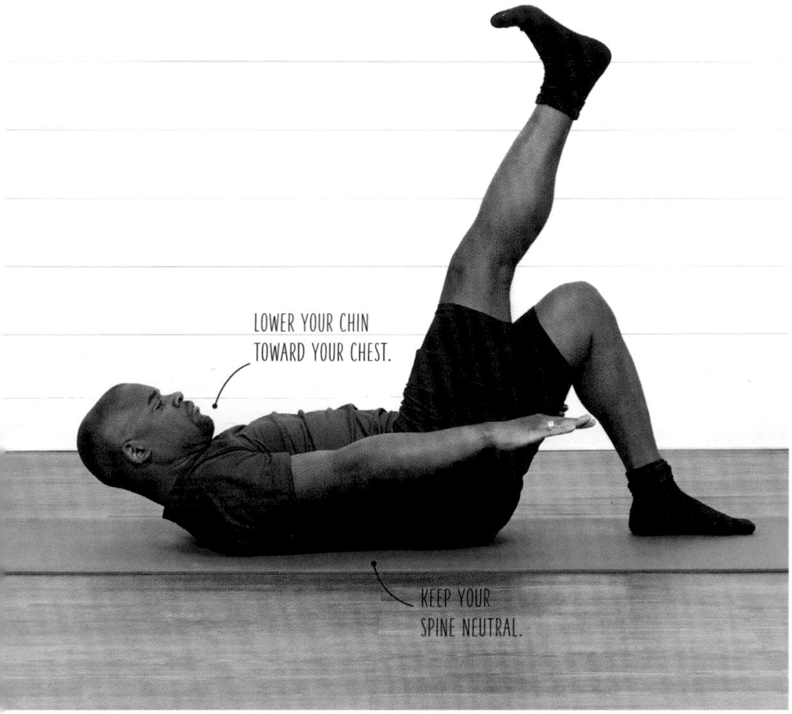

LOWER YOUR CHIN TOWARD YOUR CHEST.
KEEP YOUR SPINE NEUTRAL.

<<< WITH ONE LEG

1. Lie on your back on the floor with your knees bent and your arms relaxed at your sides.

2. Extend your right leg toward the ceiling. Raise your head and shoulders off the floor while raising your arms a few inches off the floor. Hold this position for 3 seconds. Reverse your movements to return to your starting position. Perform these steps 3 times. Repeat these steps with your left leg raised.

swimming

This is truly a full-body exercise that engages your arm, shoulder, middle and upper back, abdominal, leg, and chest muscles. Swimming is a back extension exercise that makes a great counter stretch for the many Pilates mat exercises that require forward flexion.

1 Lie on your stomach on the floor with your arms and legs extended. Raise your head slightly off the floor..

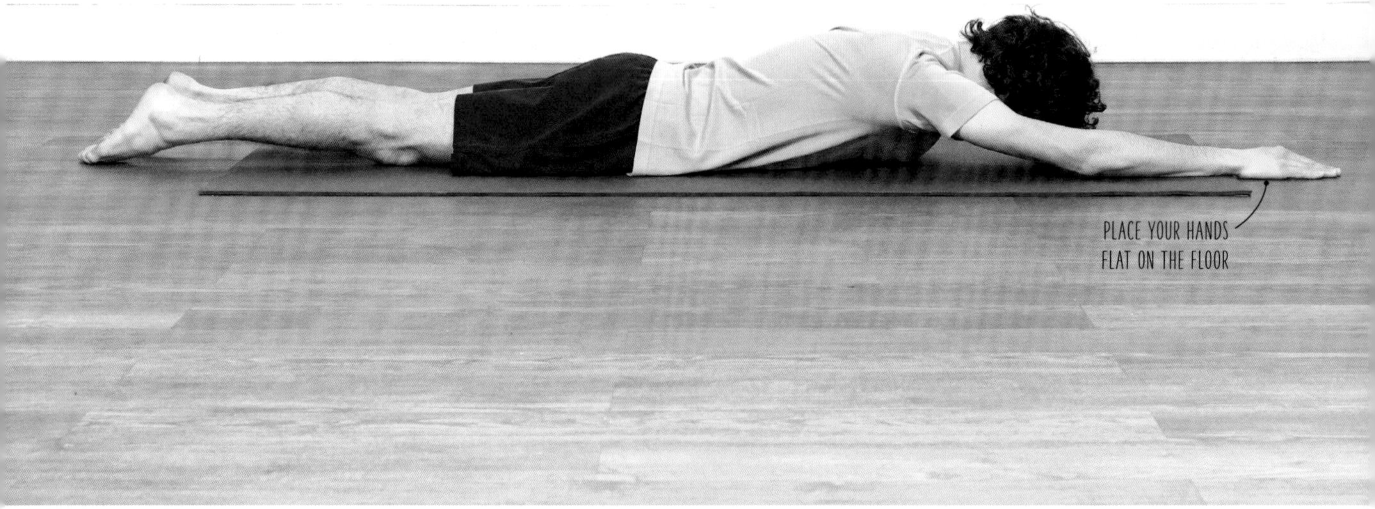
PLACE YOUR HANDS FLAT ON THE FLOOR

2 Simultaneously raise your right arm and your left leg a couple inches off the floor.

3 As you lower your right arm and left leg to the floor, simultaneously raise your left arm and right leg off the floor. Continue switching your arms and legs in a swimming motion. Perform the last two steps 10 times.

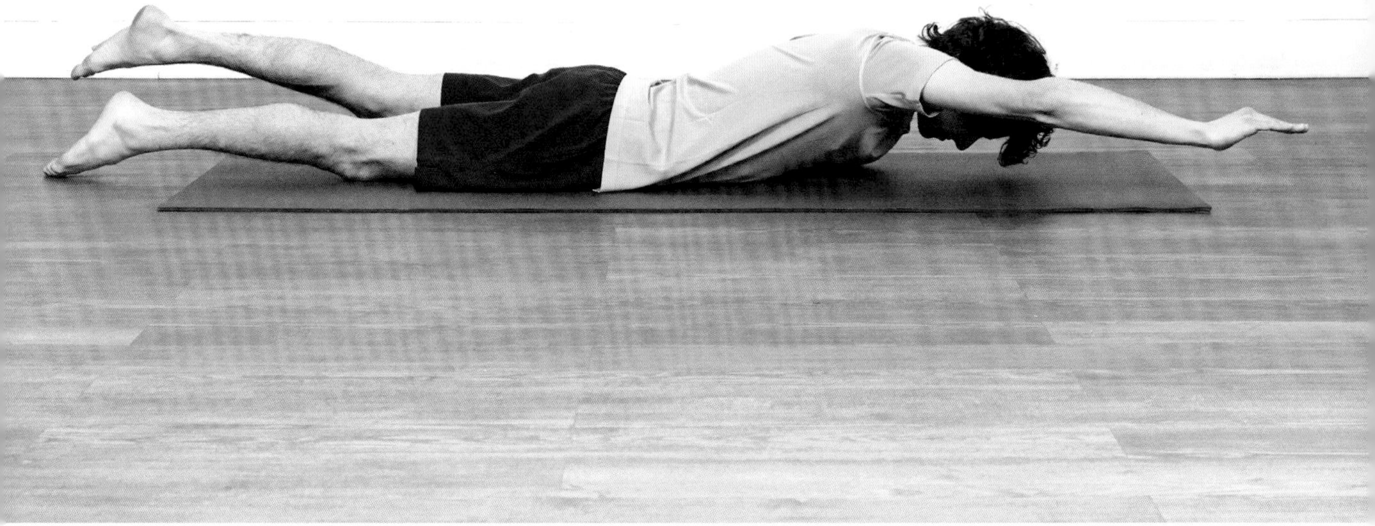

SWIMMING

VARIATIONS

If you lack core strength, using a small Pilates ball can help provide support for your lower back. The alternating and kneeling variations can help you build the core strength required to perform this exercise. The kneeling variation is also a great alternative for pregnant people.

ALTERNATING WITH LEGS ONLY

1. Lie on your stomach on the floor with your legs extended. Fold your arms on top of each other and rest your forehead on your top forearm.

2. Bend your left knee to form a 90-degree angle with your left leg. Hold this position for 2 seconds. Lower your left leg to the floor.

3. Bend your right knee to form a 90-degree angle with your right leg. Hold this position for 2 seconds. Lower your right leg to the floor. Perform the steps 3 times.

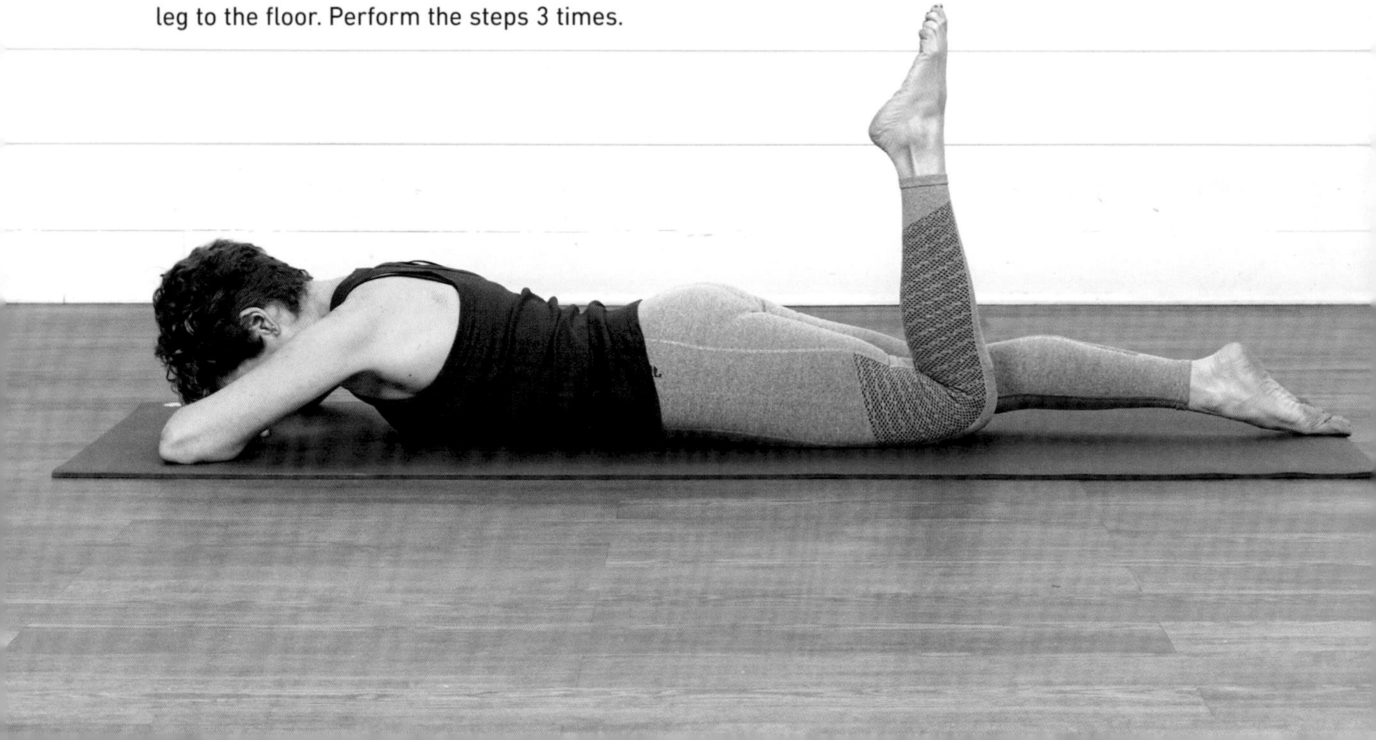

KNEELING

1. Place your hands and knees flat on the floor. Align your hands and shoulders as well as your knees and your hips.

2. Simultaneously extend your left arm forward and your right leg backward.

3. As you return your left arm and right leg to their starting positions, simultaneously extend your right arm forward and your left leg backward. As you return your right arm and left leg to their starting positions, return to step 2. Perform the last two steps 6 times.

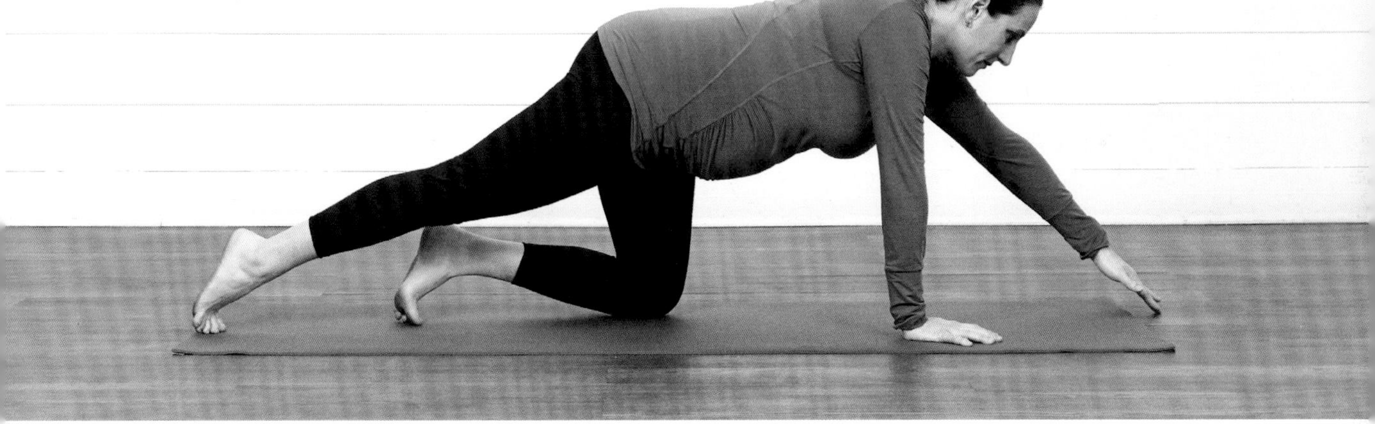

WITH A SMALL PILATES BALL

1. Lie on your stomach with your elbows and forearms flat on the floor. Place a small Pilates ball under your chest. Press your glutes and pubic bone into the floor.

2. Raise your chest off the ball and hold this position for 2 seconds. Reverse your movements to return to your starting position. Perform these steps 4 times.

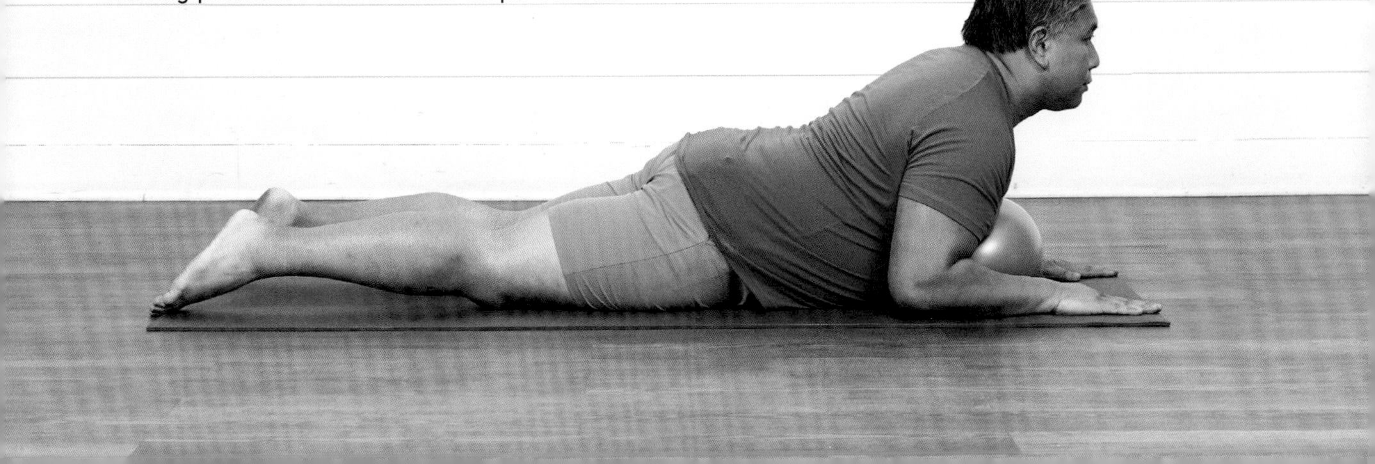

Four-Point Balance

This is one of the best Pilates balance exercises because it incorporates the strength and stability of your core in one exercise. Performing these movements helps you learn to stabilize your center while moving your limbs. You can also improve your pelvic stability and strengthen your posterior chain (the muscles of the backside of the body) with this exercise.

1 Place your hands and knees flat on the floor. Align your hands with your shoulders as well as your knees with your hips.

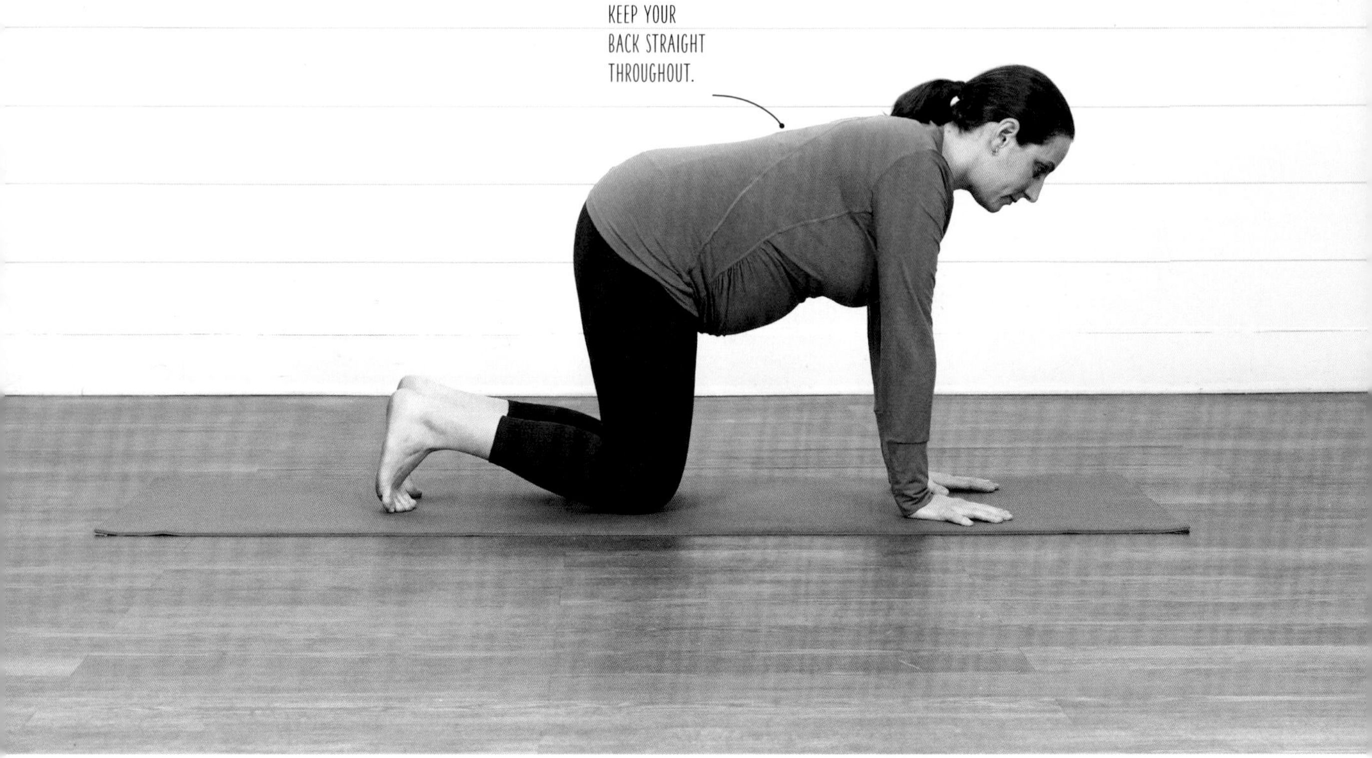
KEEP YOUR BACK STRAIGHT THROUGHOUT.

2 Extend your left arm to shoulder height while extending your right leg to hip height. Hold this position for 3 to 5 seconds.

3 As you reverse your movements, extend your right arm to shoulder height while extending your left leg to hip height. Hold this position for 3 to 5 seconds. Reverse your movements to return to your starting position. Perform these steps 6 times.

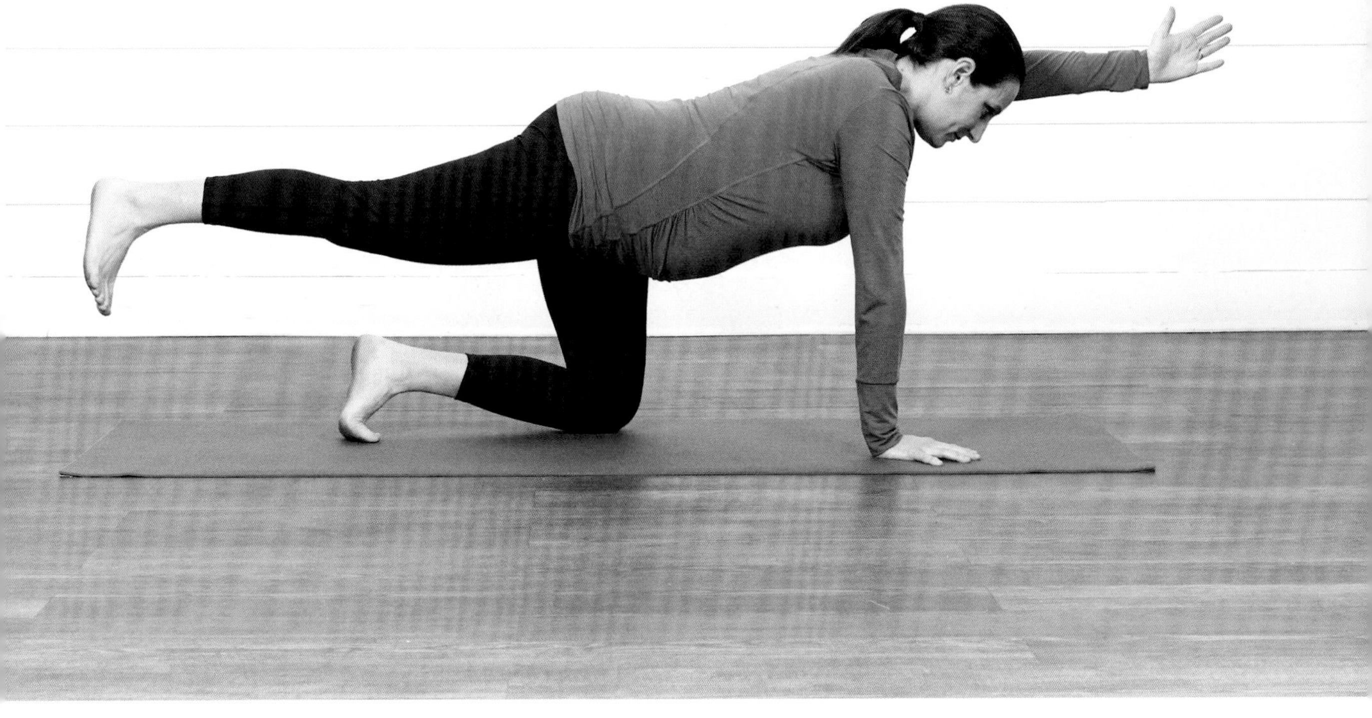

FOUR-POINT BALANCE

VARIATIONS

If you have tight shoulders or lower-back discomfort, try one of these alternative poses. Performing a variation might even help ease some of that tension and allow you to develop some strength in those areas.

ARMS AND LEGS STABLE

In steps 2 and 3, keep your arms and legs on the floor. As you inhale through your nose, pull your navel toward your spine. As you exhale through your mouth, engage your abs. Continue with the remaining text.

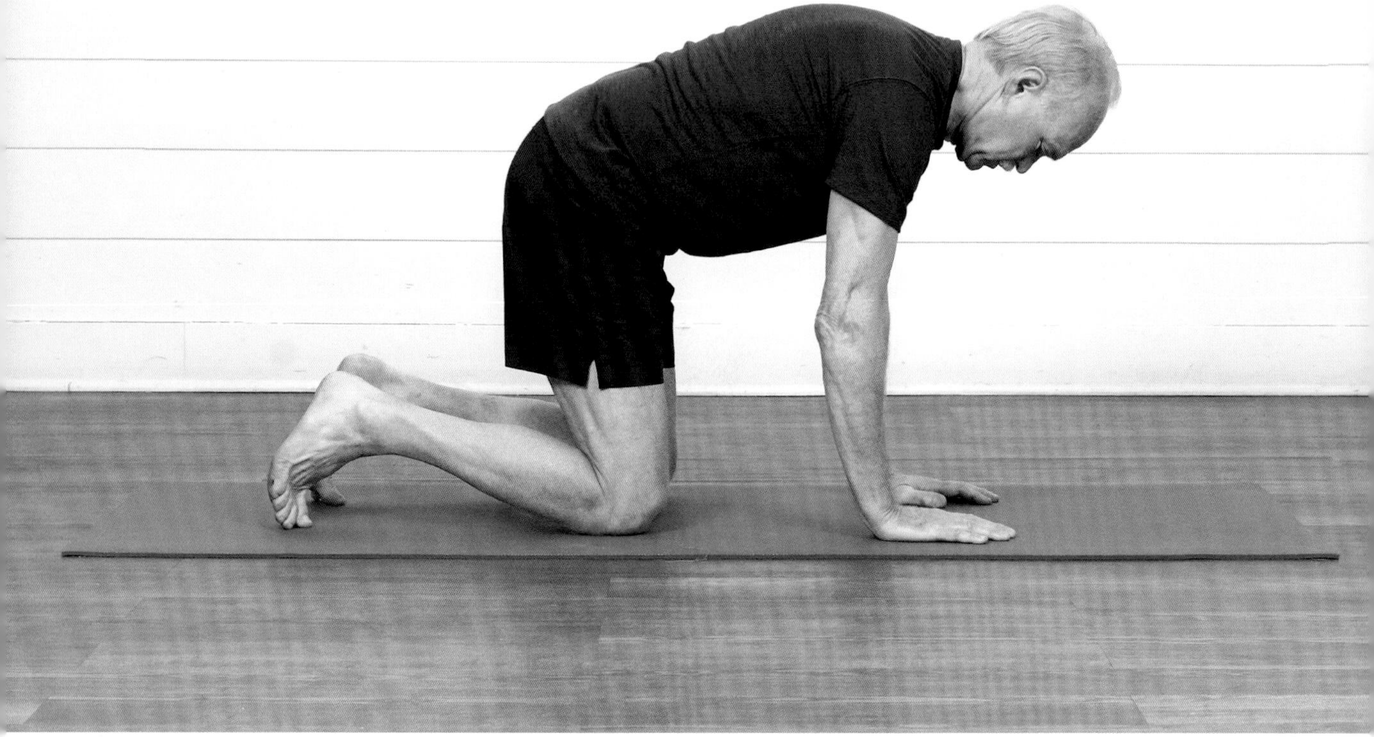

WITH A LOOP BAND

In step 1, place a loop band around your arms just below your elbows.

In steps 2 and 3, keep your arms and legs on the floor, pressing your arms against the band. As you inhale through your nose, pull your navel toward your spine. As you exhale through your mouth, engage your abs. Continue with the remaining text.

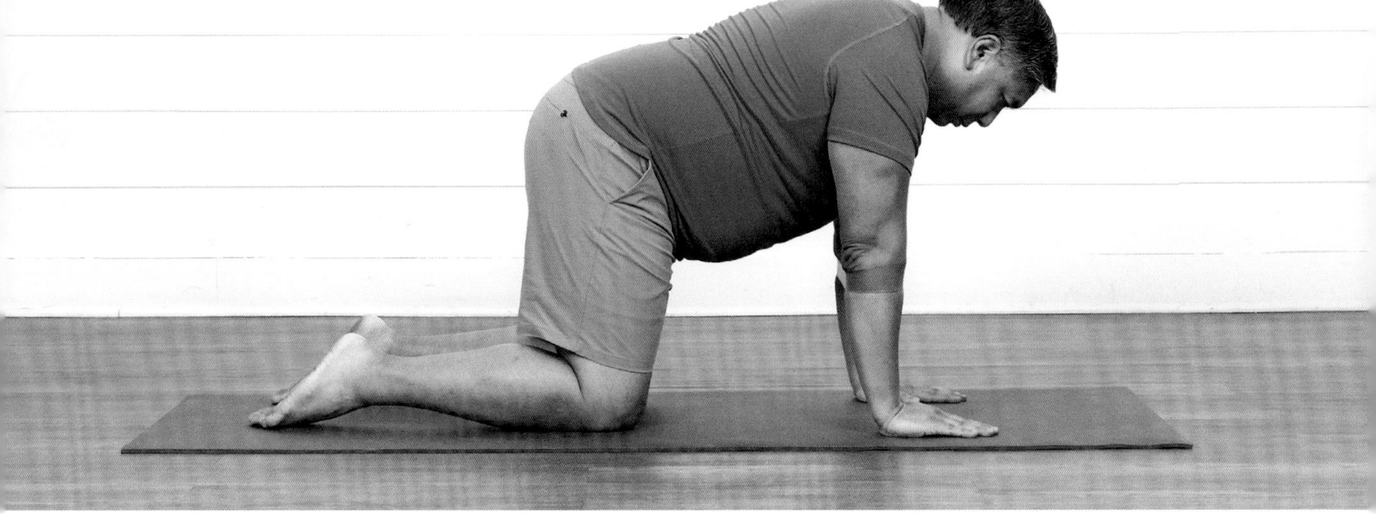

WITH A STABILITY BALL

In step 1, place a stability ball under your torso.
Continue with the remaining text.

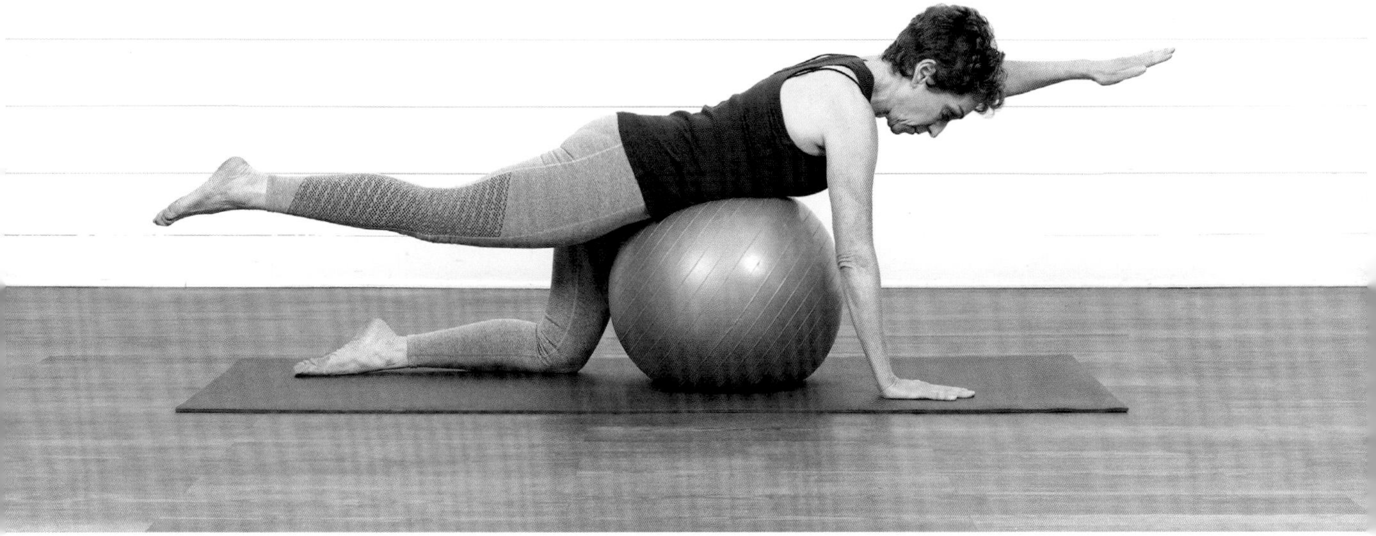

Leg Pull-Ups

This total-body exercise can help you strengthen your back, abdominal, gluteal, shoulder, and leg muscles. Plus, these movements can help improve stability in your shoulders and trunk as well as enhance your balance skills.

1 Sit on the floor with your legs extended. Place your hands shoulder width apart on the floor behind you.

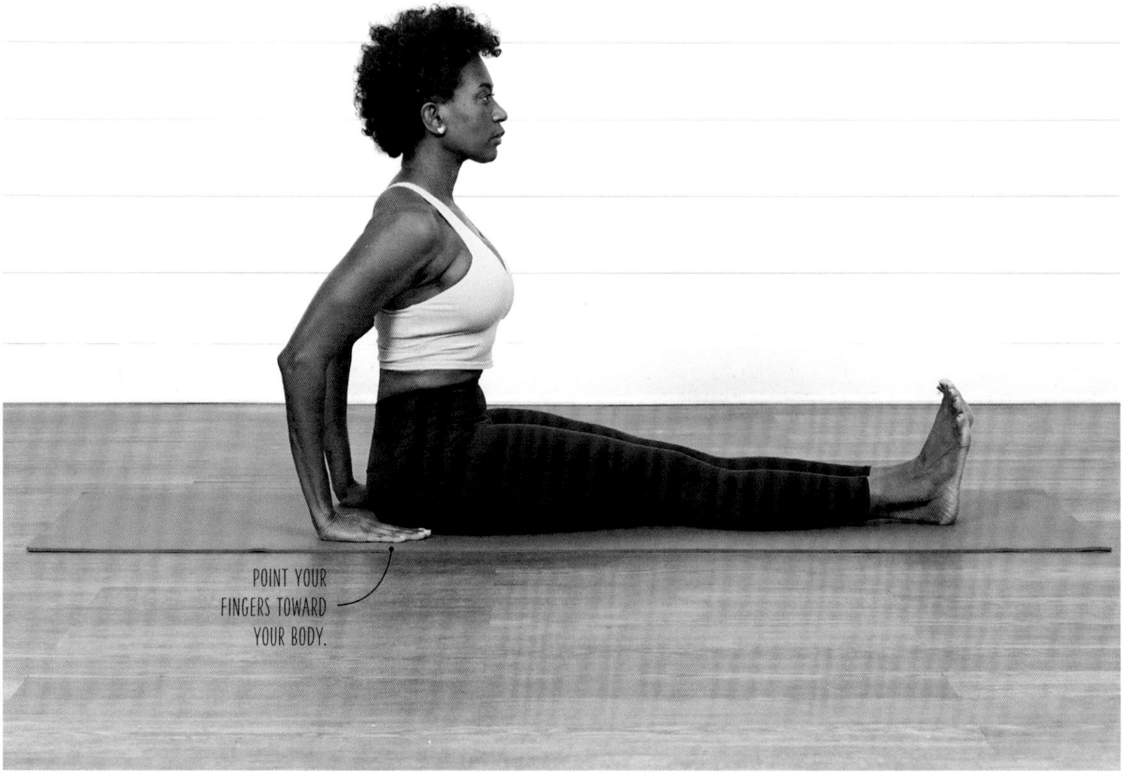
POINT YOUR FINGERS TOWARD YOUR BODY.

2 Press through your hands to raise your buttocks and upper legs off the floor.

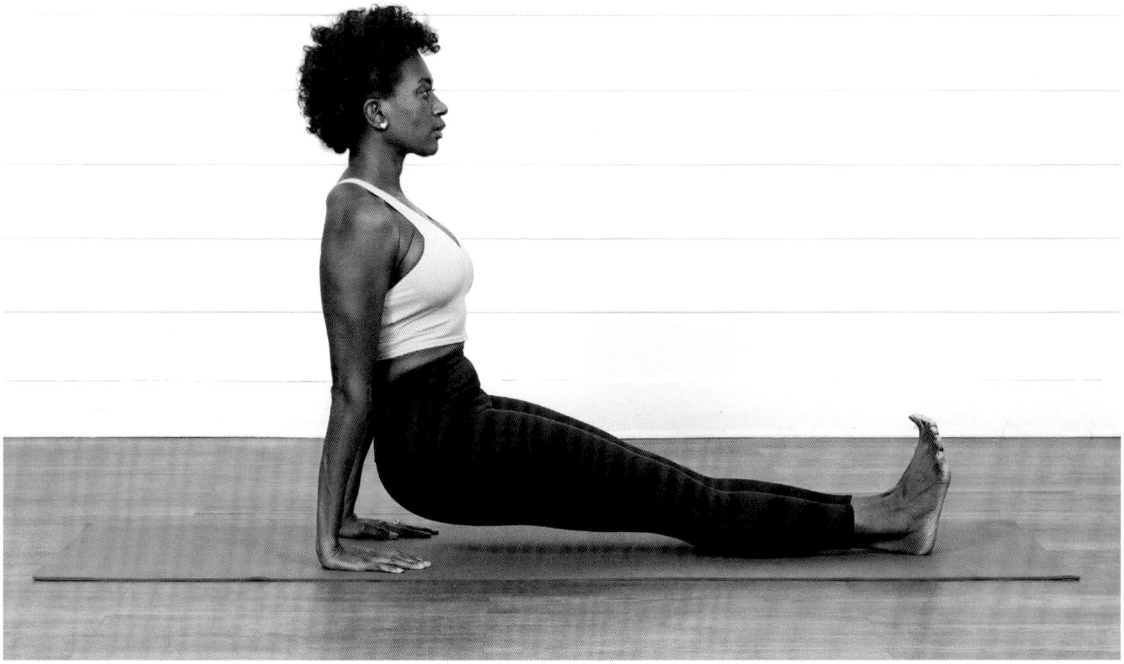

3 Extend your left leg toward the ceiling to form a 45-degree angle with the floor. Reverse your movements to return your left leg to the floor. Perform these steps 6 times. Repeat these steps with your right leg extended.

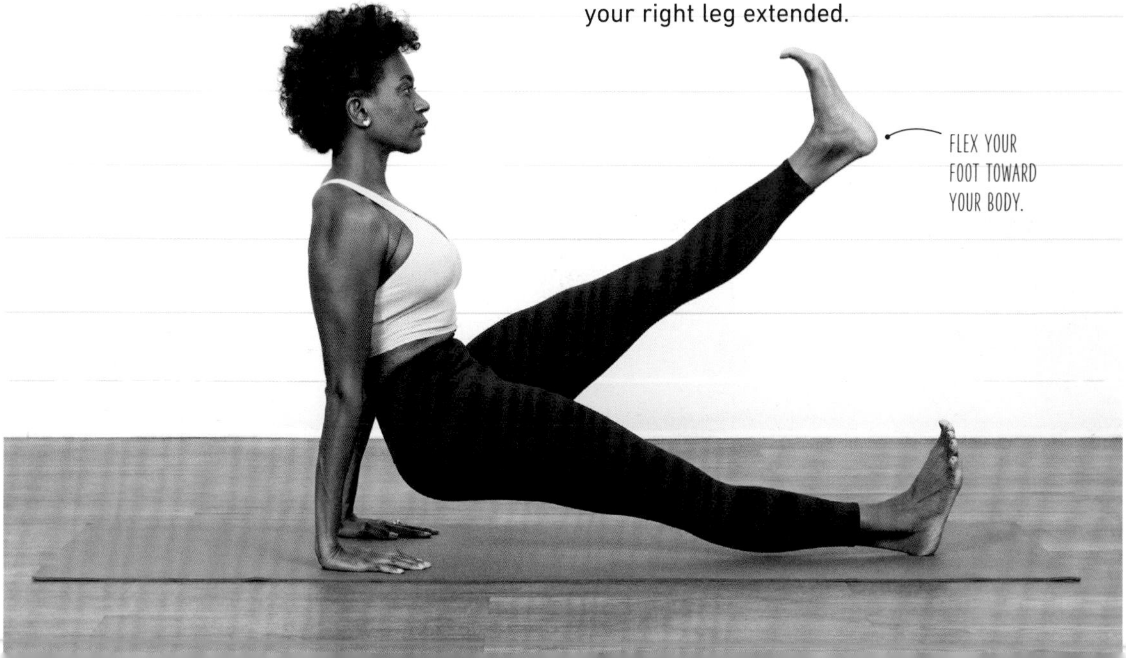
FLEX YOUR FOOT TOWARD YOUR BODY.

LEG PULL-UPS

VARIATIONS

This exercise is essentially a reverse plank with added movements. Because these movements require power in your arms, core, and legs, if you lack strength in any of these areas, these variations might help. Taking the lift out of the move and/or using a wall for support are excellent options for modifying this exercise.

ON THE FLOOR WITH ONE BENT LEG

In step 1, bend your left knee and place your left foot flat on the floor.

In step 2, keep your hips on the floor.

In step 3, raise your right leg until parallel with the floor. Continue with the remaining text.

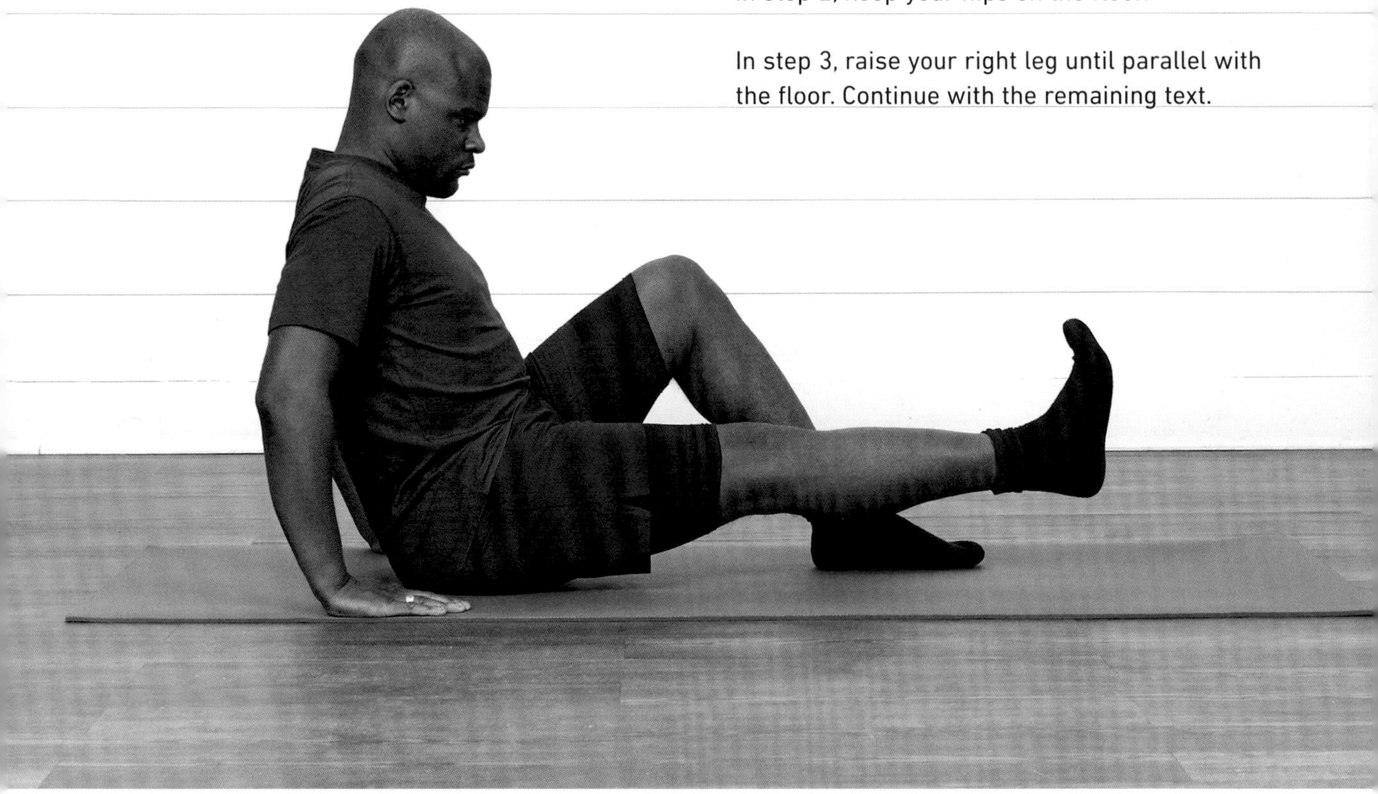

ON THE FLOOR WITH BOTH KNEES BENT

In step 1, bend both knees and place your feet flat on the floor.

In step 2, keep your hips on the floor.

In step 3, raise your right leg until your lower right leg is parallel with the floor. Continue with the remaining text.

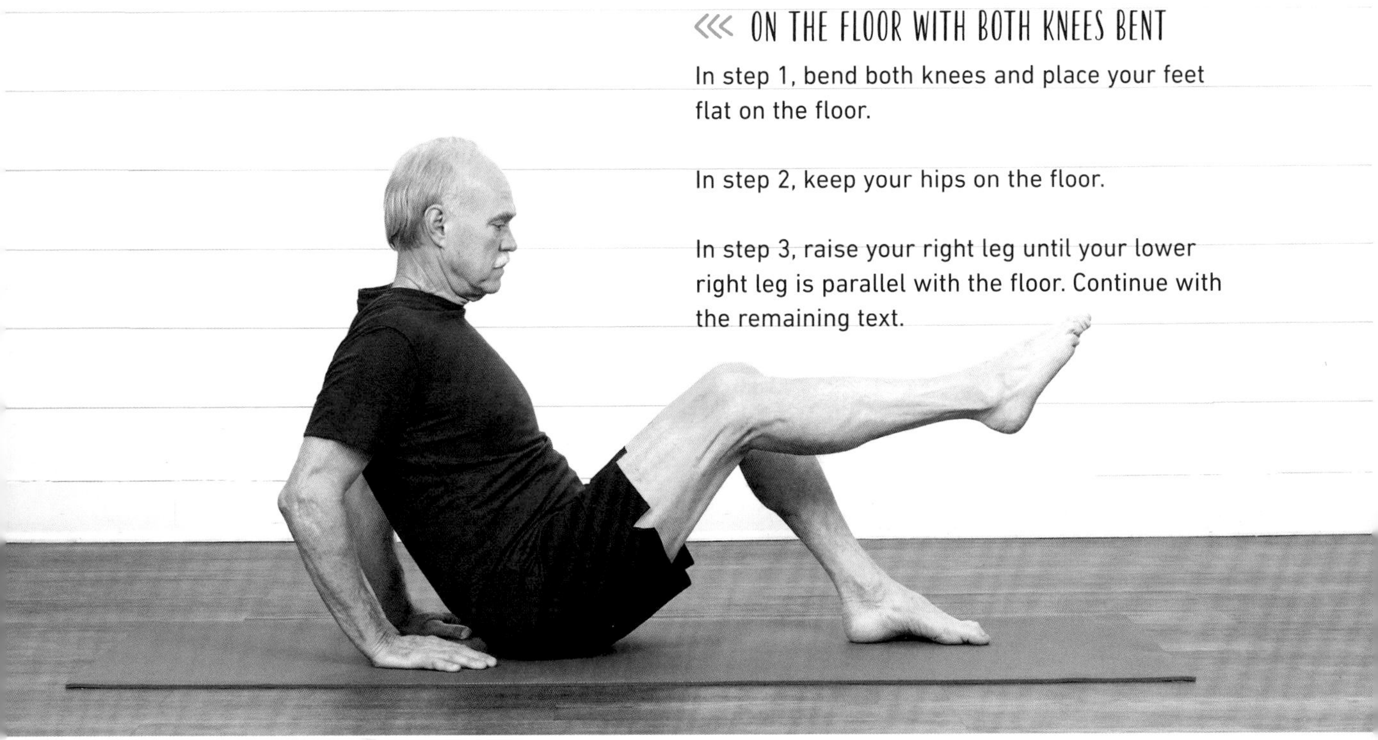

AGAINST A WALL

In step 1, lean your back into a wall. Bend your right leg and keep your hips on the floor. Continue with the remaining text.

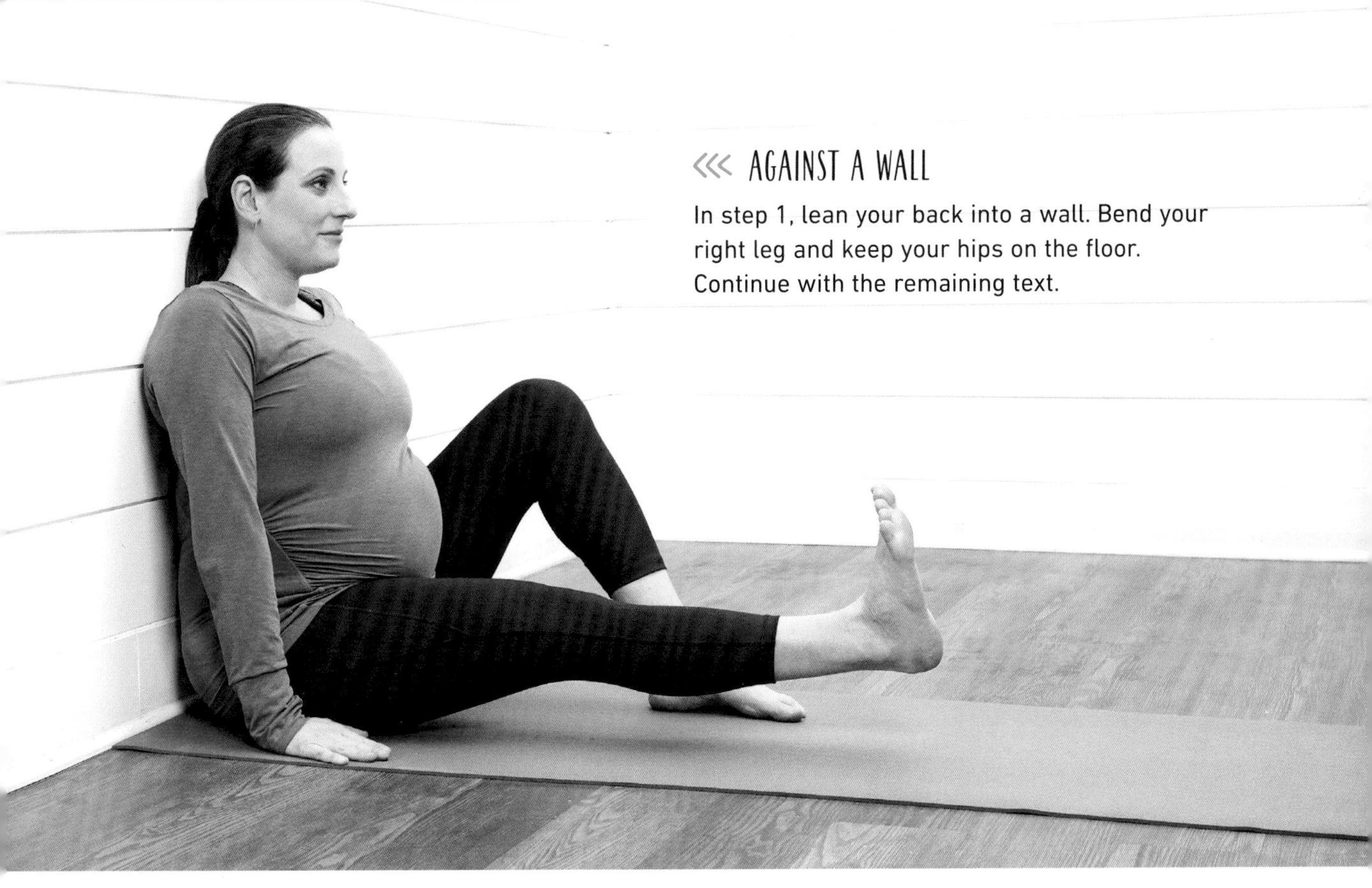

Kneeling Side Kicks

Primarily targeting your hip flexors, abs, and spinal muscles, this exercise also addresses your groin, hamstrings, lower back, obliques, and outer thighs. These movements can strengthen your hips and shoulders while you work on pelvic stability, hamstring flexibility, and balance.

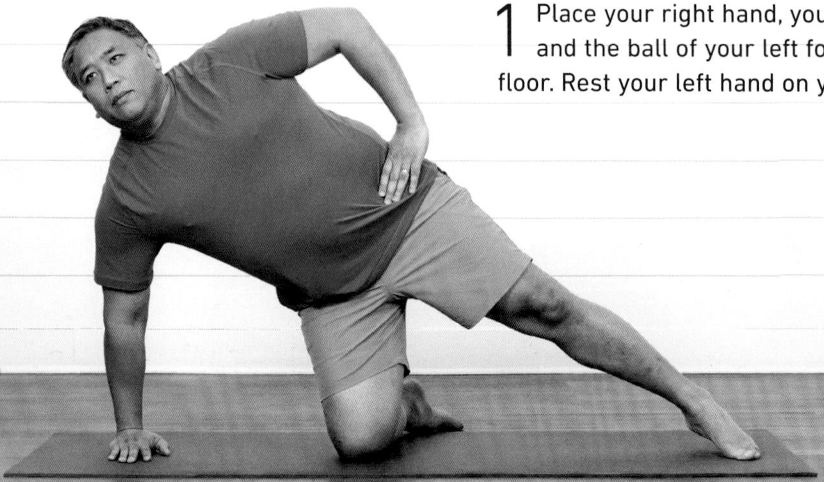

1 Place your right hand, your right knee, and the ball of your left foot flat on the floor. Rest your left hand on your left hip.

2 Extend your left leg to your left side until parallel with your hip or the floor.

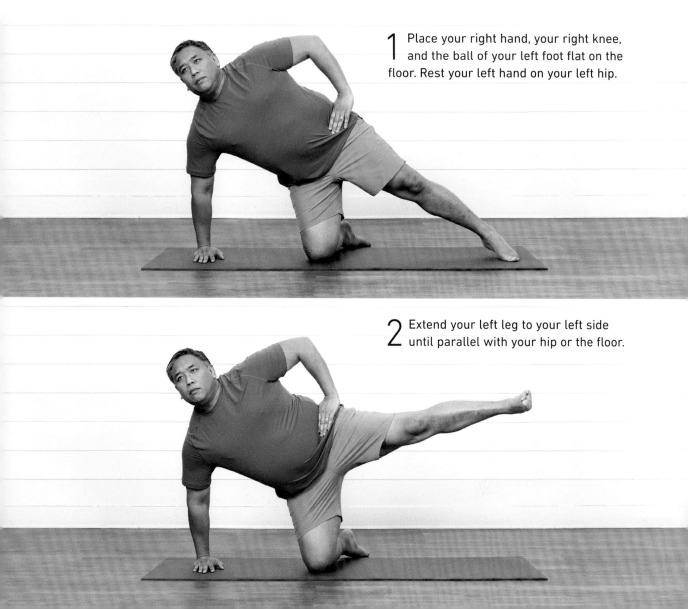

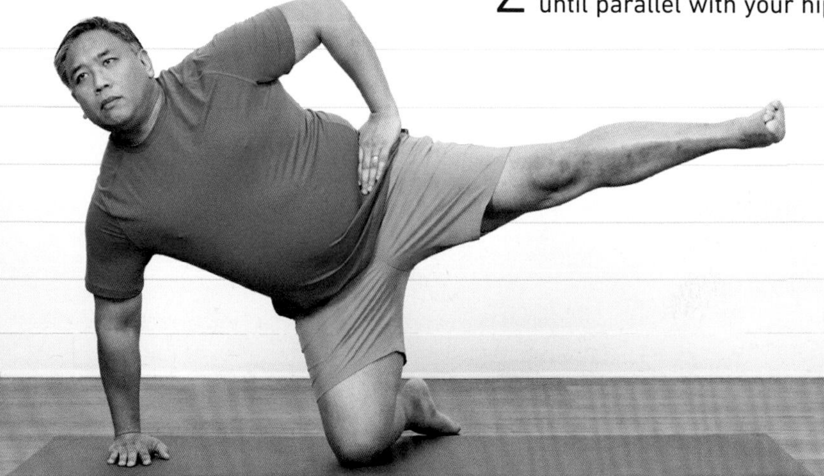

3 Slowly sweep your left leg backward, flexing your left foot toward your body.

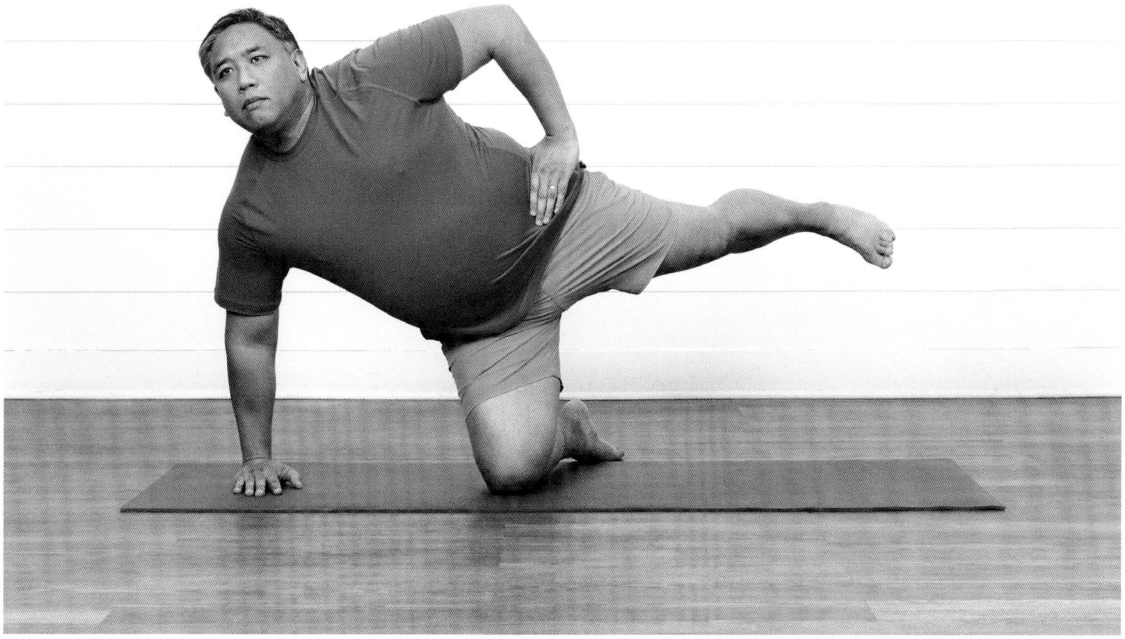

4 Slowly sweep your left leg forward, keeping your toes flexed. Perform the last two steps 5 times. Repeat these steps with your right leg sweeping.

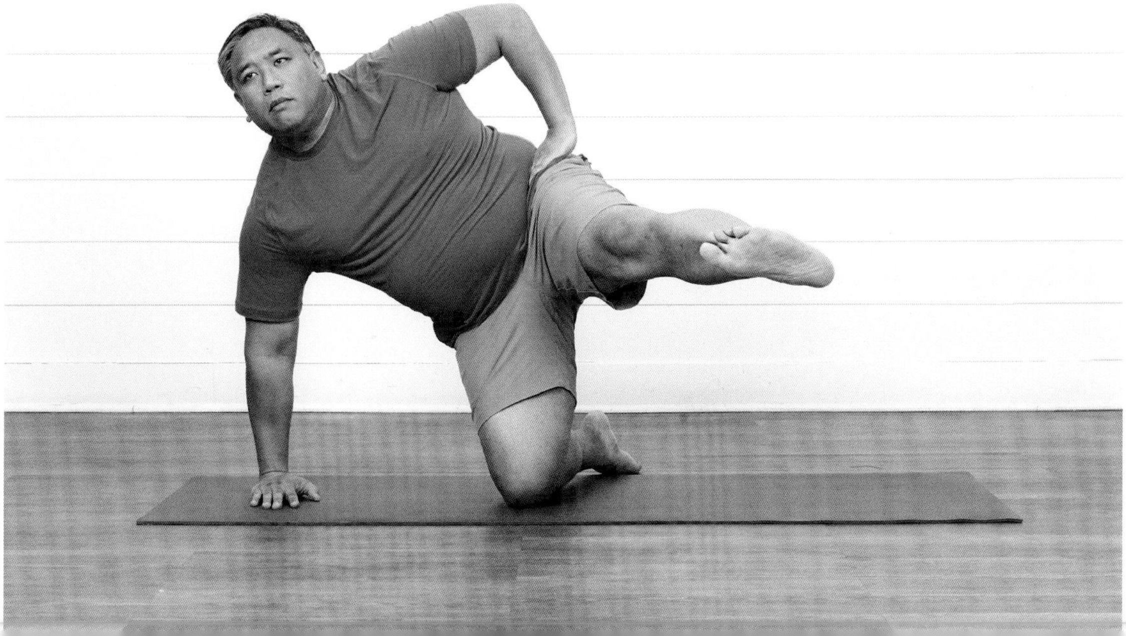

KNEELING SIDE KICKS

VARIATIONS

If you have tight shoulders or lower-back discomfort, try one of these alternative poses. Performing a variation might even help ease some of that tension and allow you to develop some strength in those areas.

<<< ON YOUR SIDE

1. Lie on your right side with your legs stacked. Place your right elbow flat on the floor and rest your head in your right hand. Place your left hand flat on the floor or relax your left arm at your side.

2. Extend your left leg backward as far as comfortable.

3. Extend your left leg forward as far as comfortable. Perform the last two steps 5 times. Repeat these steps on your left side.

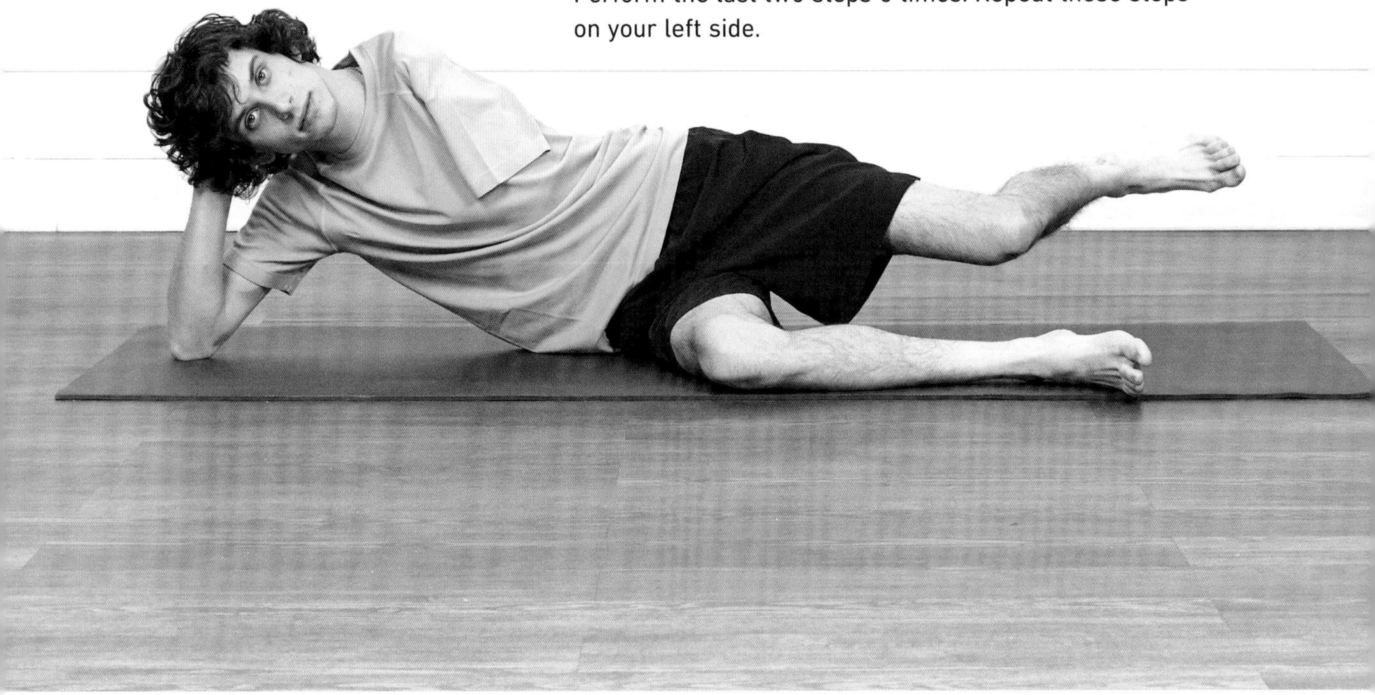

WITH A SMALL PILATES BALL >>>

In step 1 of the variation on page 140, place a small Pilates ball between your ribs and hips. Continue with the remaining text.

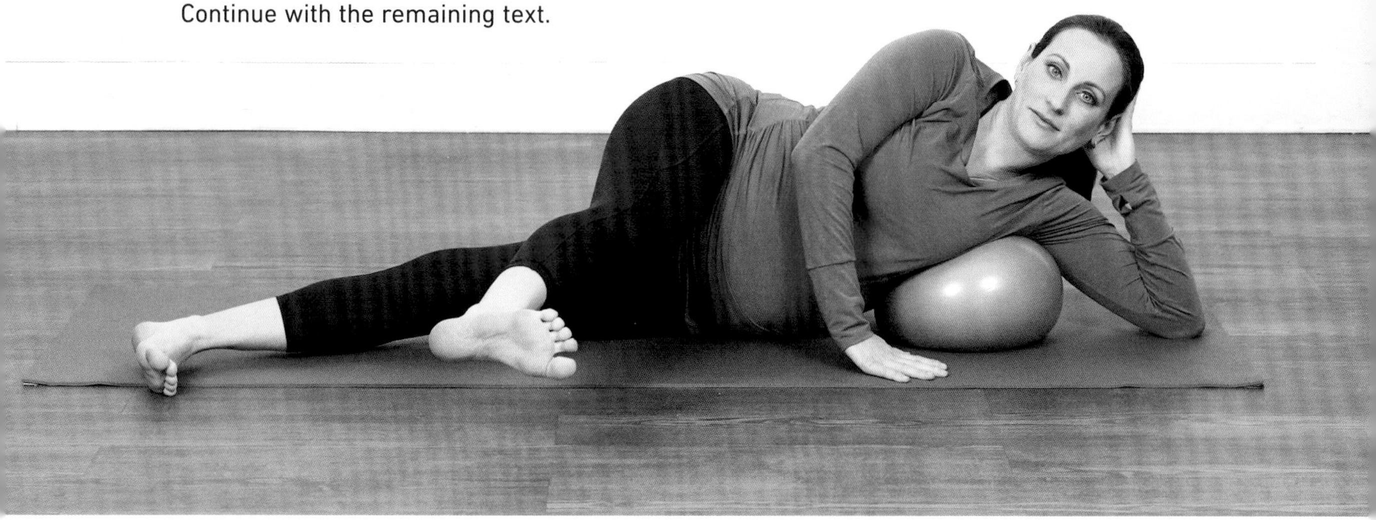

<<< ON A FOREARM

In step 1 of the variation on page 140, place your right forearm flat on the floor. Continue with the remaining text.

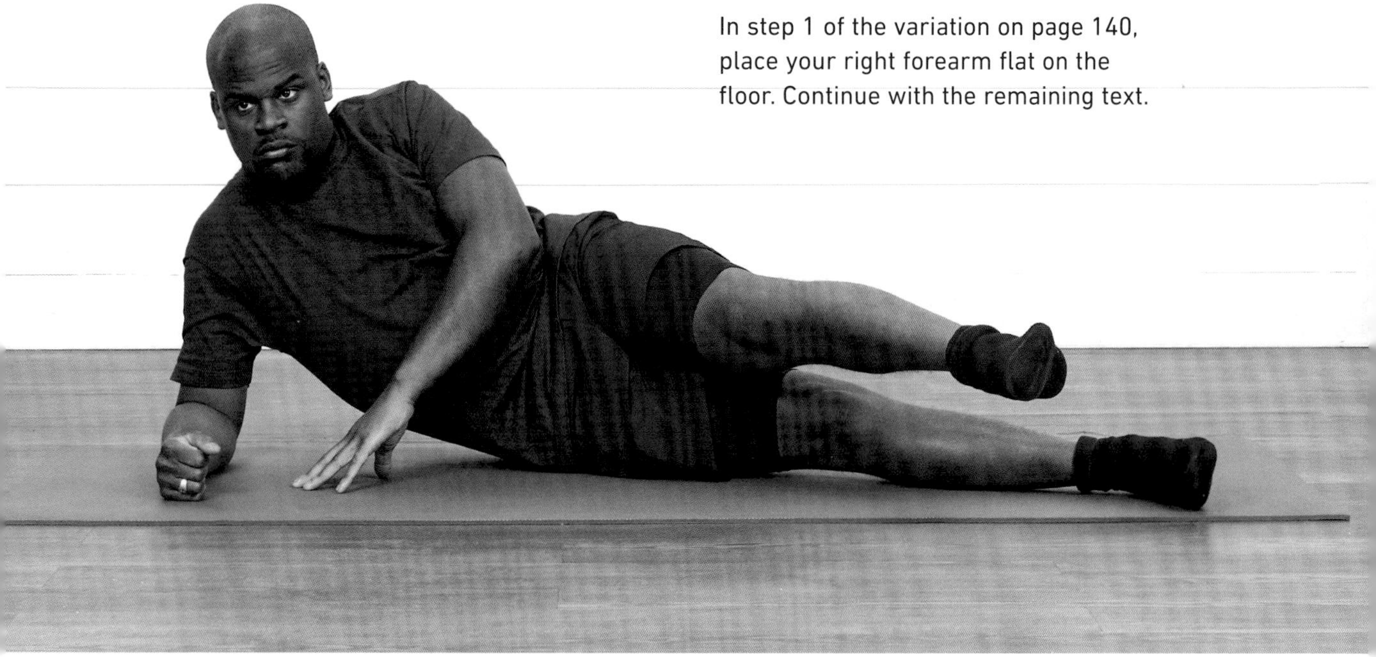

JERRY DENYS

I'm an active, young 70-year-old. I've been practicing Pilates for more than 12 years. My first introduction to Pilates was when a friend talked me into taking a mat class at the National Institute for Fitness and Sports in Indianapolis. Feeling a little intimidated at first, I found the class to be fun and physically challenging. I continued to go to classes and started incorporating Pilates into a golf-specific training program. I began to increase my strength, flexibility, and concentration. The Pilates method helped me train my mind and body—and hopefully extend my years playing golf.

I'm still learning. Using Pilates equipment, I continue to take studio and private classes. In fact, I have more Pilates equipment in my home than golf clubs. I've been fortunate to have excellent instructors over the years to help motivate and inspire me to step out of my comfort zone. My goal is to "keep moving." Pilates is not only an exercise method—it's also a lifestyle. I believe no matter what age you are, Pilates is a lifelong journey.

Note: Jerry was also a model for Linda Paden's Idiot's Guides: Pilates *(Alpha Books, 2014).*

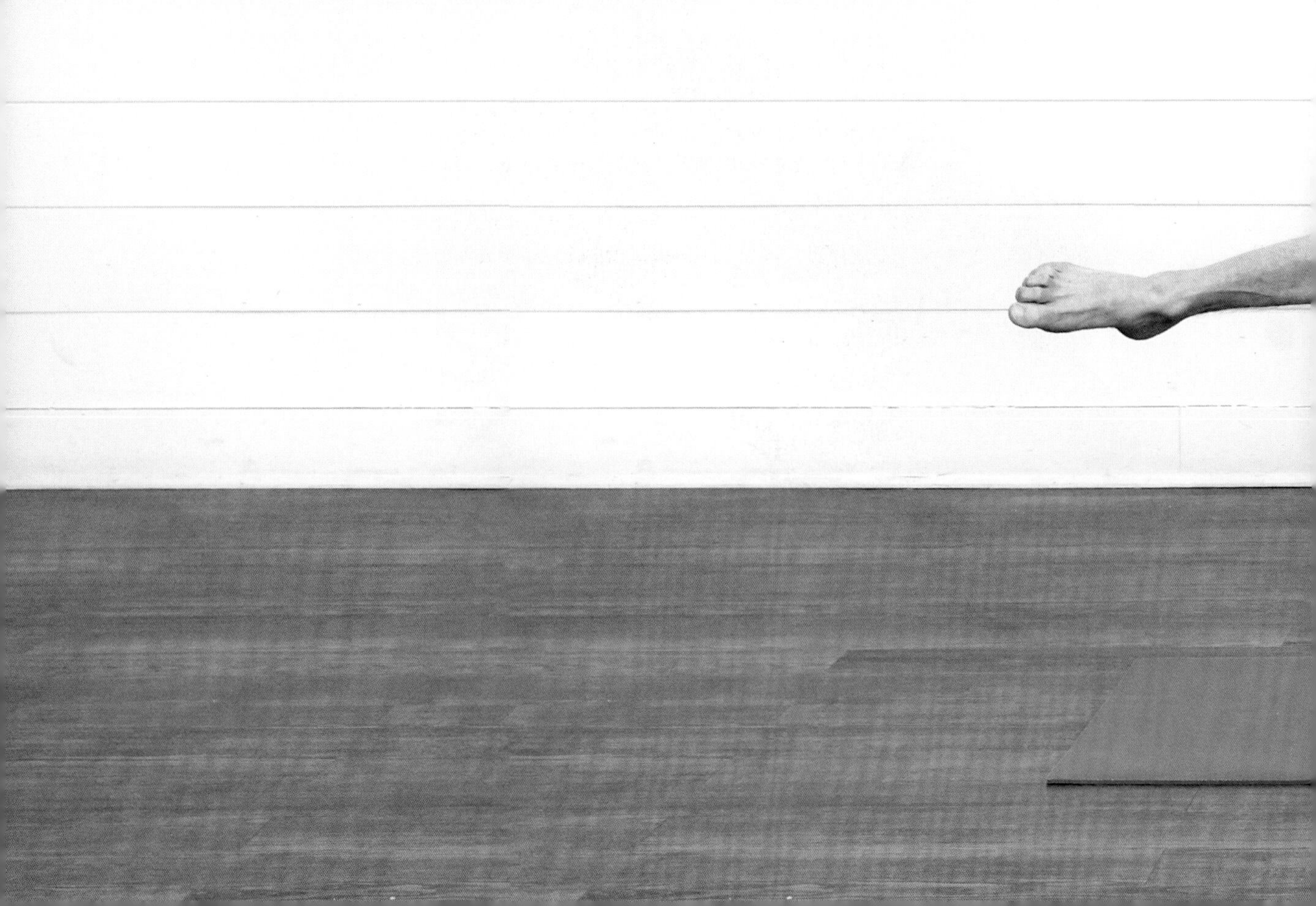

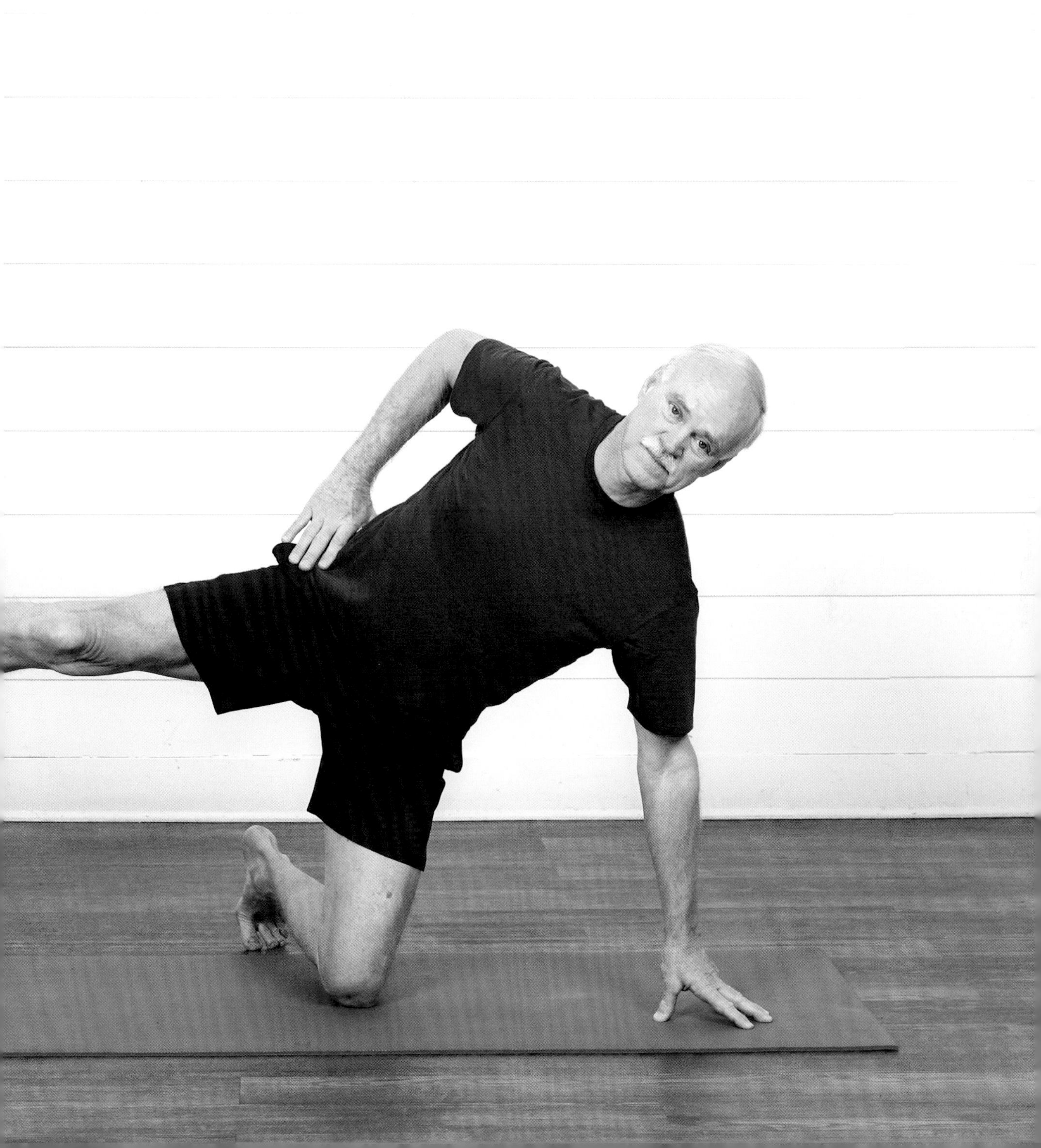

Side Bends

This exercise strengthens your core muscles, scapular stabilizers, glutes, and legs—truly a total-body move. These movements can also help improve lumbo-pelvic stability and provide lower back pain relief by strengthening your abdominal and back muscles.

1 Sit on the floor with your legs extended toward your left side and your left foot just in front of your right foot. Place your right hand flat on the floor and rest your left hand on your left thigh.

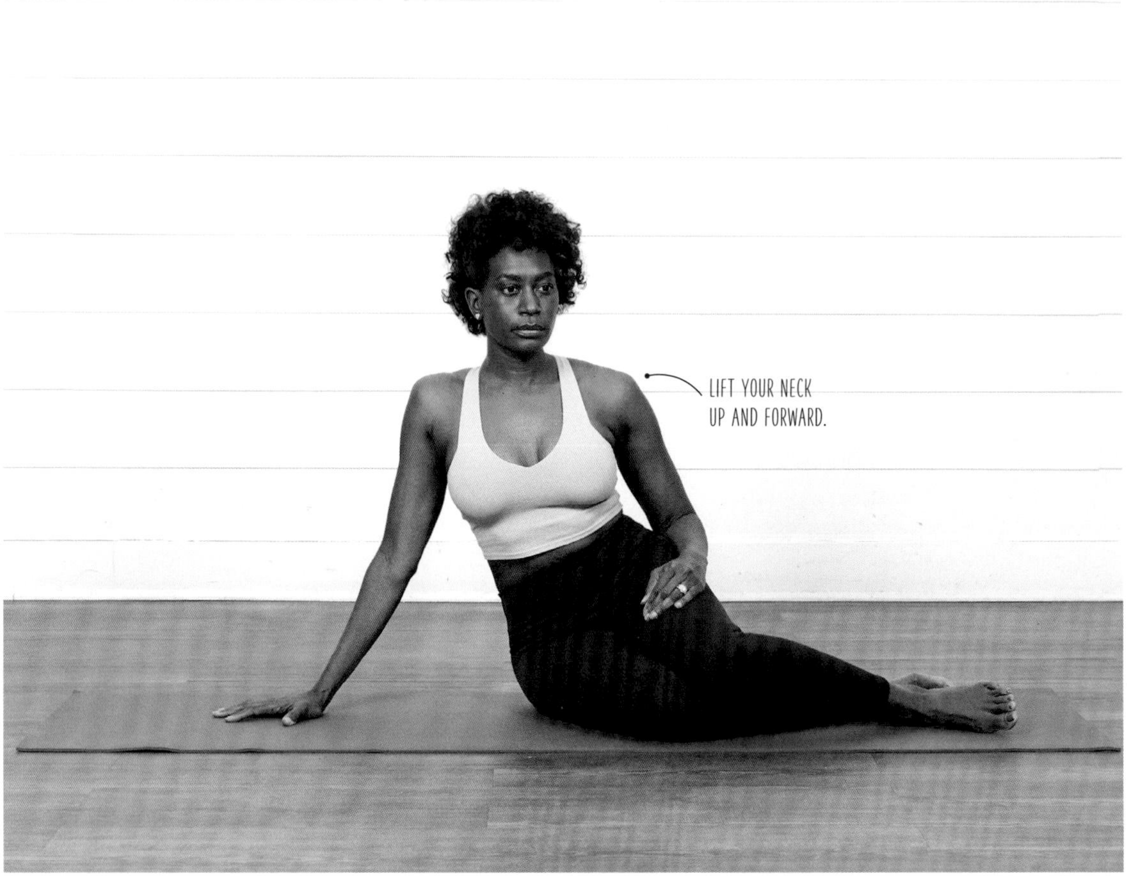
LIFT YOUR NECK
UP AND FORWARD.

2 Press into your right hand and raise your hips off the floor until your legs are straight. Reverse your movements to return to your starting position. Perform these steps 3 times. Repeat these steps with your legs extended to your right side.

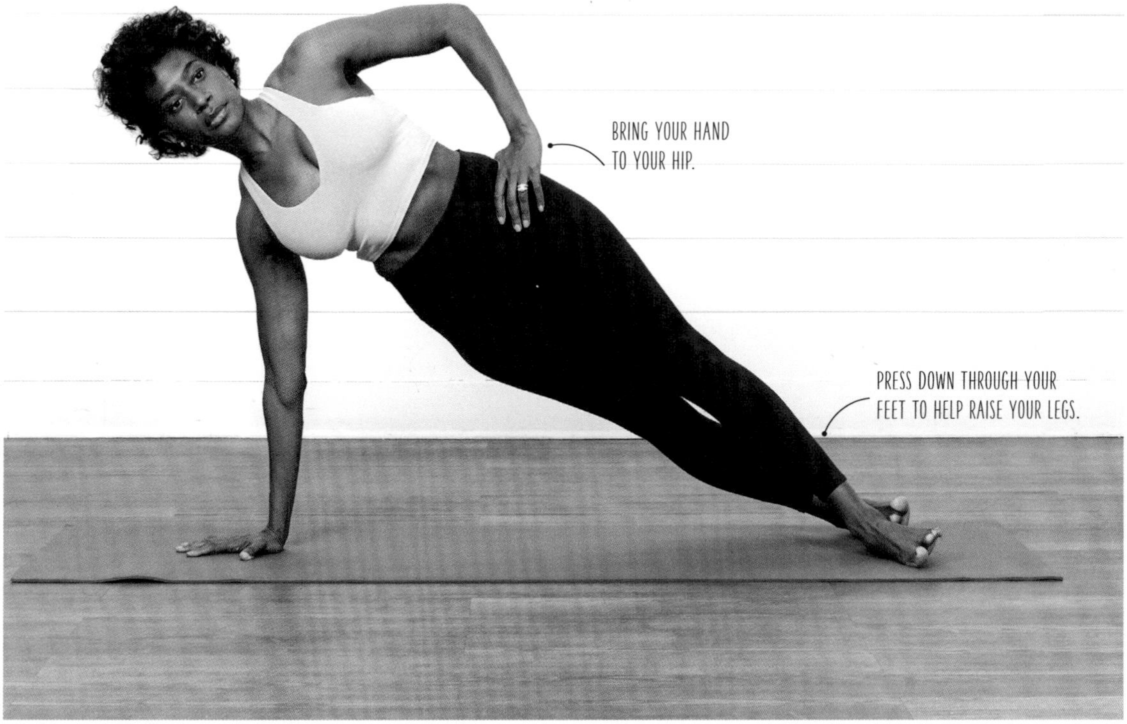
BRING YOUR HAND TO YOUR HIP.
PRESS DOWN THROUGH YOUR FEET TO HELP RAISE YOUR LEGS.

SIDE BENDS

VARIATIONS

Traditional side bends require lateral flexion of the trunk—movement of the trunk to your right or left side accompanied by movement of the shoulder toward the hip on either side. If you have limited mobility of the spine, these variations can help with improved mobility and flexibility.

STANDING >>>

1. Stand with your feet shoulder width apart. Relax your arms at your sides.

2. Extend your left arm alongside your head. Reach your left arm over the top of your head toward your right side as you bend toward your right. (Bend as far as you're comfortable.) Reverse your movements to return to your starting position.

3. Extend your right arm alongside your head. Reach your right arm over the top of your head toward your left side as you bend toward your left. (Bend as far as you're comfortable.) Reverse your movements to return to your starting position. Perform these steps 6 times.

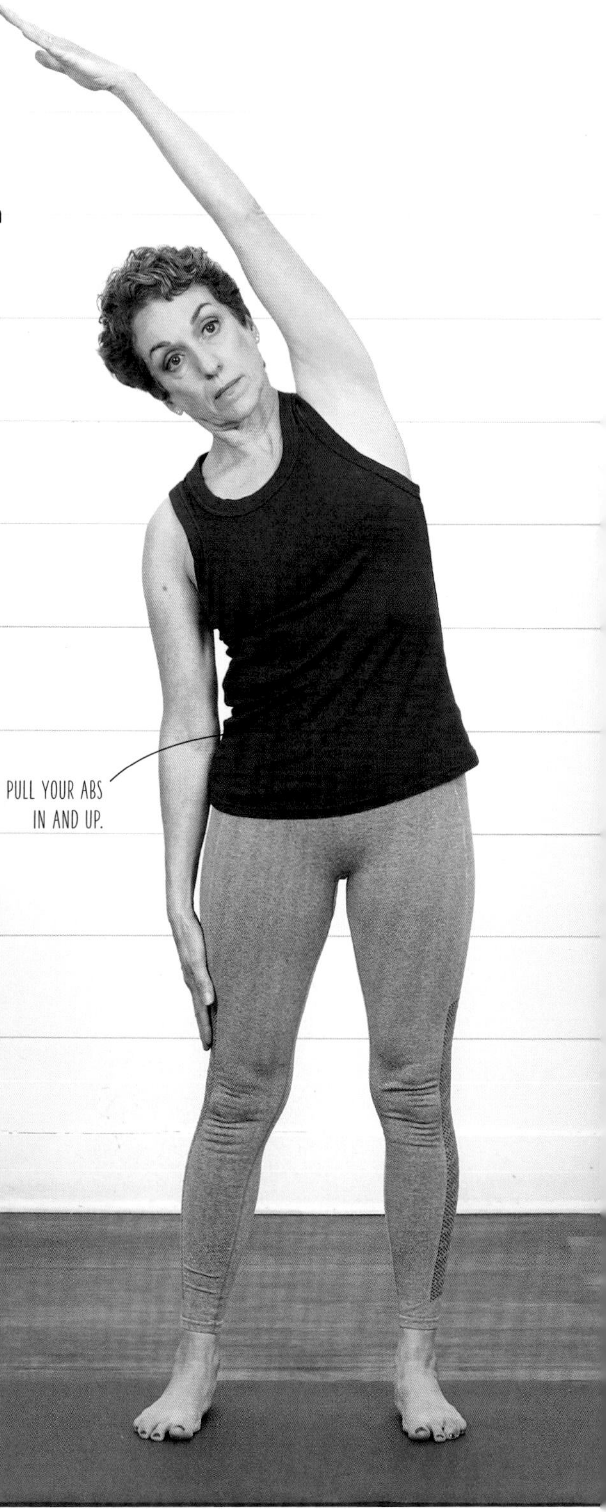

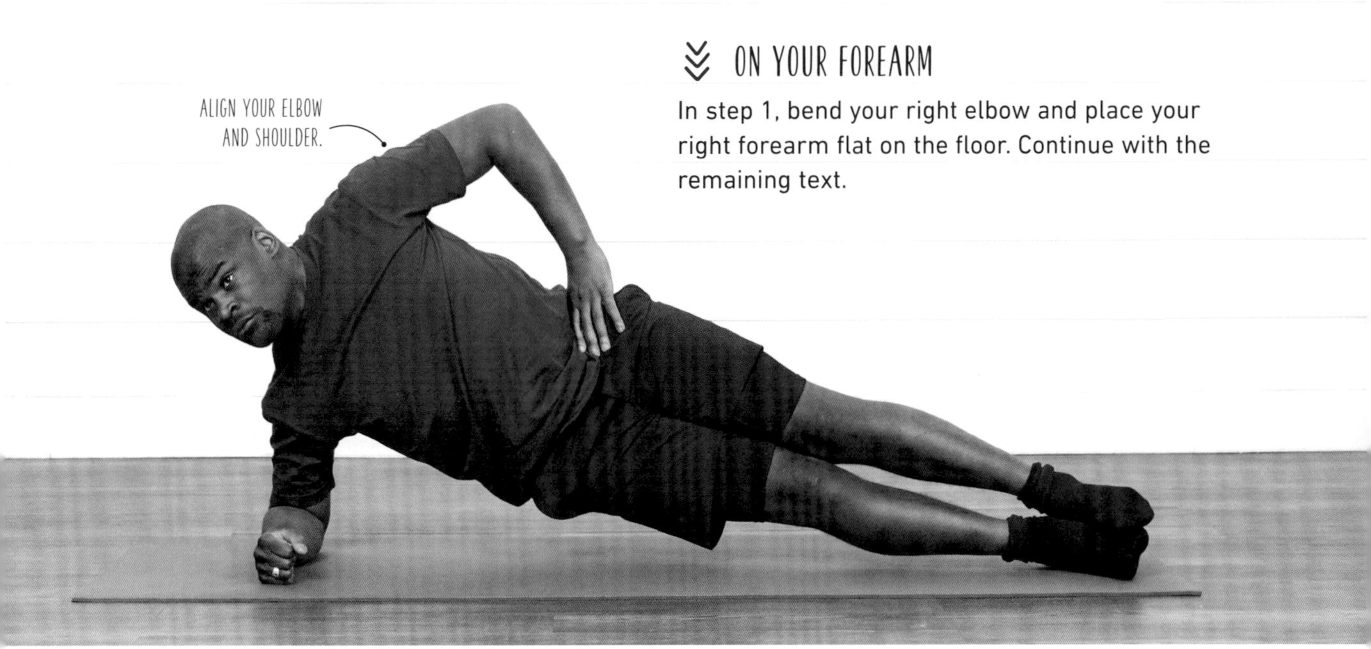

ALIGN YOUR ELBOW
AND SHOULDER.

ON YOUR FOREARM

In step 1, bend your right elbow and place your right forearm flat on the floor. Continue with the remaining text.

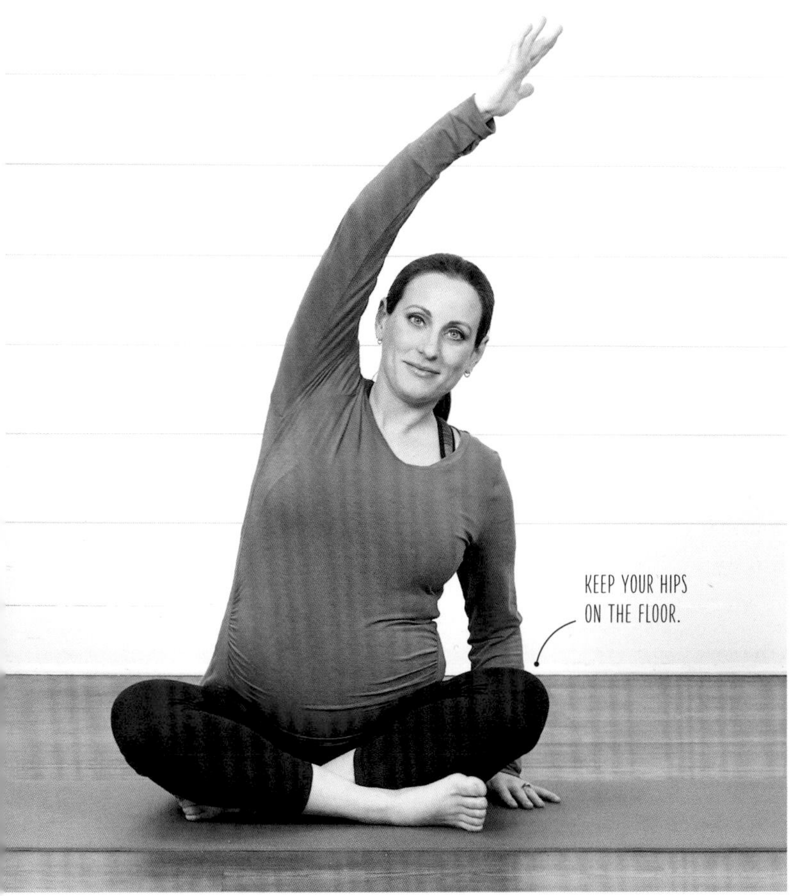

KEEP YOUR HIPS
ON THE FLOOR.

SITTING ON THE FLOOR

1. Sit on the floor with your knees bent and your ankles stacked, forming a meditation pose. Relax your arms at your sides.

2. Extend your right arm alongside your head. Reach your right arm over the top of your head toward your left side as you bend toward your left. Reverse your movements to return to your starting position.

3. Extend your left arm alongside your head and toward the ceiling. Reach your left arm over the top of your head toward your right side as you bend toward your right. Reverse your movements to return to your starting position. Perform these steps 5 times.

Hip Circles

This exercise focuses on your abs, hip flexors, and shoulder stabilizers. These movements can strengthen your obliques, promote shoulder stabilization, and stretch your back and hamstrings. This challenging exercise teaches lift in your upper body while providing a stretch across your chest.

1 Sit on the floor with your legs extended to form a V with your body. Place your hands flat on the floor behind you—a little wider than shoulder width apart.

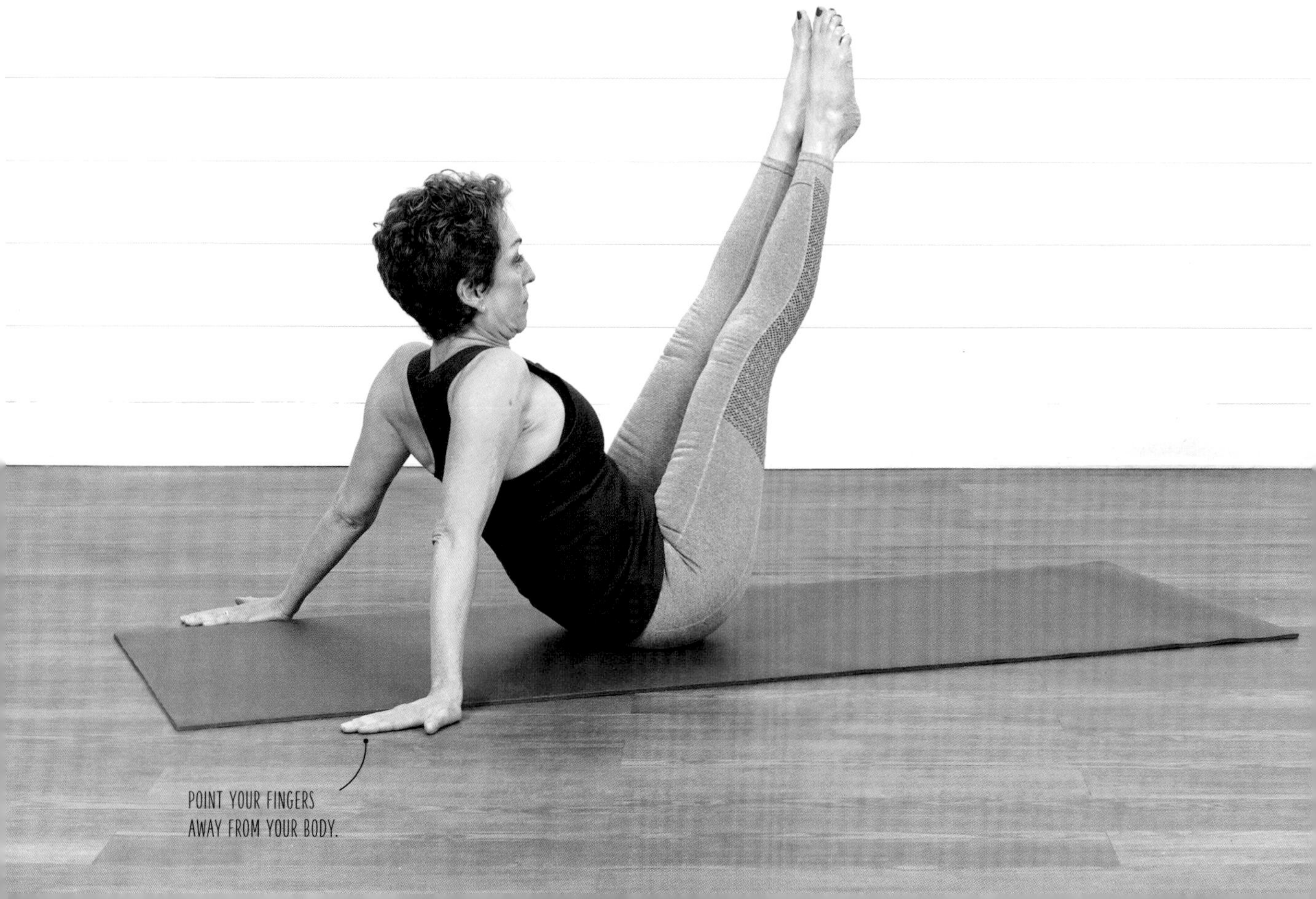

POINT YOUR FINGERS AWAY FROM YOUR BODY.

2 On an inhale, begin to trace a large clockwise circle. Exhale at the bottom and complete the circle.

3 On an inhale, begin to trace a large counterclockwise circle. Exhale at the bottom and complete the circle. Perform the last two steps 6 times.

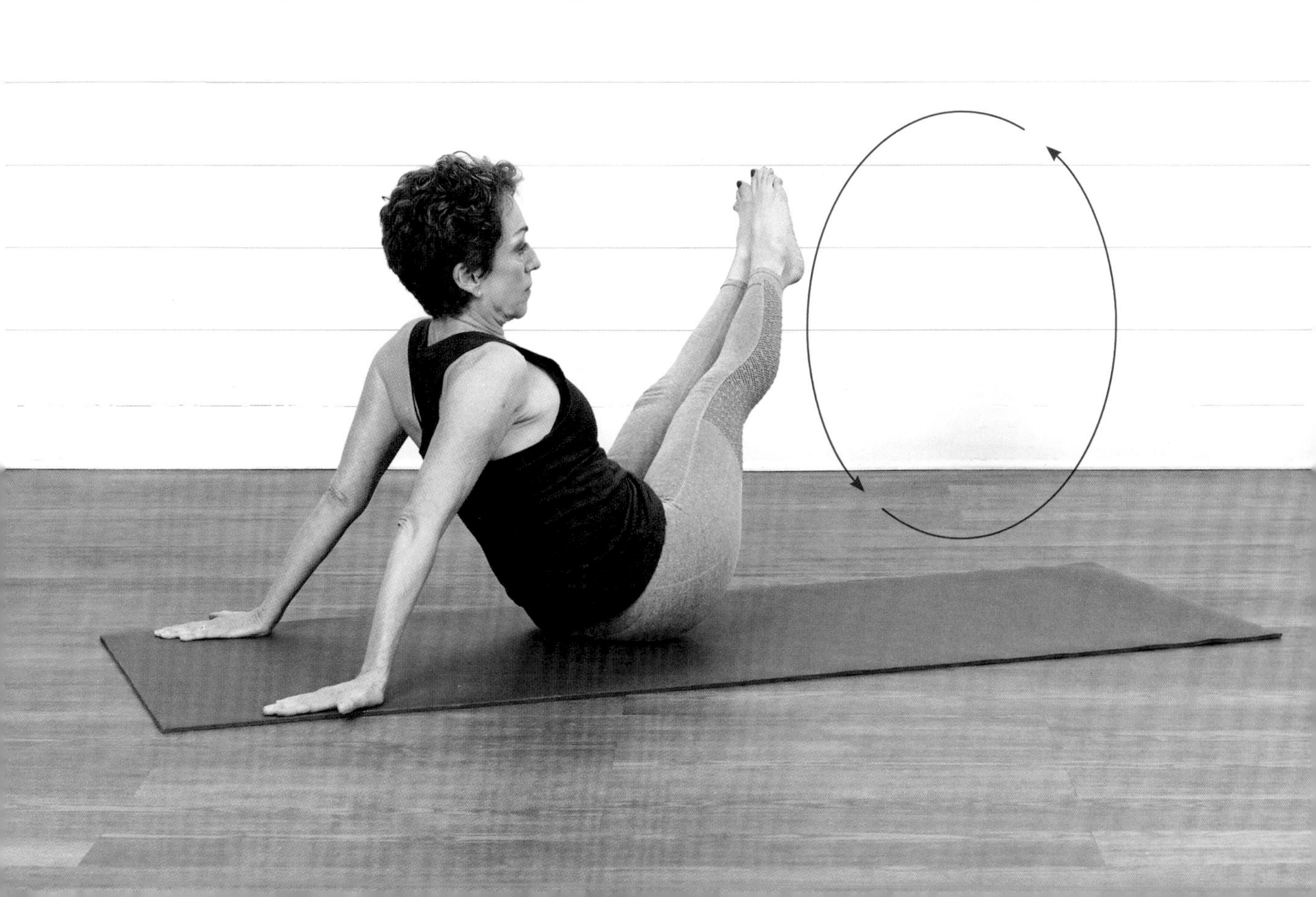

HIP CIRCLES

VARIATIONS

Moving the weight of your legs (your heaviest body part) with the strength of your core while stabilizing your trunk is quite the task. If stability is a challenge, using a small Pilates ball can add some support. If you have difficulty coming down to the floor, the standing variation might suit you best.

WITH A SMALL PILATES BALL AND ON YOUR FOREARMS

In step 1, place a small Pilates ball at your lower back. Raise your legs to form a 90-degree angle with your legs. Lower yourself backward to place your forearms flat on the floor. Continue with the remaining text.

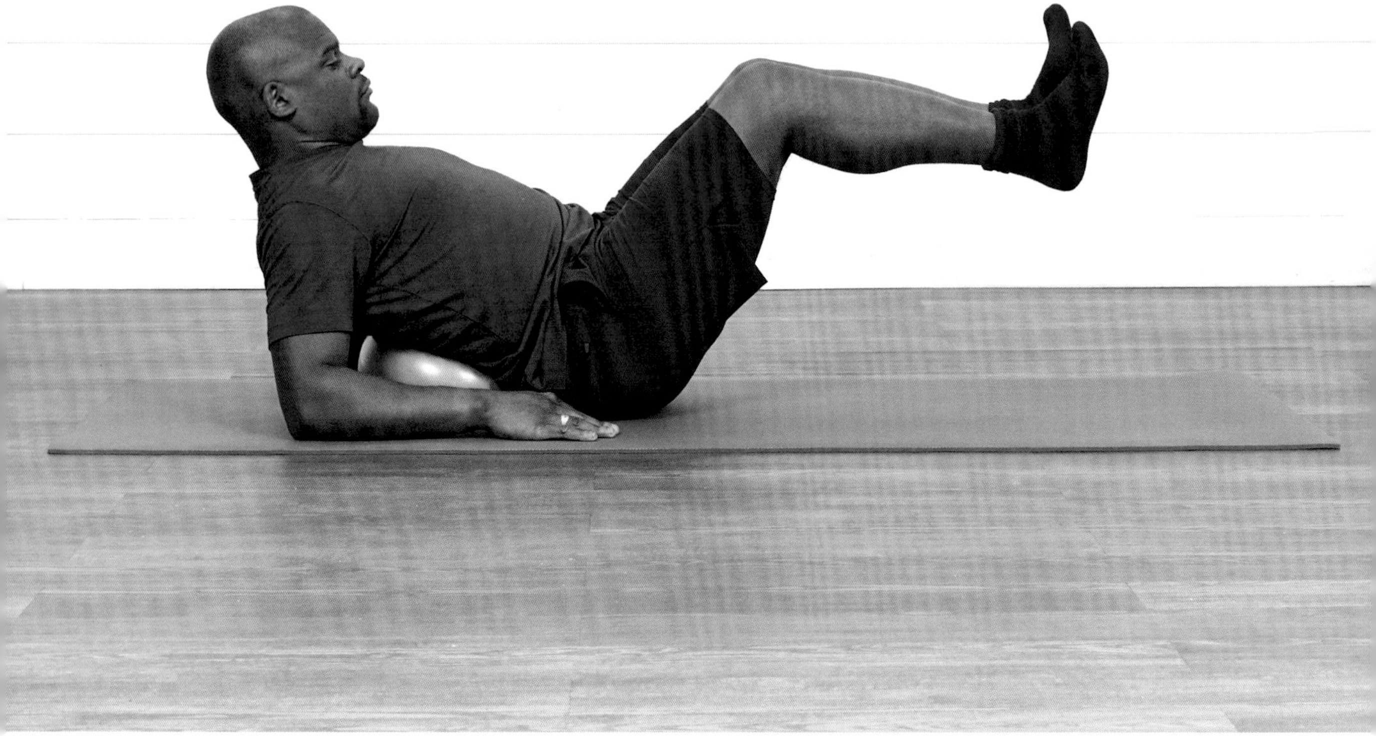

WITH ONE LEG

1. Lie on your back on the floor with your right leg extended toward the ceiling. Relax your arms at your sides.

2. Trace a clockwise basketball-sized circle with your toes for 3 seconds.

3. Trace a counterclockwise basketball-sized circle with your toes for 3 seconds. Repeat these steps with your left leg extended.

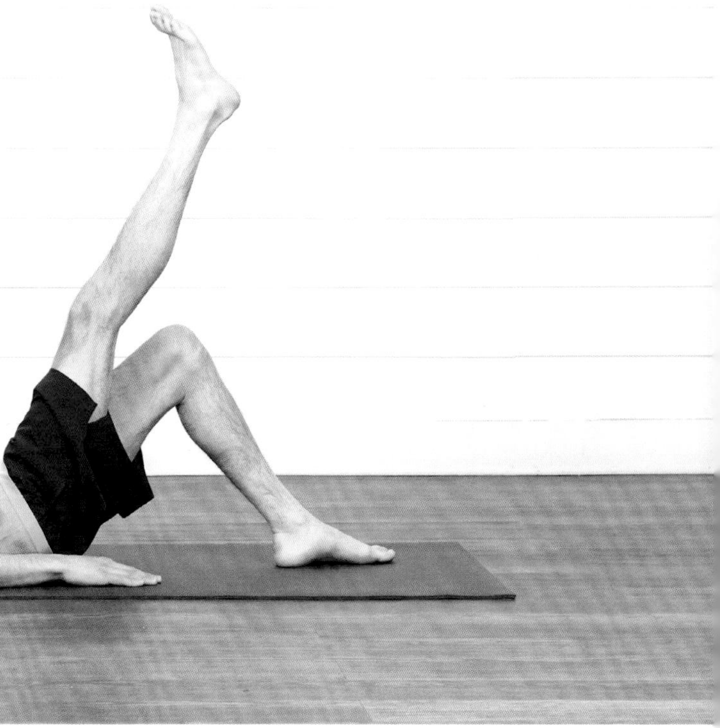

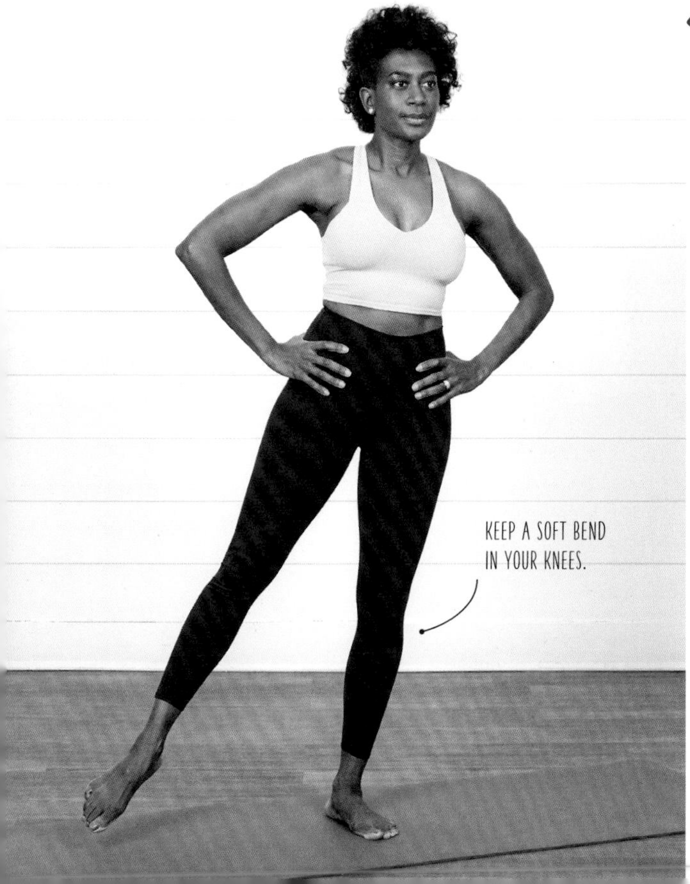
KEEP A SOFT BEND IN YOUR KNEES.

STANDING

1. Stand with your feet shoulder width apart and your hands resting on your hips.

2. Extend your right leg to your right side. Trace a clockwise basketball-sized circle with your leg for 4 seconds.

3. Reverse your movements to trace a counterclockwise basketball-sized circle with your leg for 4 seconds. Repeat these steps with your left leg.

Single-Leg Stretches

The purpose of this exercise is to engage your abdominal muscles with the movement of your legs while stabilizing your upper body. Performing these movements can strengthen your abs, hip flexors, and gluteal muscles as well as stretch your hip flexors. You can also improve coordination and torso stability by practicing this stretch.

1 Lie on your back on the floor with your head and shoulders raised off the floor. Extend your legs toward the ceiling to form a 90-degree angle with your body. Relax your arms at your sides and place your hands flat on the floor.

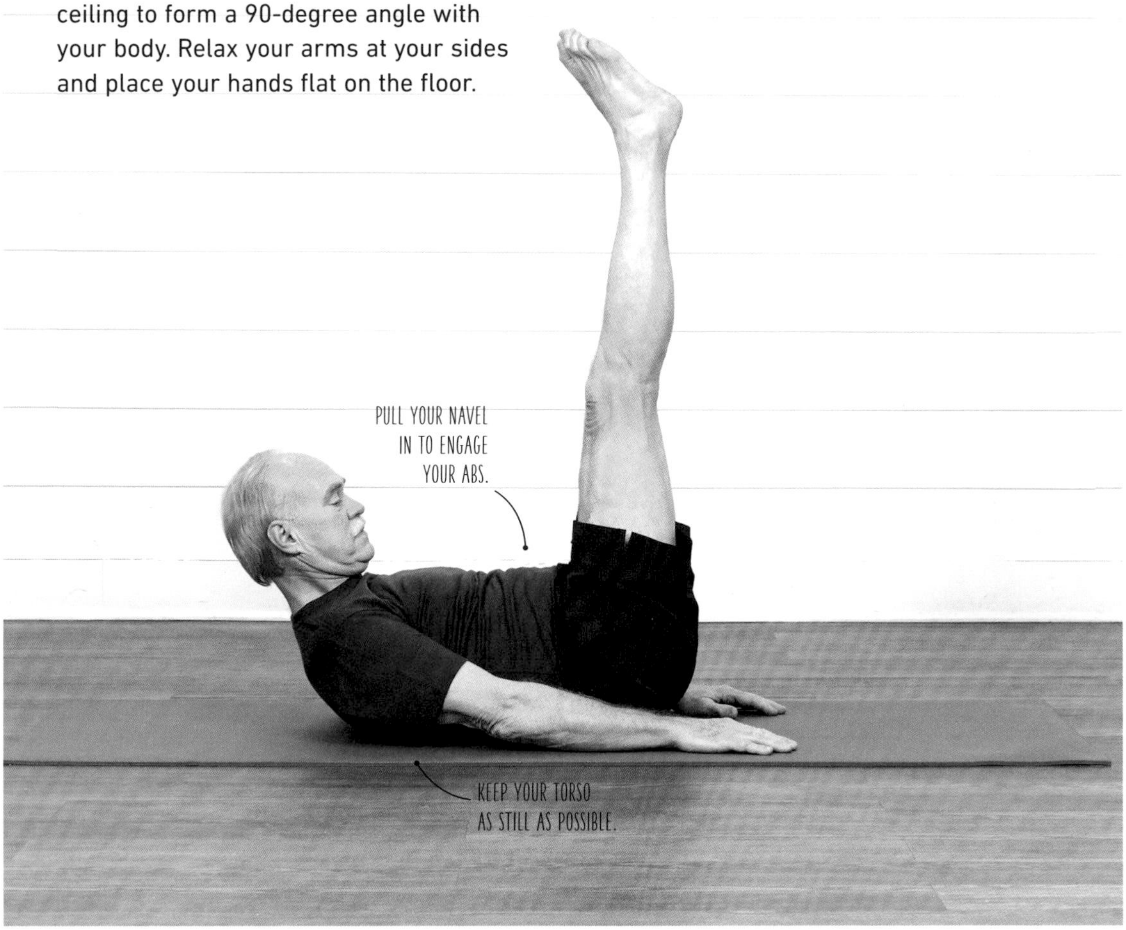
PULL YOUR NAVEL IN TO ENGAGE YOUR ABS.
KEEP YOUR TORSO AS STILL AS POSSIBLE.

2 Bend your right knee and grasp your right shin with both hands as you pull your right knee toward your chest. Simultaneously lower your left leg to form a 45-degree angle with the floor. Reverse your movements to return to your starting position.

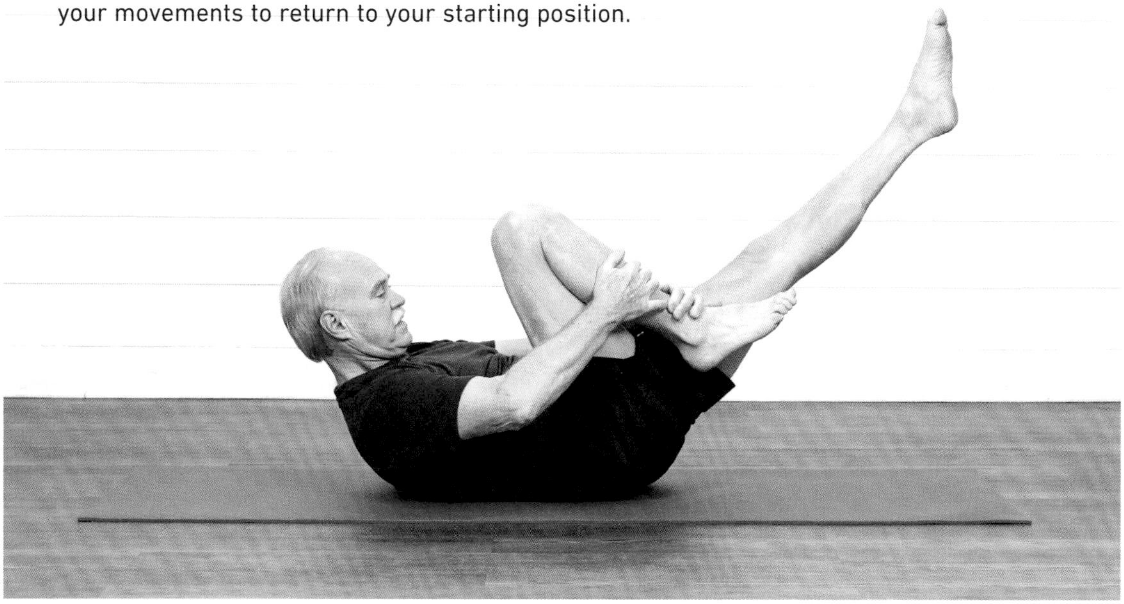

3 Bend your left knee and grasp your left shin with both hands as you pull your left knee toward your chest. Simultaneously lower your right leg to form a 45-degree angle with the floor. Reverse your movements to return to your starting position. Perform these steps 8 times.

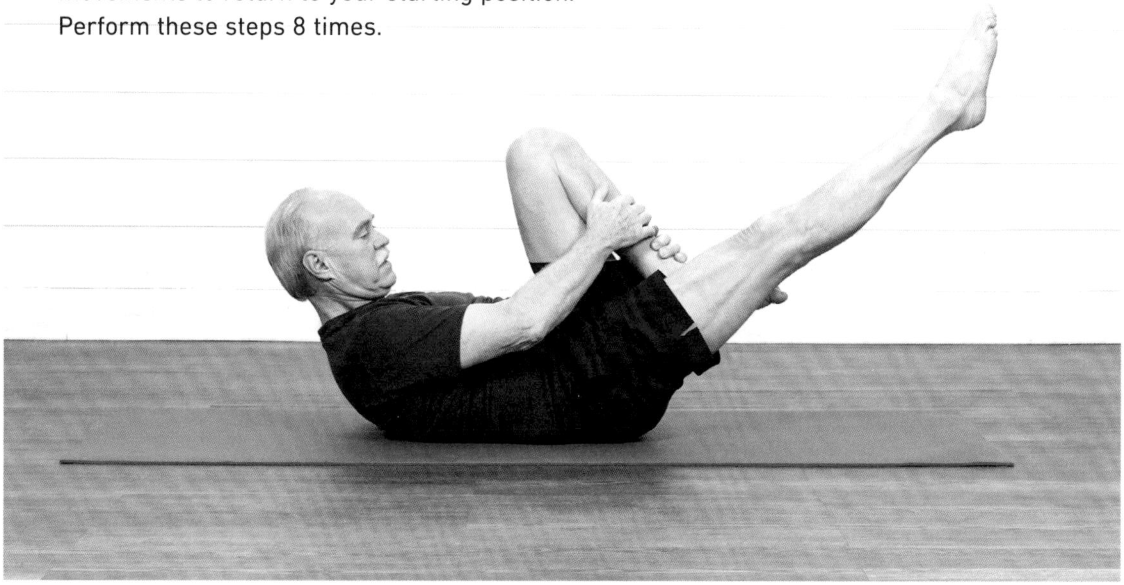

SINGLE-LEG STRETCHES

VARIATIONS

If you feel a strain when lifting your head, keeping your head on the floor can provide relief. When your neck and shoulders aren't properly supported in an exercise, they take on too much work. Using a small Pilates ball or resistance band can also support your lower back.

WITH A SMALL PILATES BALL

1. Sit on the floor with your legs extended. Place a small Pilates ball at your lower back. Lower your upper body backward until your forearms and hands are flat on the floor.

2. Raise your left leg to form a 90-degree angle with your body. Bend your right knee and raise your right foot a few inches off the floor. Reverse your movements to return to your starting position.

3. Raise your right leg to form a 90-degree angle with your body. Bend your left knee and raise your left foot a few inches off the floor. Reverse your movements to return to your starting position. Perform these steps 8 times.

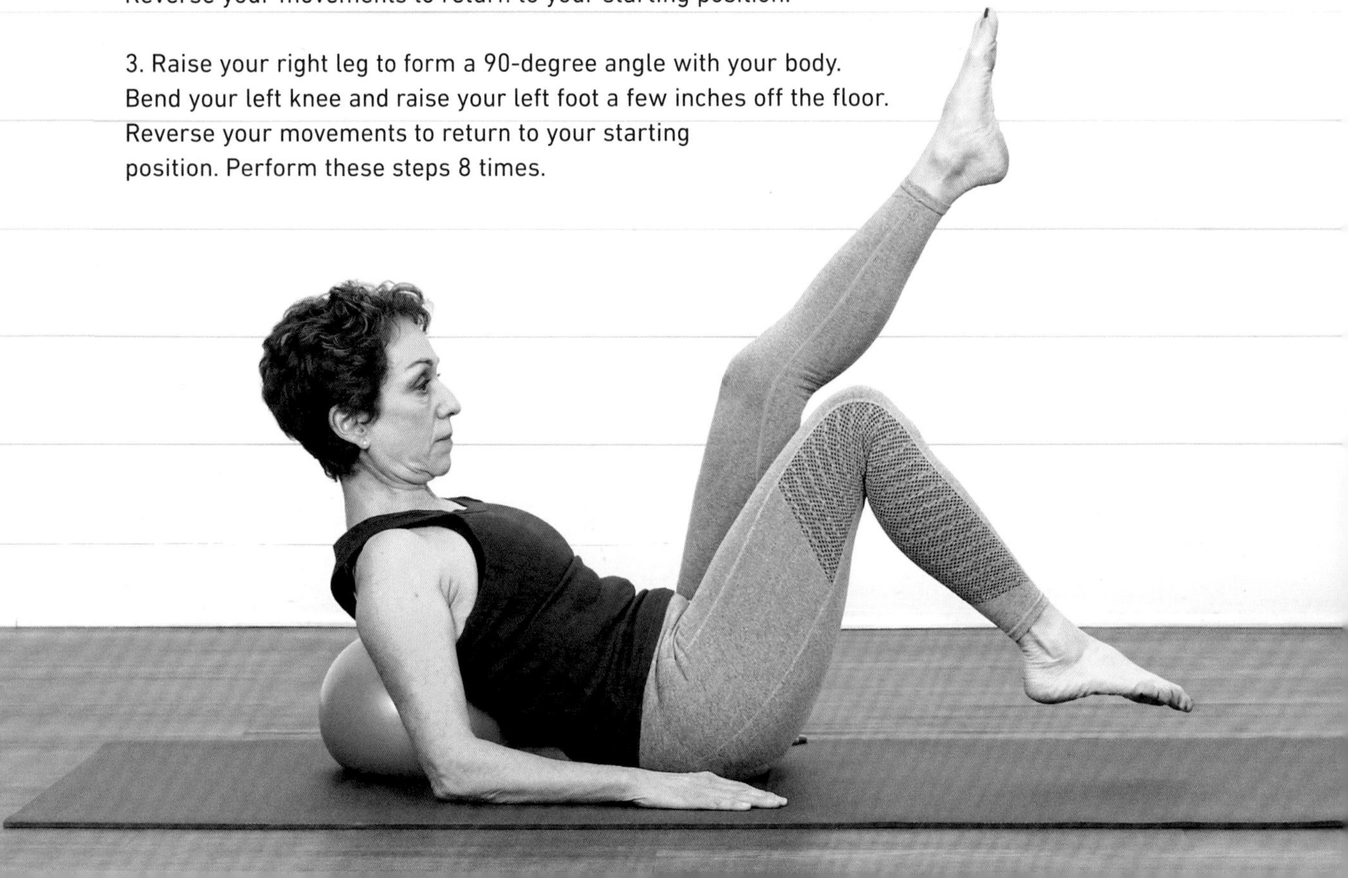

WITH A SMALL PILATES BALL AND DIFFERENT HAND PLACEMENTS

In step 1, place a small Pilates ball at your lower back. Keep your legs extended.

In steps 2 and 3, when you bend your knee toward your body, place your hands just below your bent knee. Continue with the remaining text.

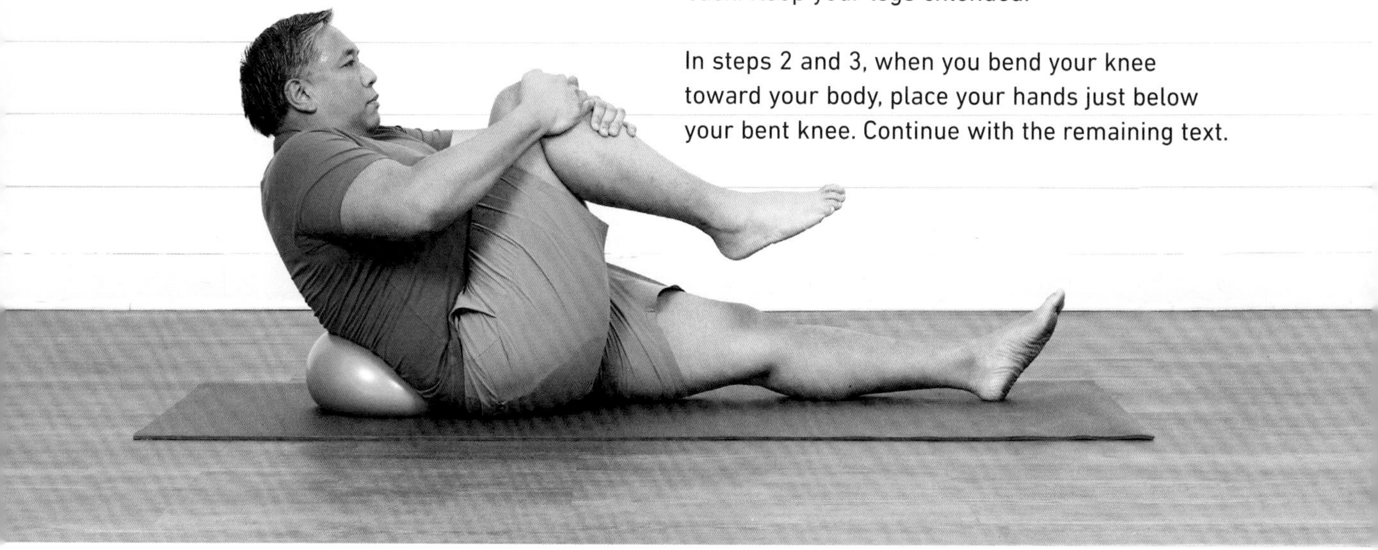

WITH A STABILITY BALL AND YOUR UPPER BACK ON THE FLOOR

In step 1, place your lower legs on top of a stability ball. Keep your head, shoulders, and hands flat on the floor.

In steps 2 and 3, lift your leg off the ball. Continue with the remaining text.

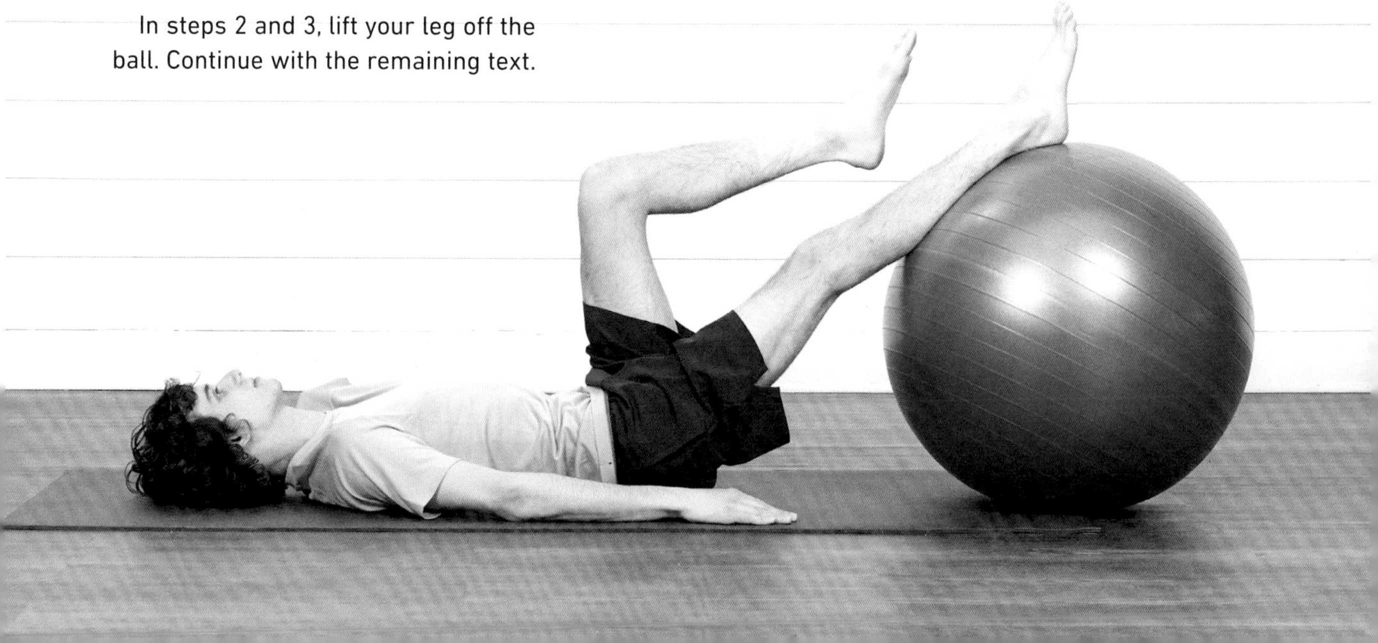

Single Straight-Leg Stretches

This exercise provides a stretch for the back of your legs while engaging your abdominal, gluteal, and hip muscles. Practicing these movements can improve spinal flexor, abdominal, and hip flexor strength as well as increase hamstring and lower back flexibility.

1 Lie on your back on the floor and bend your knees to form a 90-degree angle with your body. Relax your arms at your sides.

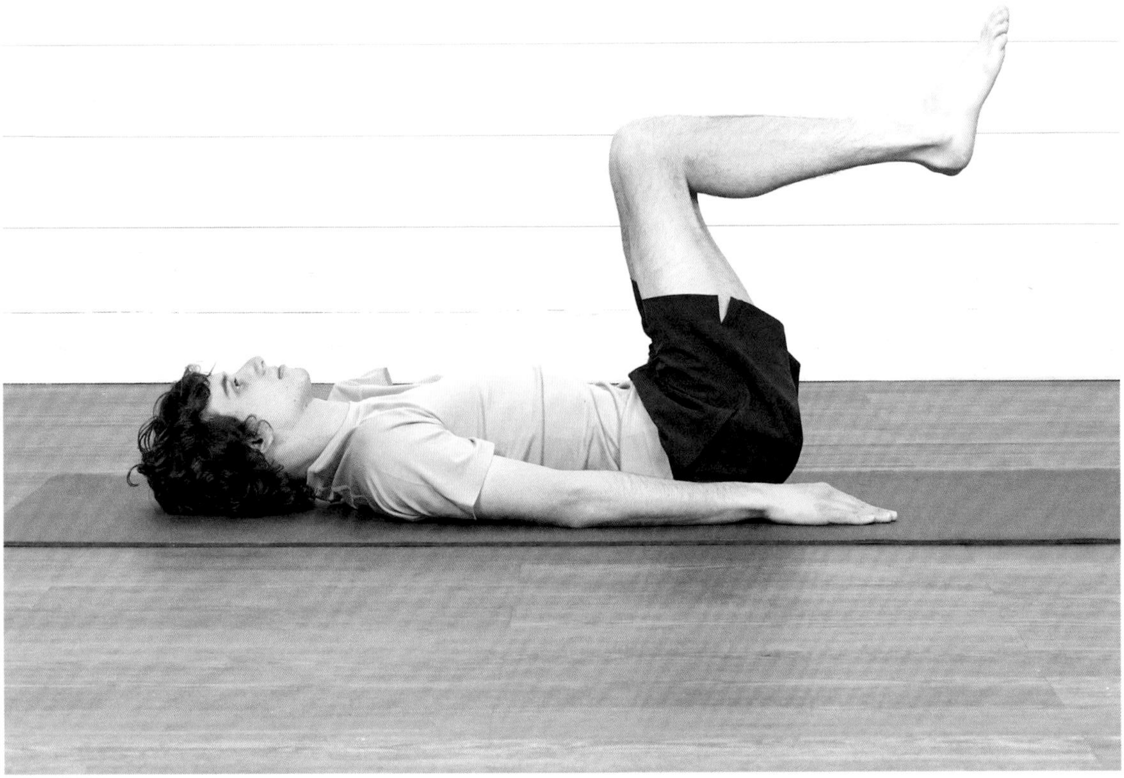

2 Press through your hands to raise your head and shoulders off the floor.

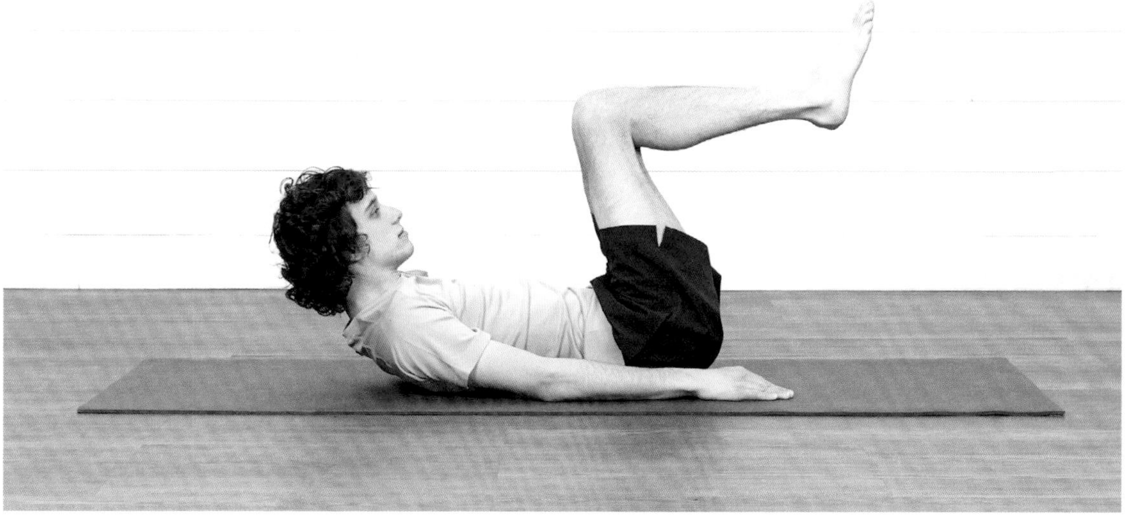

3 Extend your right leg toward the ceiling and lower your left leg to almost parallel with the floor. Reverse your movements to extend your left leg toward the ceiling and lower your right leg to almost parallel with the floor. Perform this step 8 times.

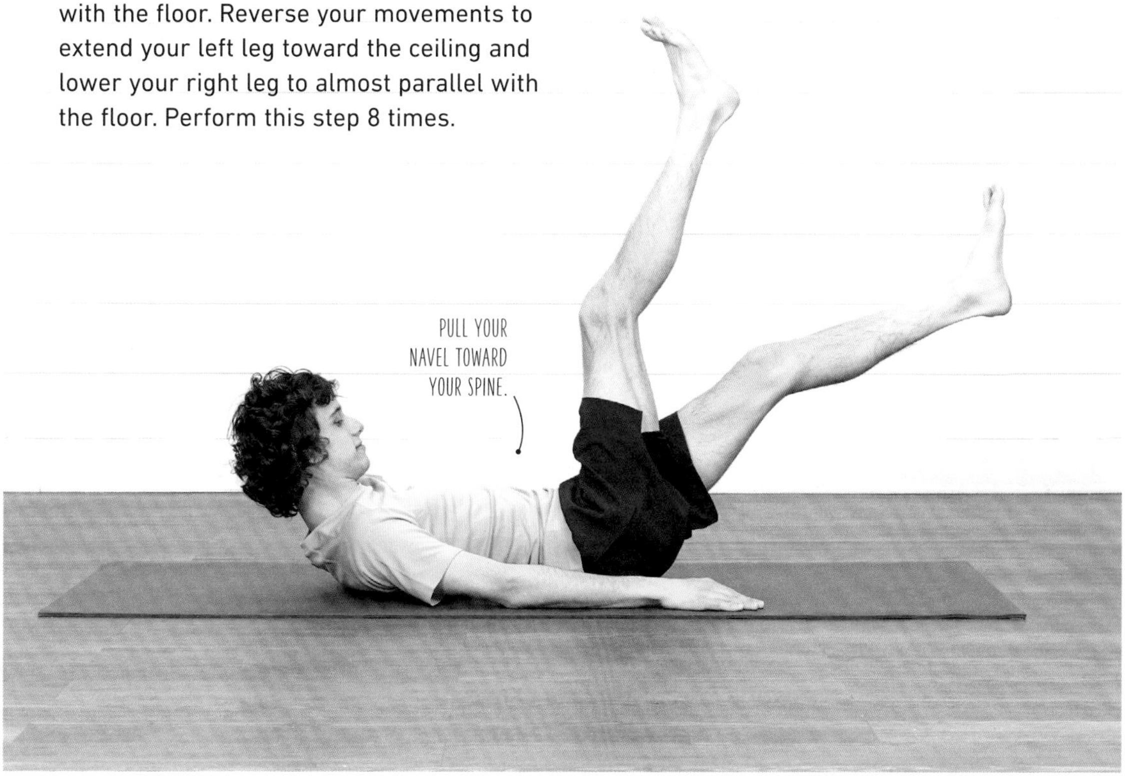
PULL YOUR NAVEL TOWARD YOUR SPINE.

SINGLE STRAIGHT-LEG STRETCHES

VARIATIONS

When your neck and shoulders aren't properly supported in an exercise, you could strain them. These variations can help prevent that. Using the Magic Circle can also assist with the proper alignment of your arms and shoulders.

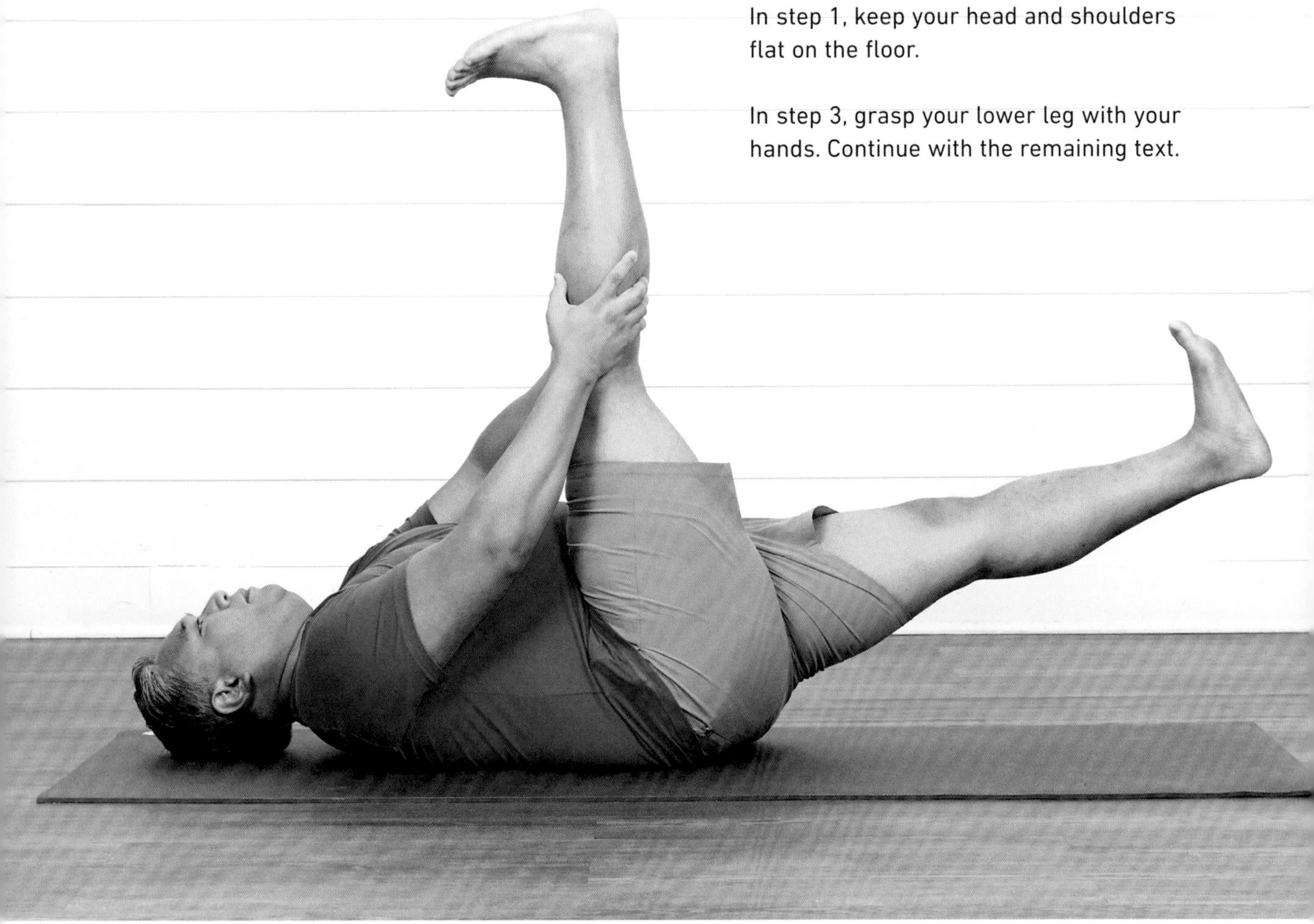

WITH YOUR HEAD ON THE FLOOR

In step 1, keep your head and shoulders flat on the floor.

In step 3, grasp your lower leg with your hands. Continue with the remaining text.

WITH YOUR HEAD ON THE FLOOR AND KNEES BENT

In step 1, keep your head flat on the floor.

In step 3, bend your knees more deeply. Continue with the remaining text.

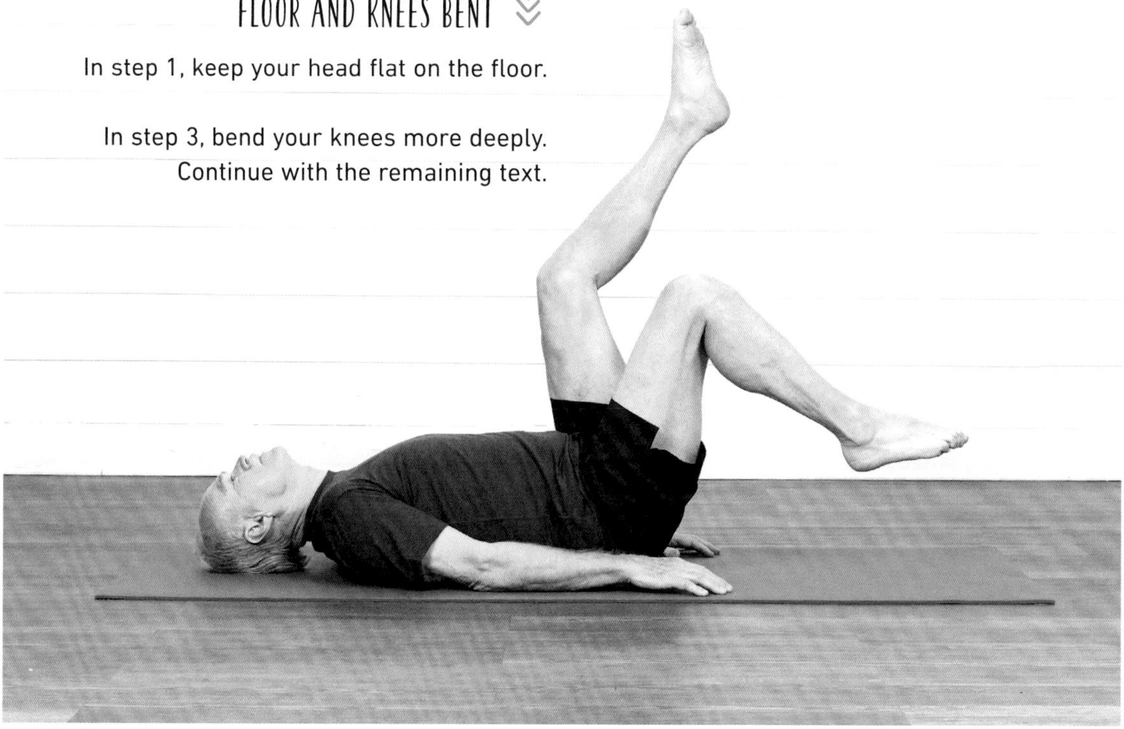

WITH THE MAGIC CIRCLE

In step 1, hold the Magic Circle between the heels of your hands. Keep your head flat on the floor. (You can also bend your knees where needed).

In steps 2 and 3, keep the Magic Circle stable. Continue with the remaining text.

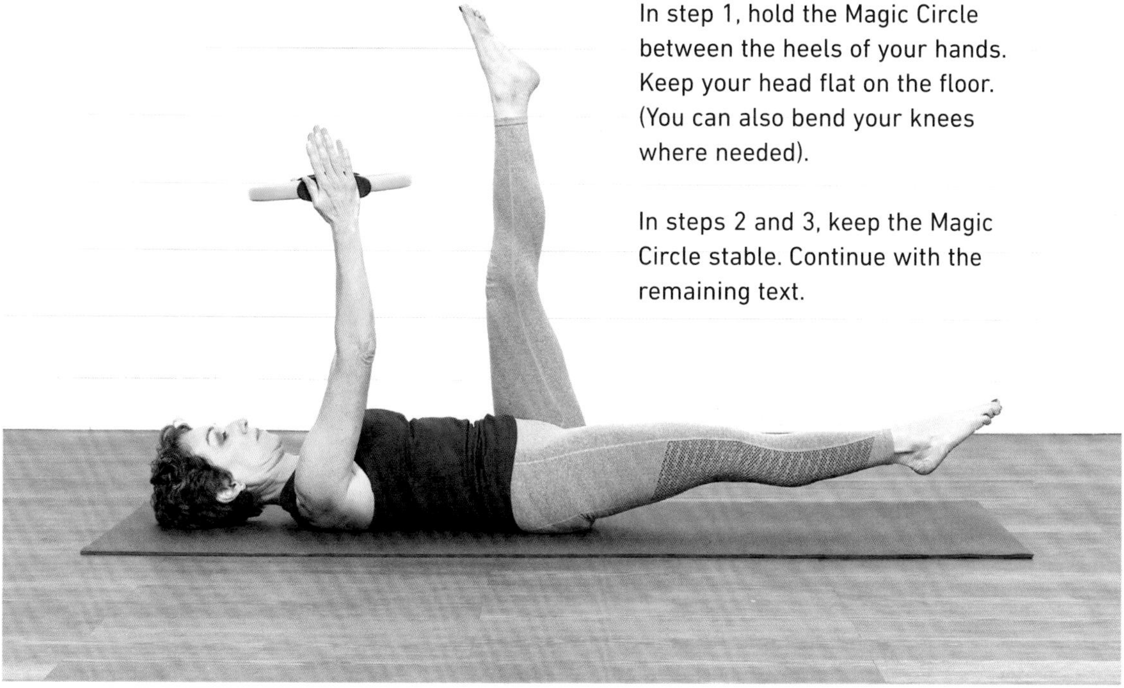

Double-Leg Stretches

This stretch works your abs as well as your hip flexors and quadriceps. It uses the extension of your arms and legs as an added weighted challenge for the abs. This exercise also helps build endurance, increases coordination, and encourages the development of a greater mind–body connection.

1 Lie on your back on the floor and bend your knees to form a 90-degree angle with your legs. Place your hands on your shins.

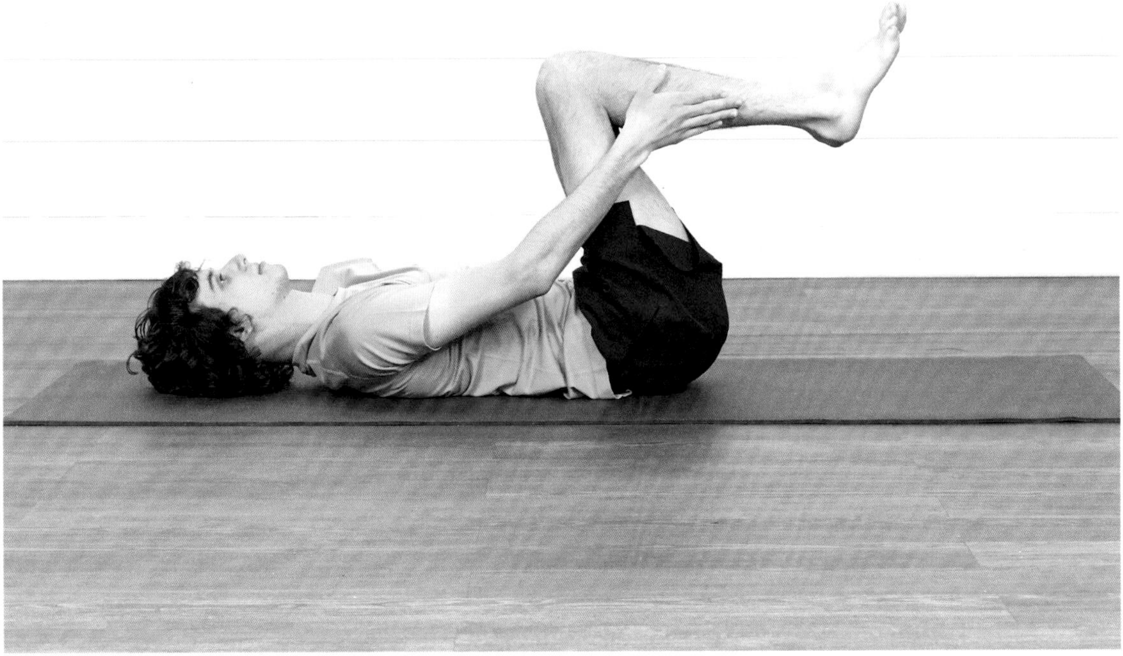

2 Raise your head and shoulders off the floor.

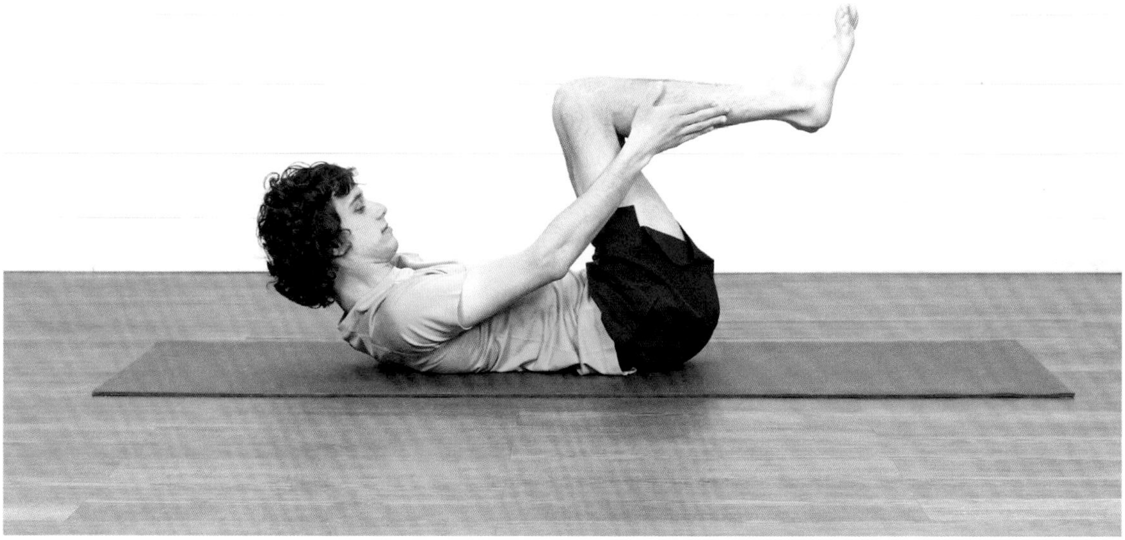

3 Extend your legs a few inches more toward the ceiling. Extend your arms backward until parallel with your ears. Reverse your movements to return to your starting position. Perform these steps 8 times.

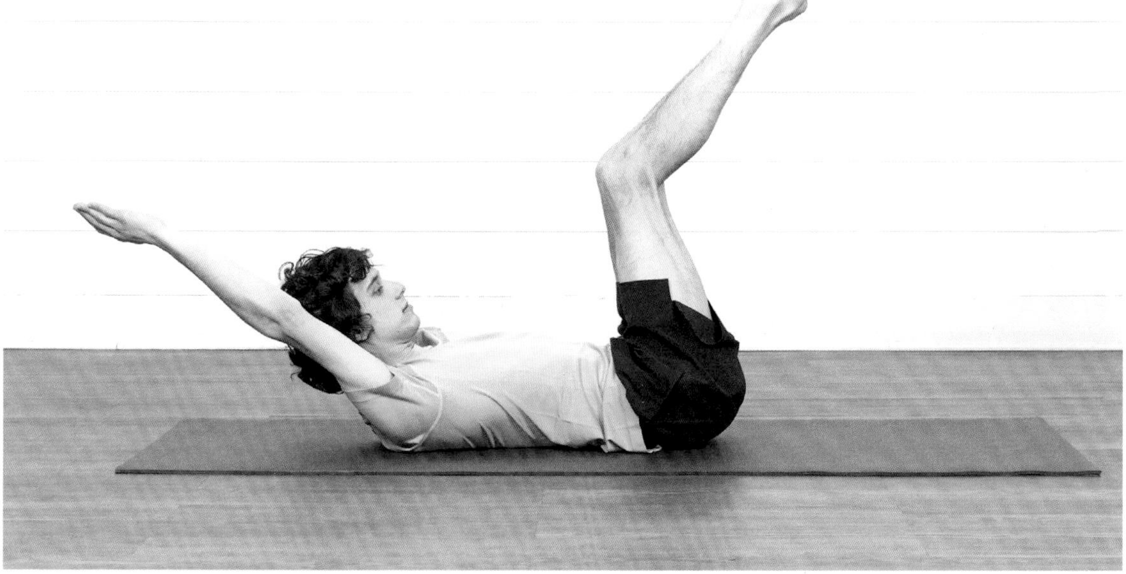

DOUBLE-LEG STRETCHES

VARIATIONS

The weight of your head, arms, and legs makes these movements extremely challenging. Keeping your head on the floor can help prevent neck strain. Placing your legs on a stability ball can help you connect more with your abs. The chair variation is a good option for pregnant people and/or anyone who has difficulty coming down to the floor.

WITH A STABILITY BALL

In step 1, place your legs on top of a stability ball. Keep your legs on the ball throughout. Continue with the remaining text.

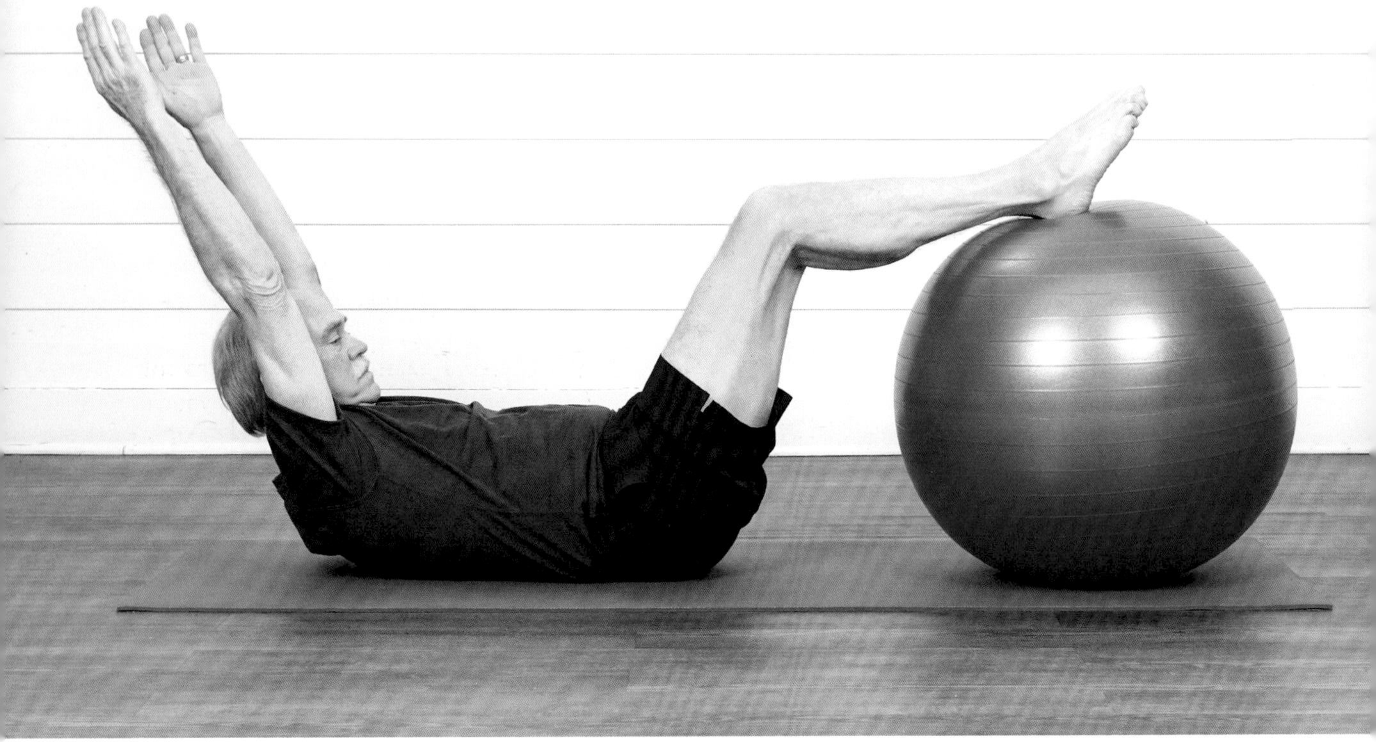

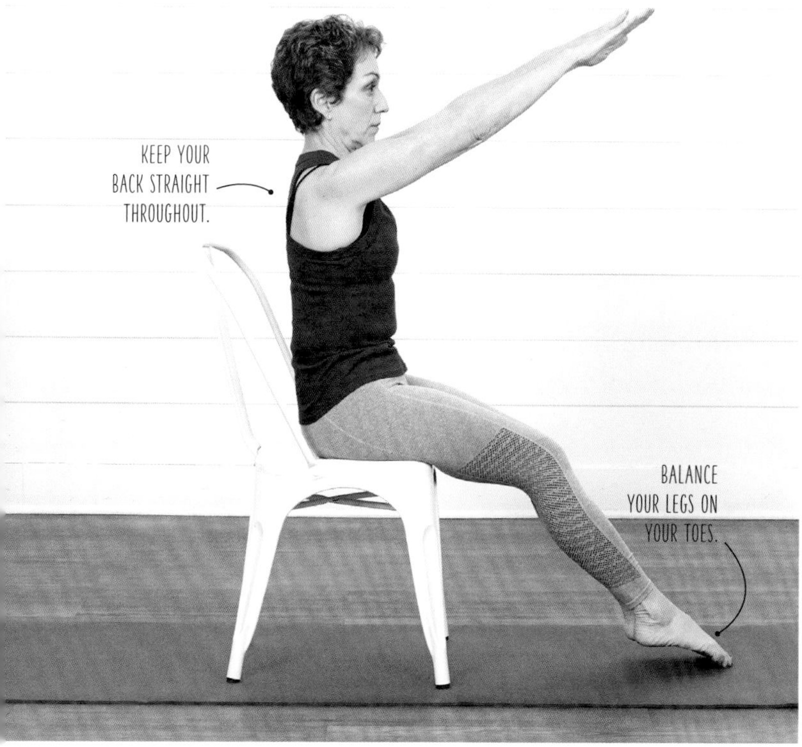
KEEP YOUR BACK STRAIGHT THROUGHOUT.
BALANCE YOUR LEGS ON YOUR TOES.

SITTING IN A CHAIR

1. Sit in a chair with your feet flat on the floor and your hands resting on your thighs.

2. Extend your legs forward while extending your arms toward the ceiling. Face your hands toward your feet. Reverse your movements to return to your starting position. Perform these steps 6 times.

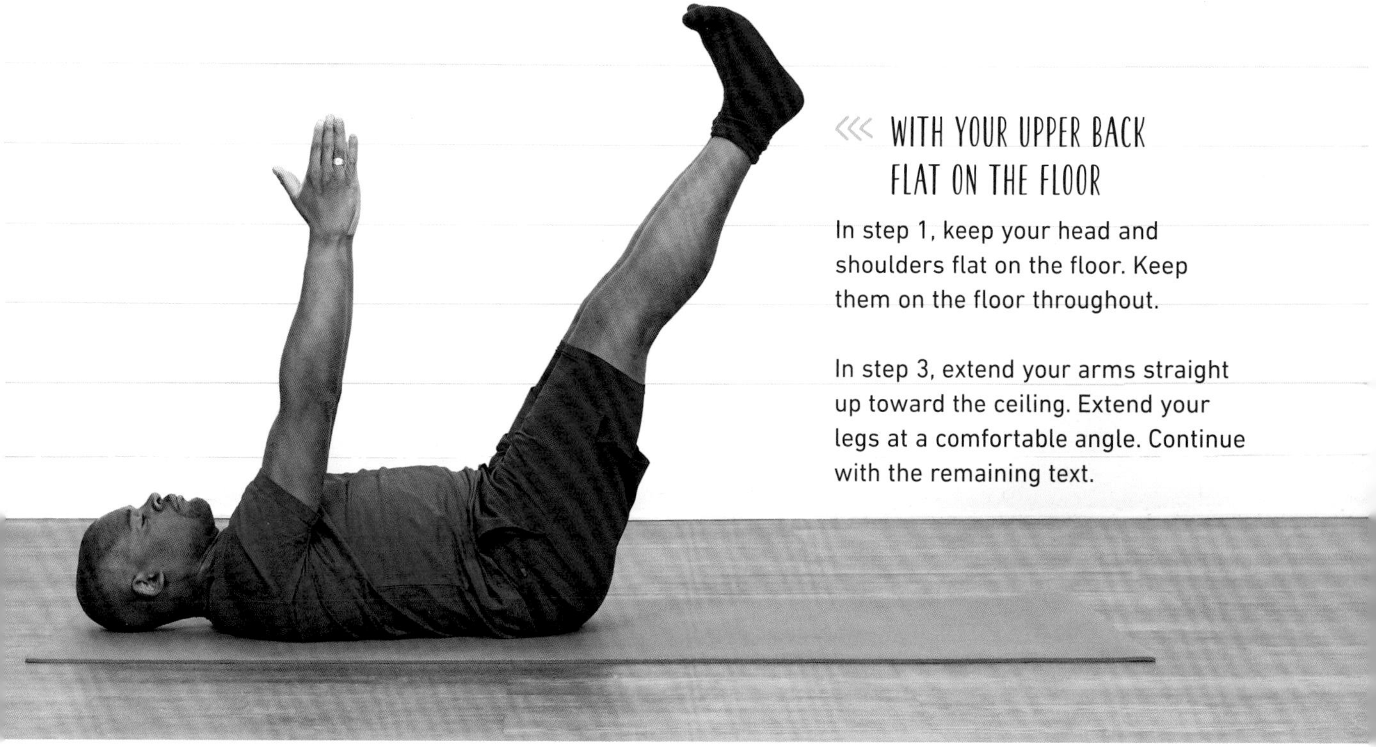

WITH YOUR UPPER BACK FLAT ON THE FLOOR

In step 1, keep your head and shoulders flat on the floor. Keep them on the floor throughout.

In step 3, extend your arms straight up toward the ceiling. Extend your legs at a comfortable angle. Continue with the remaining text.

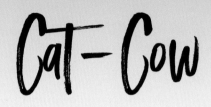

Cat-Cow

This stretch is a simple move that acts as a warm-up for your entire back and switches between a back stretch and a back extension. It can decrease lower back pain and increase lower back flexibility and mobility. Practicing these movements can help you release tension in your lower back after performing back extension work.

1 Place your hands and knees flat on the floor with your knees shoulder width apart. As you inhale, keep your back straight and pull your navel in and up. As you exhale, maintain this position.

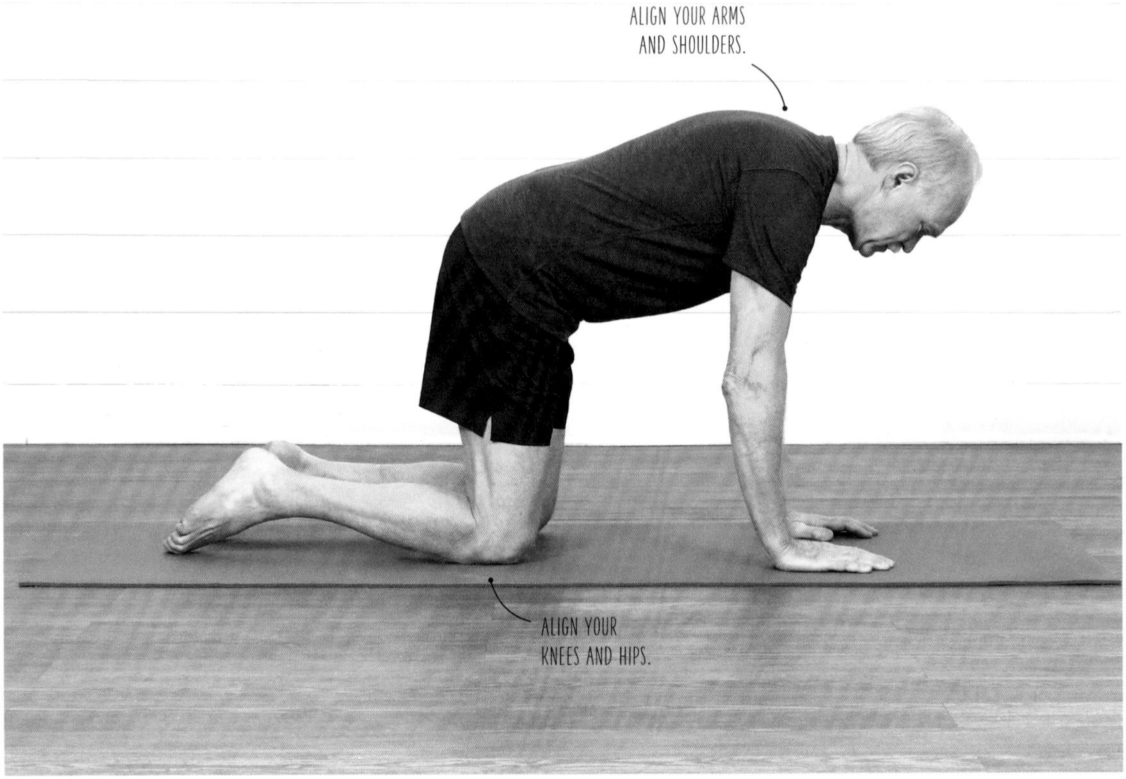

ALIGN YOUR ARMS AND SHOULDERS.
ALIGN YOUR KNEES AND HIPS.

2 As you inhale, you lower your stomach toward the floor. Raise your chin and chest to gaze forward as you increase the space between your shoulder blades.

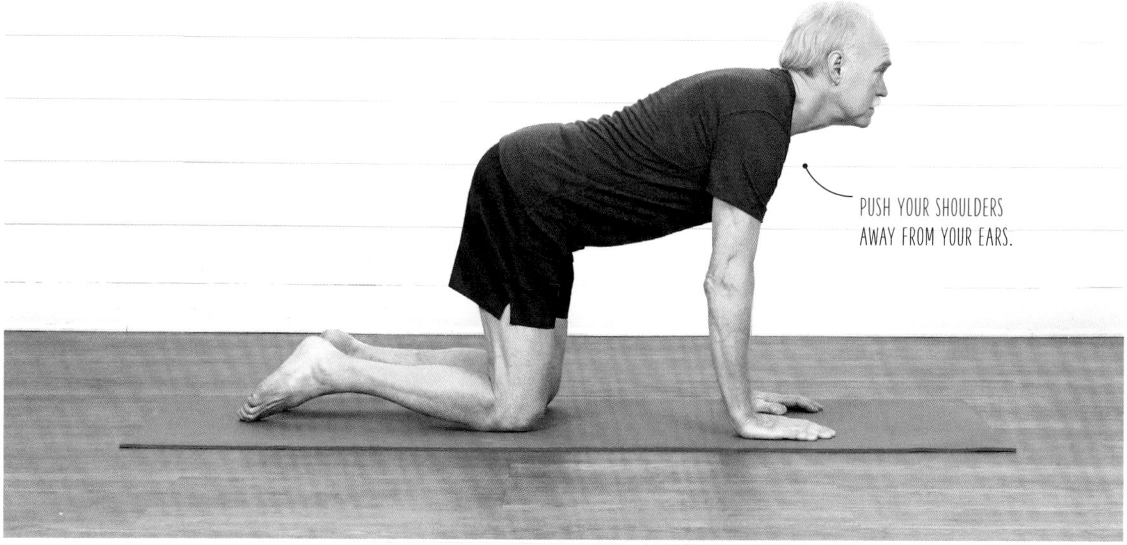

PUSH YOUR SHOULDERS AWAY FROM YOUR EARS.

3 As you exhale, you pull your navel toward your spine and round your back toward the ceiling. Reverse your movements to return to your starting position. Perform these steps 8 times.

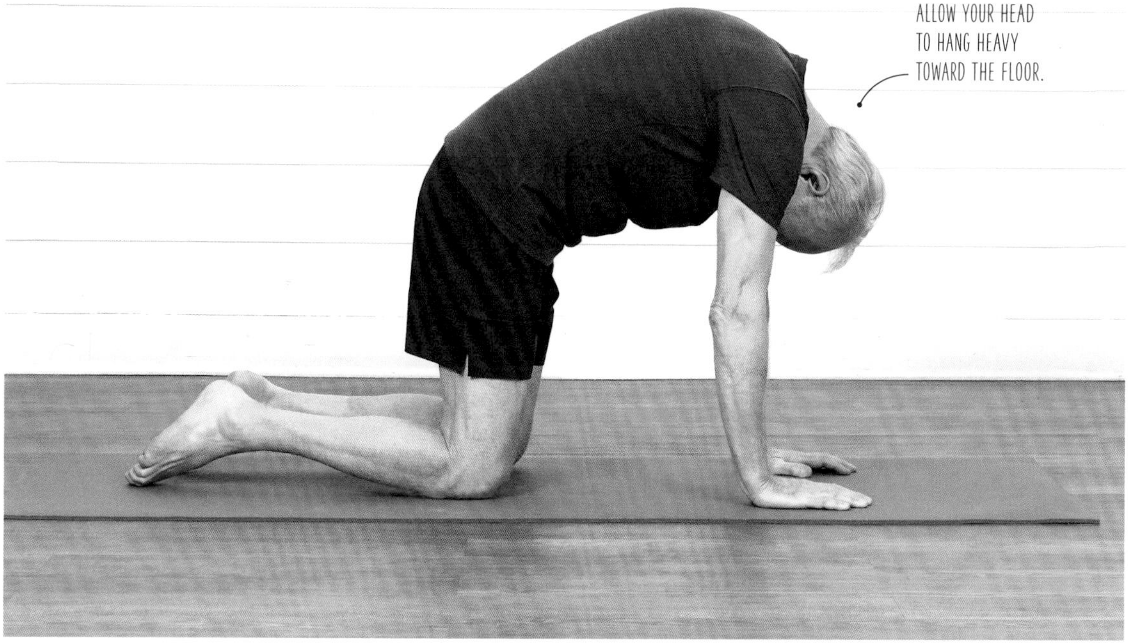

ALLOW YOUR HEAD TO HANG HEAVY TOWARD THE FLOOR.

CAT-COW

VARIATIONS

If you're experiencing wrist or shoulder pain or if you have carpal tunnel syndrome, coming down to your forearms or using a bolster can help take some pressure off your shoulders and wrists. If you have difficulty coming down to the floor, the seated option is also effective and beneficial.

ON YOUR FOREARMS

In step 1, place your forearms flat on the floor. Continue with the remaining text.

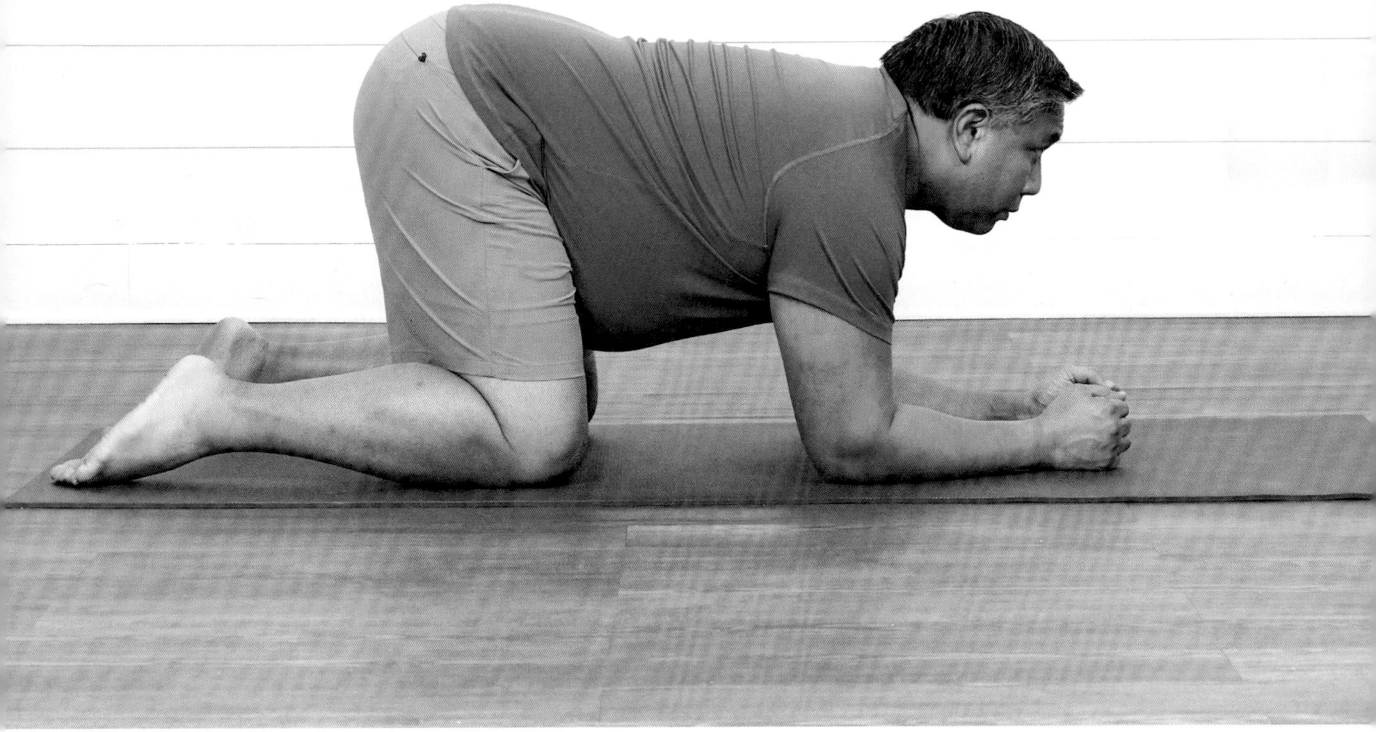

WITH A BOLSTER

In step 1, place your forearms on a bolster or a stack of firm blankets to raise your torso more upright. (This variation is especially useful for people who are pregnant.) Continue with the remaining text.

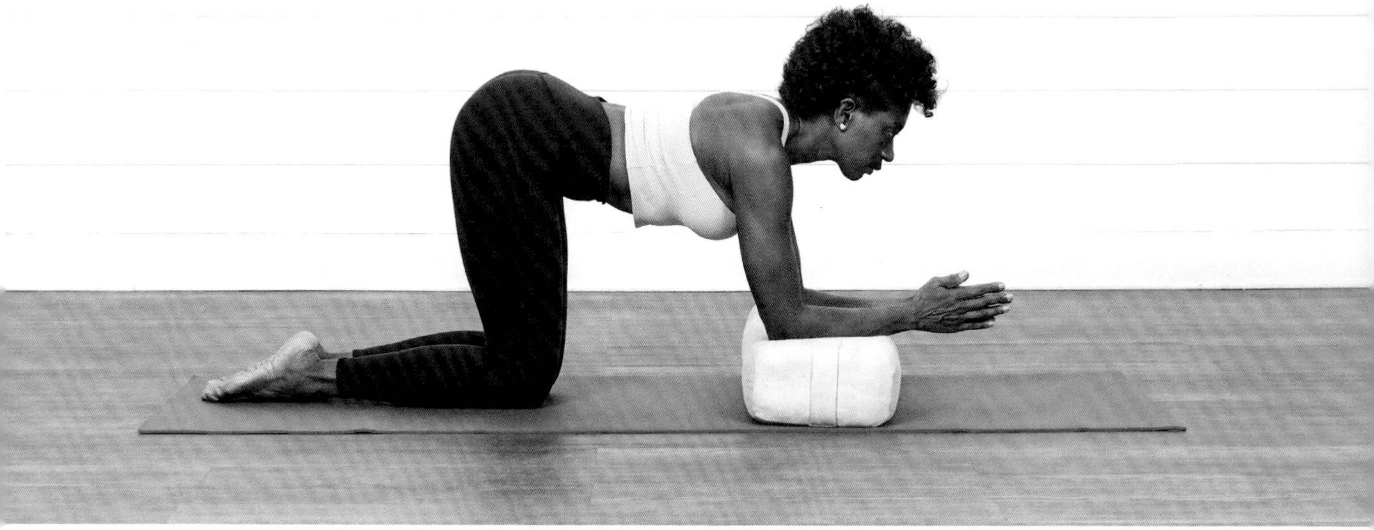

SITTING IN A CHAIR

1. Sit on the front edge of a chair with your feet shoulder width apart and your hands resting on your thighs.

2. Inhale as you raise your chin and chest to gaze toward the ceiling.

3. Exhale as you round your spine toward the wall behind you. Reverse your movements to return to your starting position. Perform these steps 8 times.

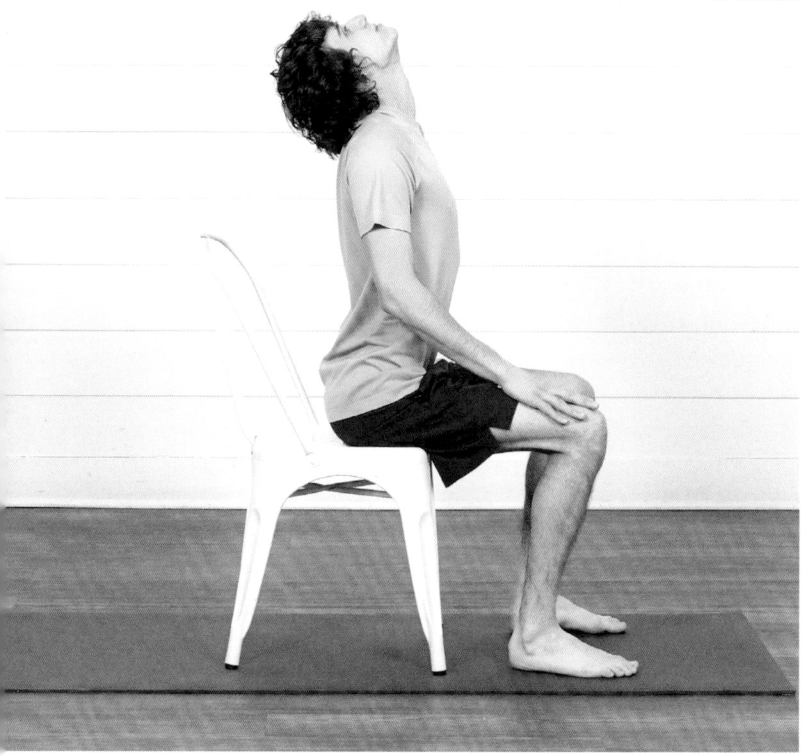

JEROME PASCUA

My name is Jerome Pascua. I'm a 46-year-old software developer and church musician from Louisville, Kentucky. My wife, Melissa, and I have been married for 22 years. We have two children, Alan and Sophia. Alan is a junior at the University of Cincinnati. Sophia is a senior in high school who'll be attending Northwestern University in the fall of 2021.

My journey of health and fitness has been a roller coaster of success and failure. I was a high school and college athlete in my younger days. When I graduated, I entered the world of software development and, unfortunately, a sedentary lifestyle. My weight has always been a struggle, but entering my forties posed an entirely new challenge. I was raised in a food-centric Filipino culture, which is to say my family LOVES to eat. Health issues related to lifestyle and genetics—specifically, a recent diagnosis of type 2 diabetes—led me to make sustainable healthy living a way of life.

My goal now is to find fun ways to stay active while making food choices that are delicious, healthy, and filling. My personal trainer, Tanika Owens, helped me prepare for the Pilates exercises. Like Micki, she holds certifications in Pilates instruction. That preparation showed me how much Pilates is a foundation for so many other forms of exercise. Working with Micki, I found that after just the first session, Pilates exercises are effective for my body. The exercises are doable despite my having some knee and shoulder issues. When I finish, I have that "good kind of tired." I can even throw in a few reps during downtime at work or when lounging around the house.

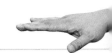

After spending time with Micki, I've now made Pilates a part of my weekly training regimen and a big reason why I'm able to keep my blood sugar under control. While I still mix failures in with my successes, I find that having good options for activity keeps me progressing in a healthy direction.

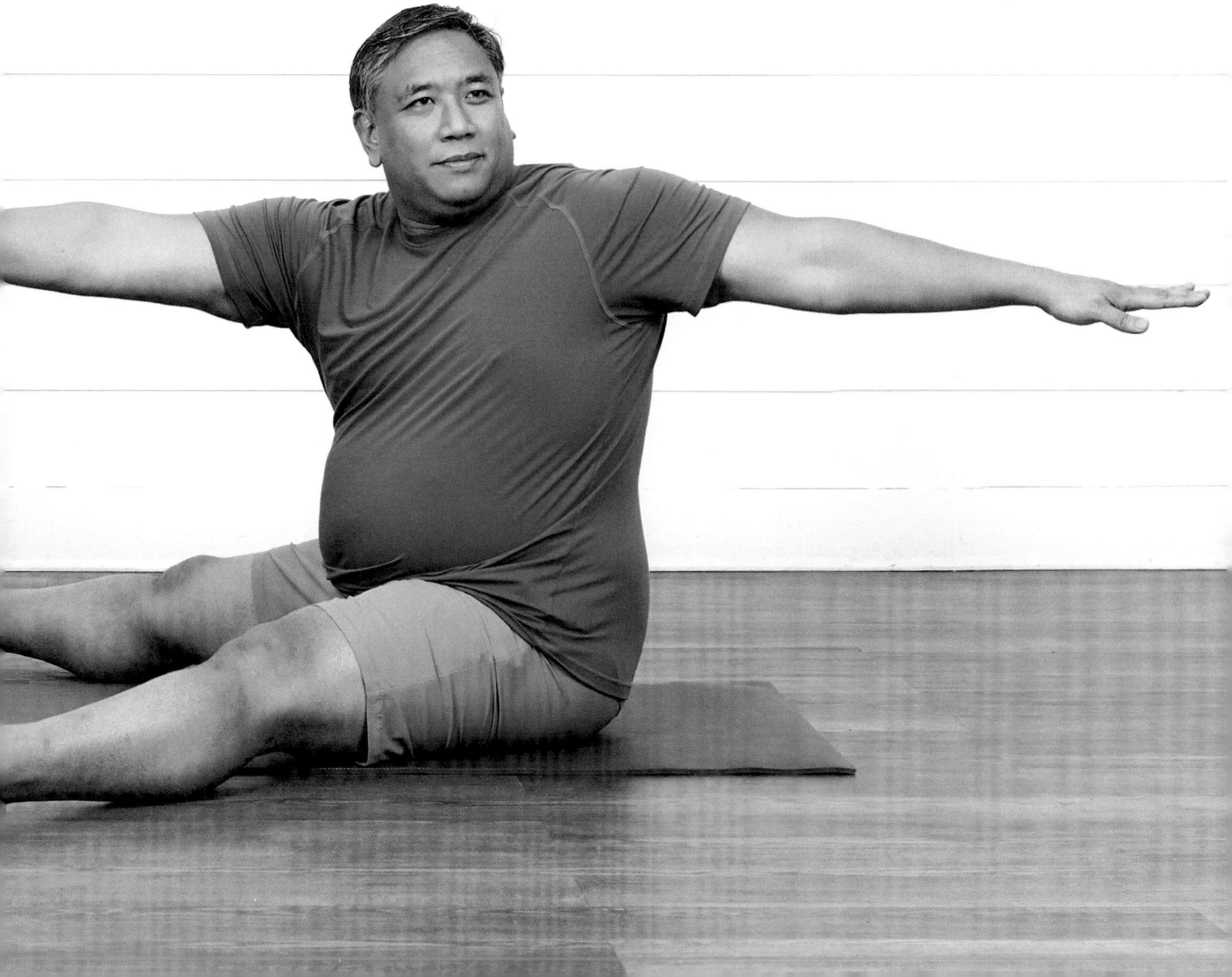

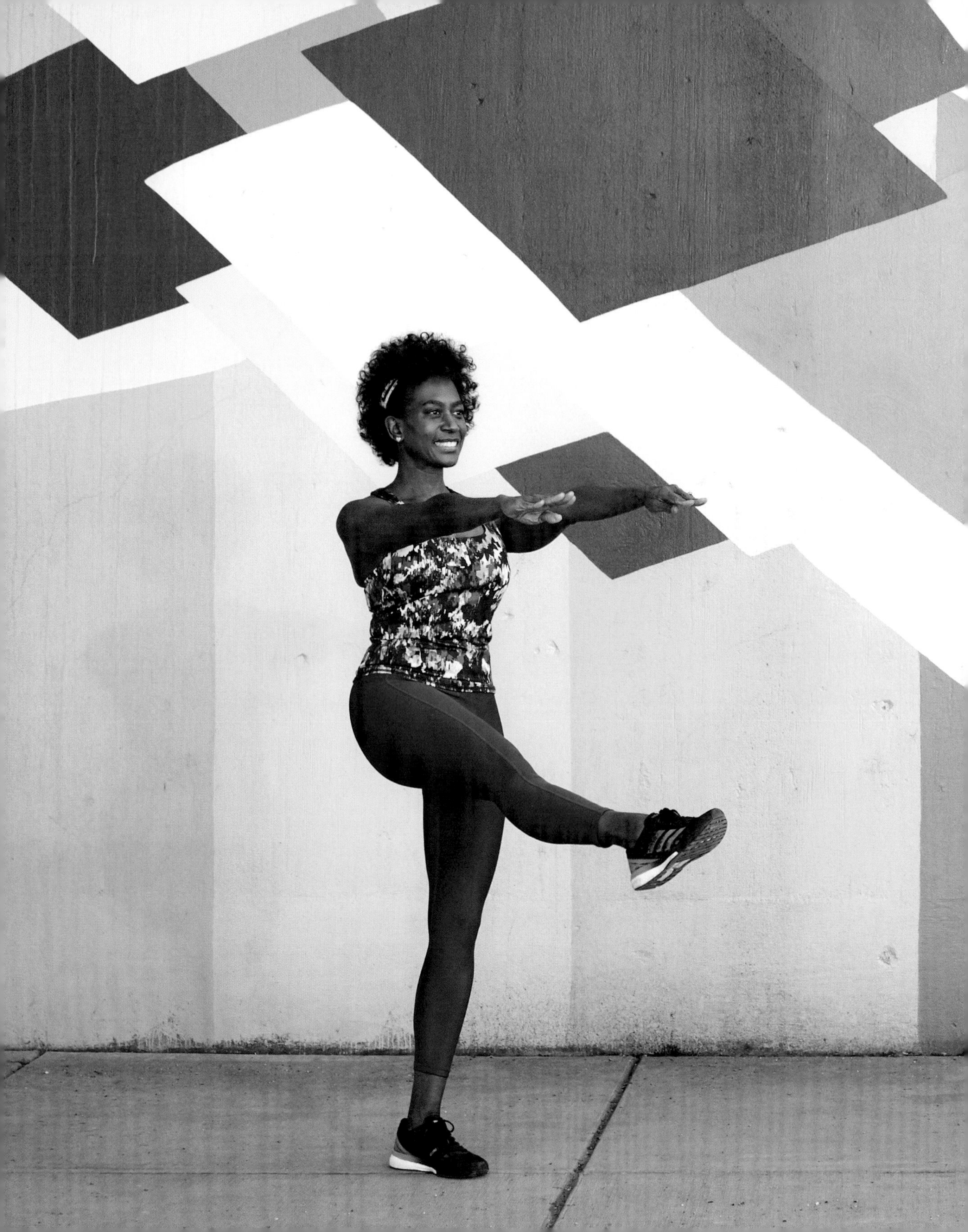

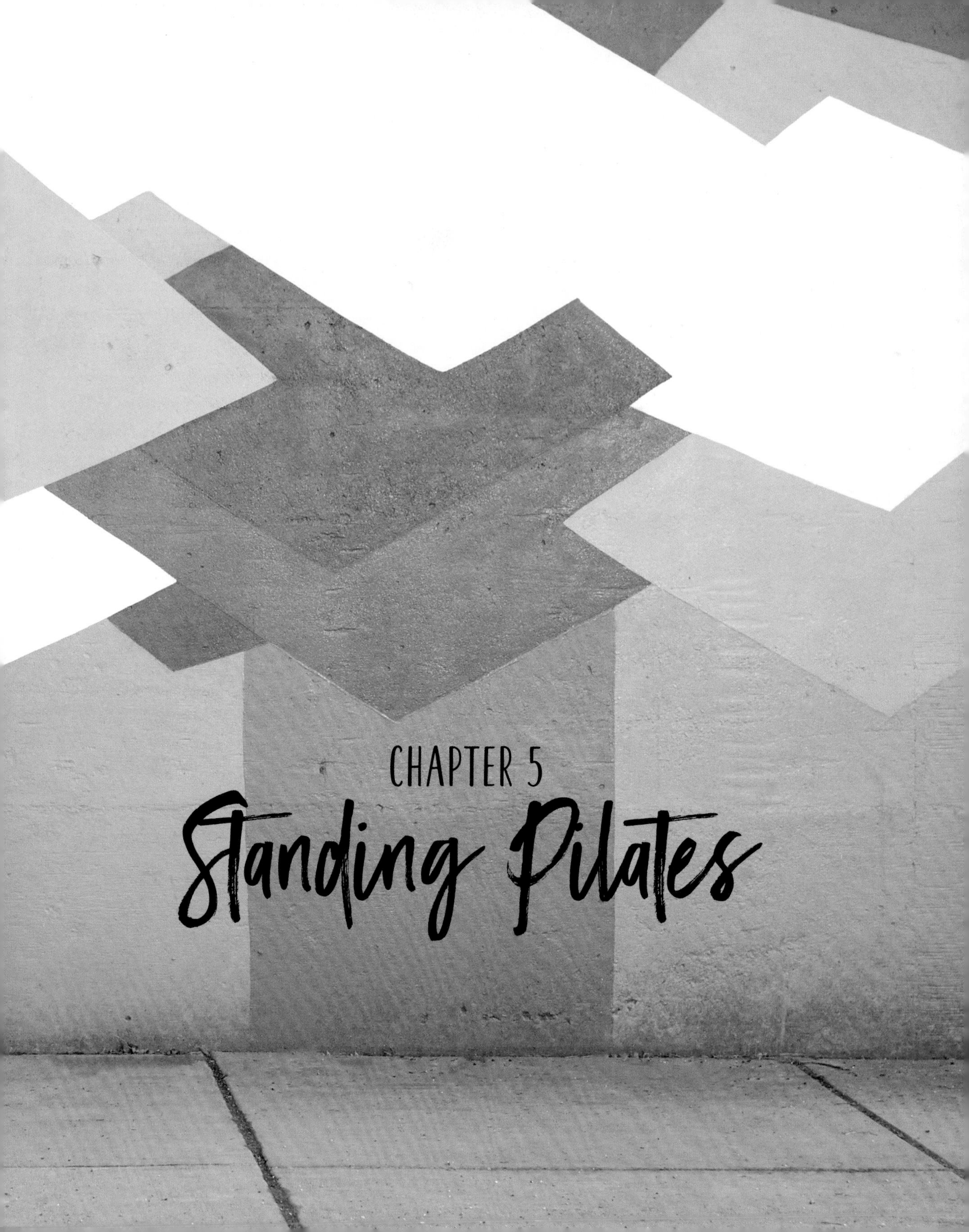

CHAPTER 5

Standing Pilates

Standing Hundred

This exercise helps build body awareness, enhance core connection, and improve your coordination. These movements can also strengthen your abs, develop scapular and trunk stability, and improve lower-body stability.

1 Stand with your heels together and your feet pointed outward, forming a V. Pull your navel toward your spine as you curl your upper body slightly forward.

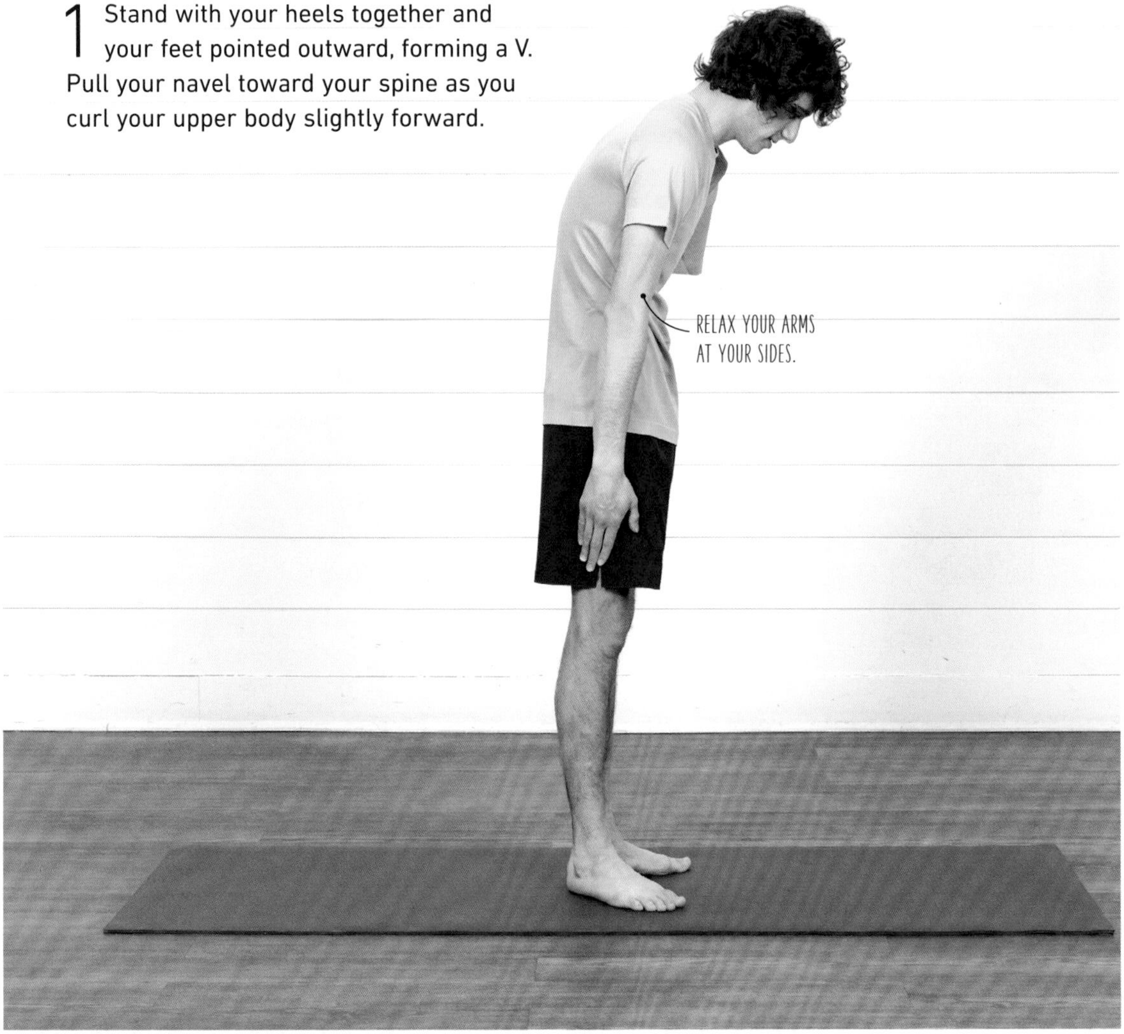
RELAX YOUR ARMS AT YOUR SIDES.

2 Slide your right leg forward. As you inhale, pulse your arms up and down for 5 seconds. Exhale for 5 seconds. Perform this step 5 times. Reverse your movements to return to your starting position. Repeat these steps with your left leg sliding forward.

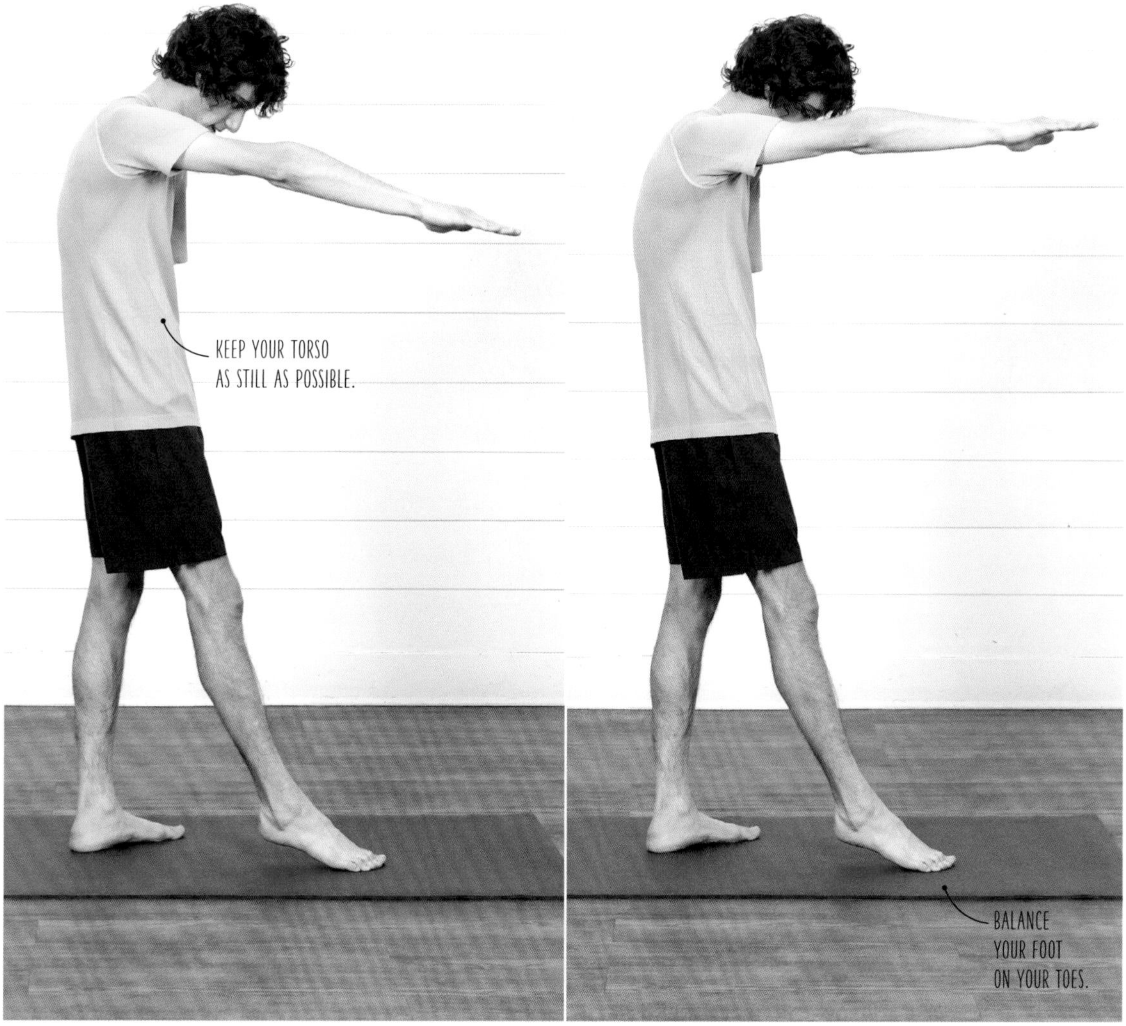

KEEP YOUR TORSO AS STILL AS POSSIBLE.
BALANCE YOUR FOOT ON YOUR TOES.

STANDING HUNDRED

VARIATIONS

These modifications are excellent alternatives for anyone who has difficulty getting down to or up from the floor or a seat. All these variations are suitable for people women over 20 weeks. After 20 weeks of pregnancy, lying on your back for extended periods of time isn't recommended.

WITH YOUR FEET PARALLEL >>>

In step 1, stand with your feet shoulder width apart. Continue with the remaining text.

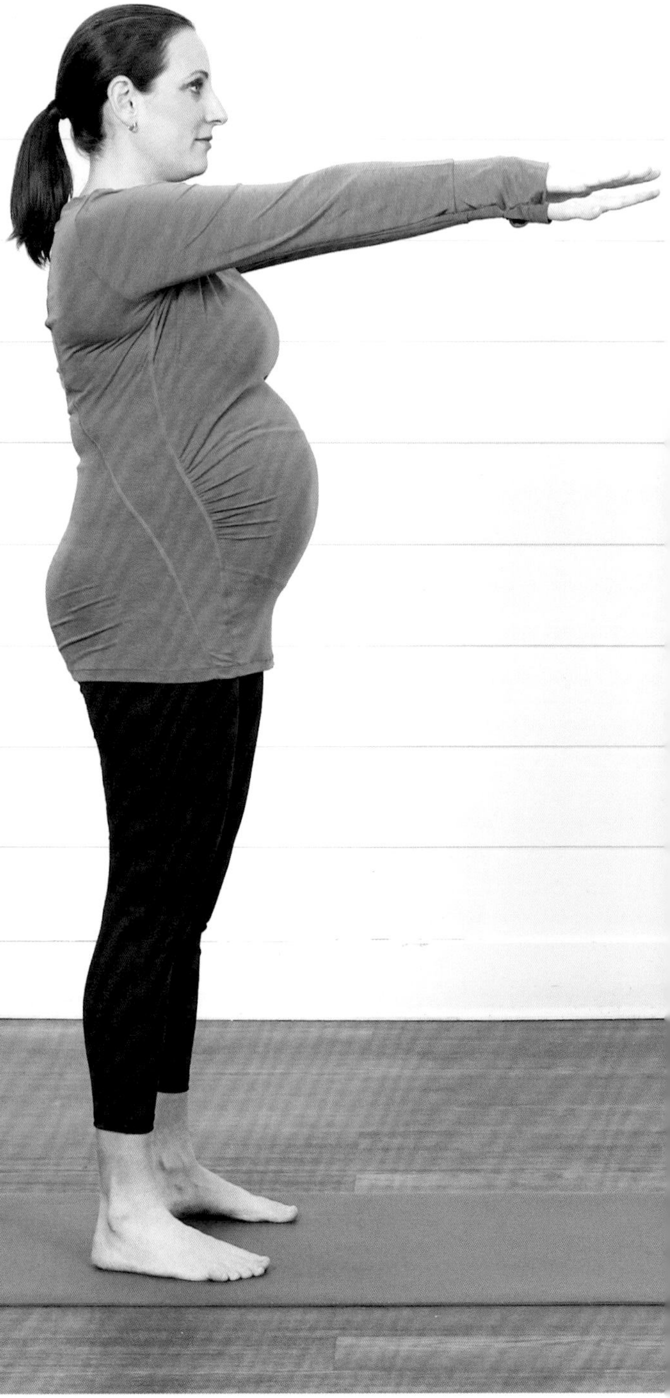

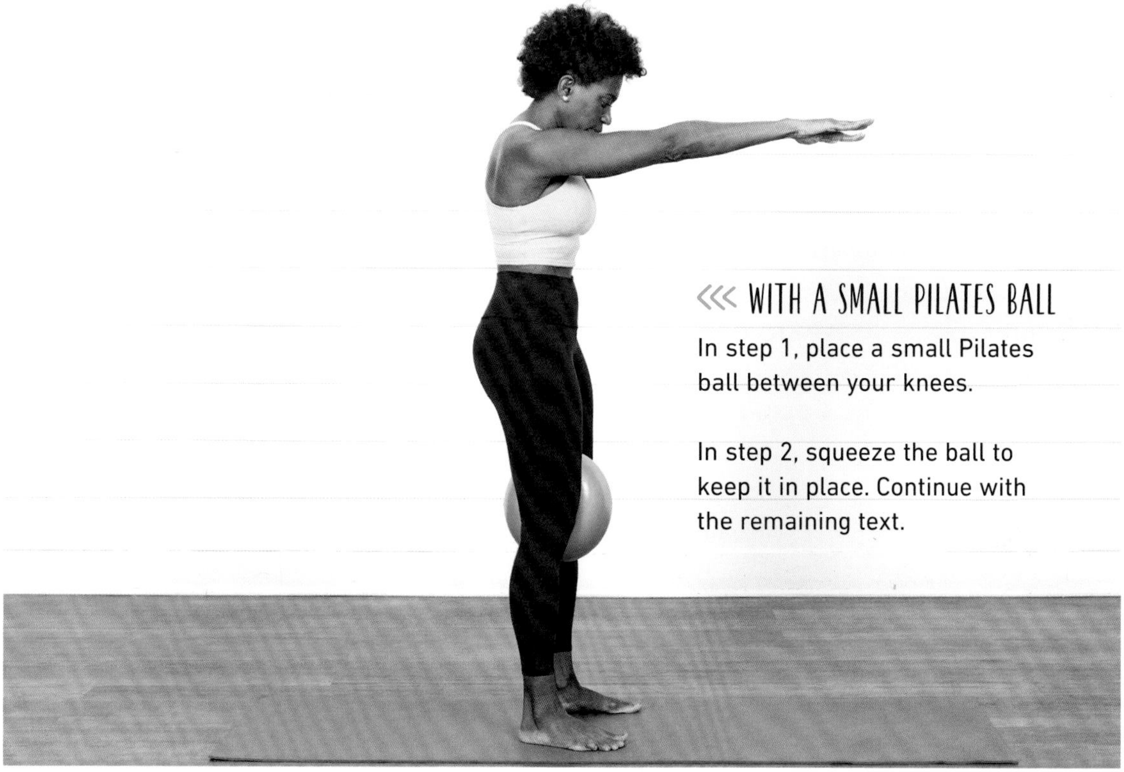

WITH A SMALL PILATES BALL

In step 1, place a small Pilates ball between your knees.

In step 2, squeeze the ball to keep it in place. Continue with the remaining text.

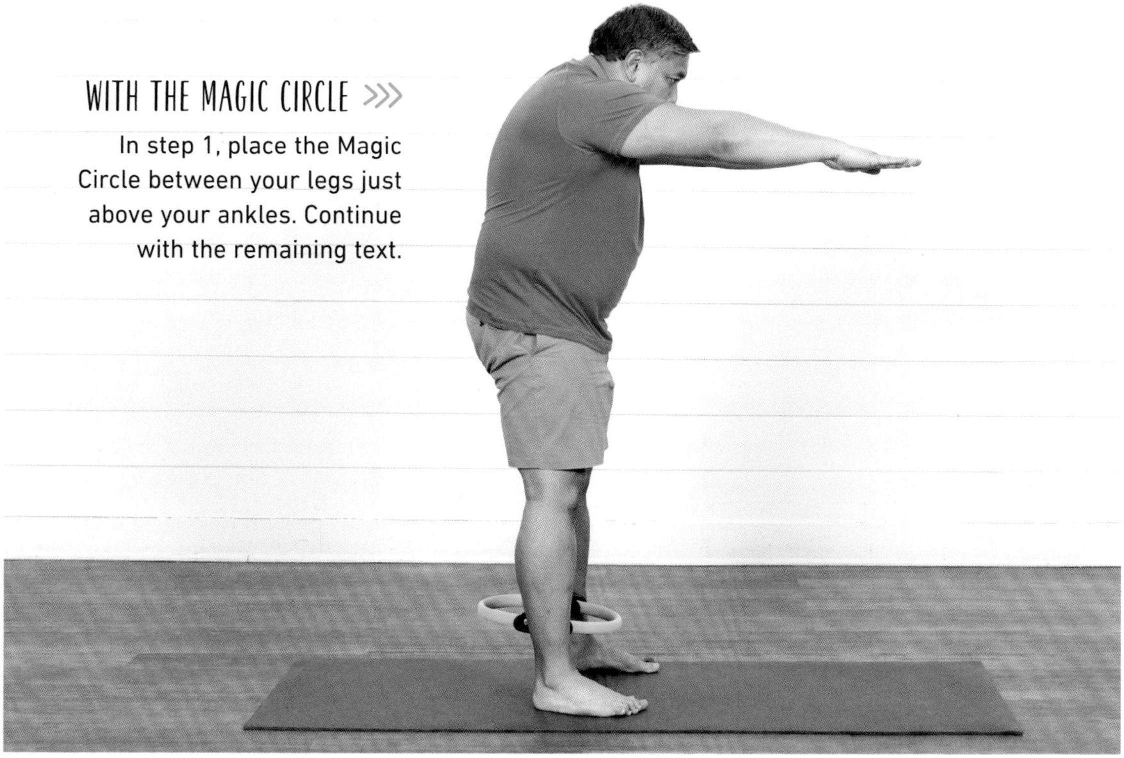

WITH THE MAGIC CIRCLE

In step 1, place the Magic Circle between your legs just above your ankles. Continue with the remaining text.

Standing Swimming

This exercise can strengthen your balance and core muscles. You can also enhance your upper-body muscles, including your back extensors. These can reduce tension in your neck and shoulders for improved posture and spinal stability.

1 Stand with your feet shoulder width apart. Extend your arms toward the ceiling, with your right arm slightly ahead of your left arm.

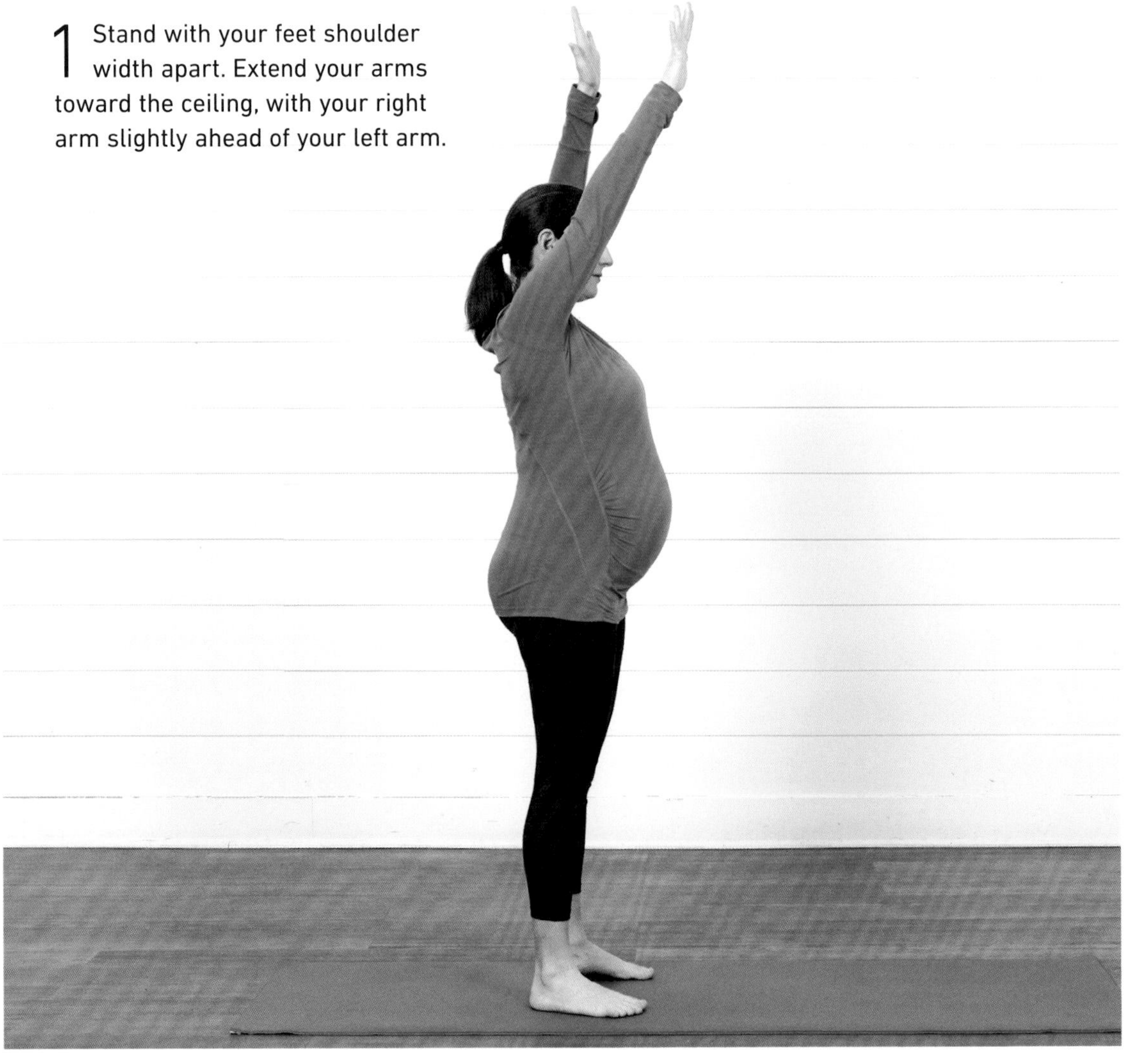

2 Pull your navel toward your spine as you flutter your arms in a swimming motion for 10 seconds.

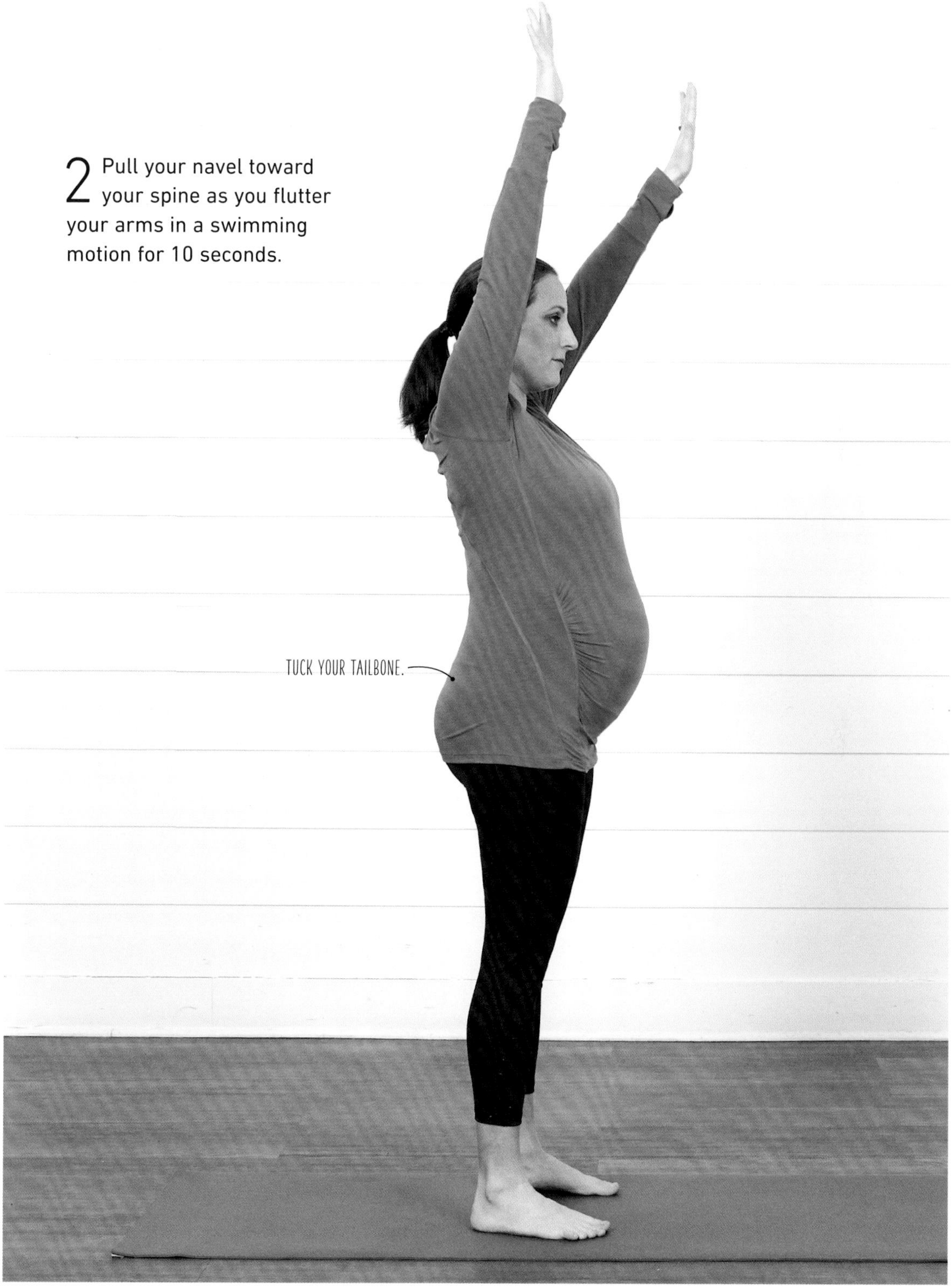

WITH ONE LEG FORWARD

In step 1, place your left foot slightly ahead of your right foot. Extend your arms at shoulder height.

In step 2, after fluttering your arms, repeat the steps with your right foot slightly ahead of your left foot.

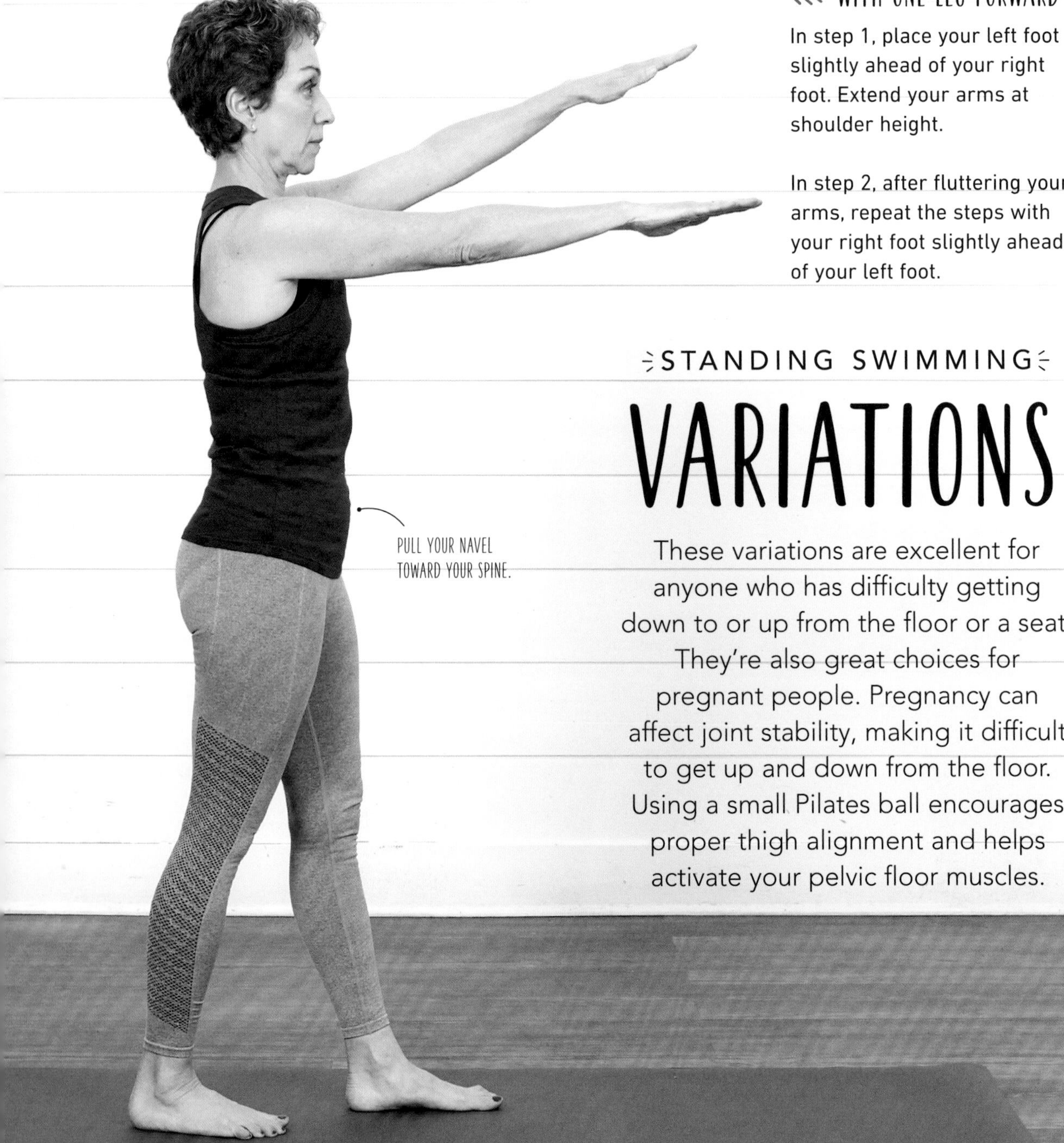
PULL YOUR NAVEL TOWARD YOUR SPINE.

STANDING SWIMMING

VARIATIONS

These variations are excellent for anyone who has difficulty getting down to or up from the floor or a seat. They're also great choices for pregnant people. Pregnancy can affect joint stability, making it difficult to get up and down from the floor. Using a small Pilates ball encourages proper thigh alignment and helps activate your pelvic floor muscles.

ARMS AT SHOULDER HEIGHT

In step 1, raise your arms to parallel with your shoulders. Continue with the remaining text.

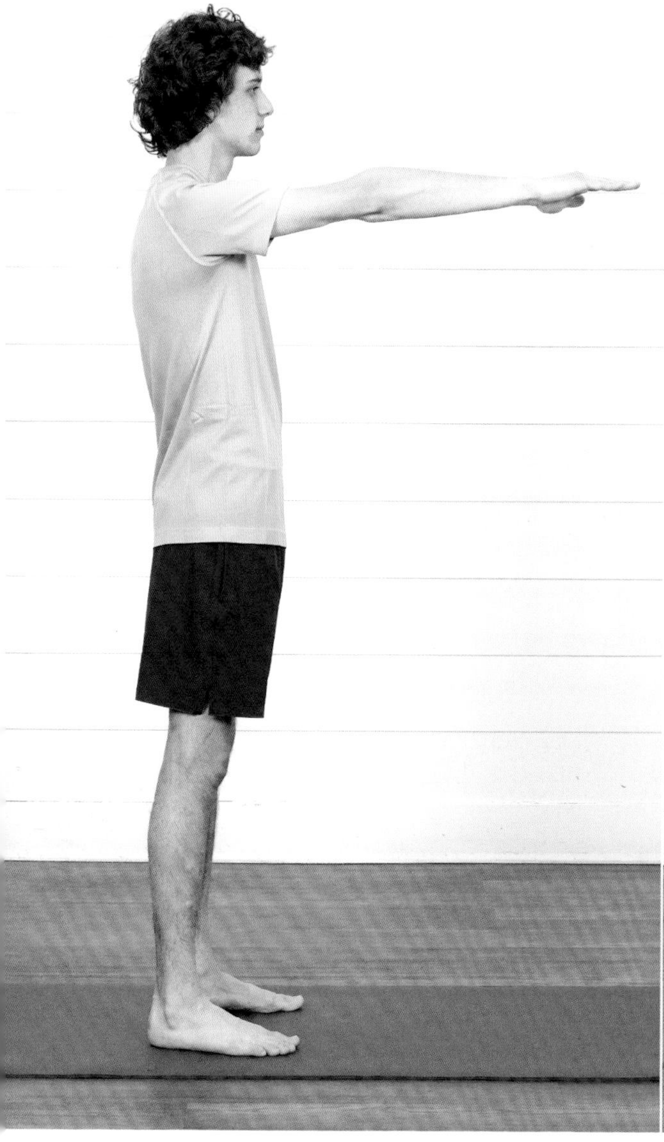

WITH A SMALL PILATES BALL

In step 1, place a small Pilates ball between your legs just above your knees.

In step 2, squeeze the ball to keep it in place. Continue with the remaining text.

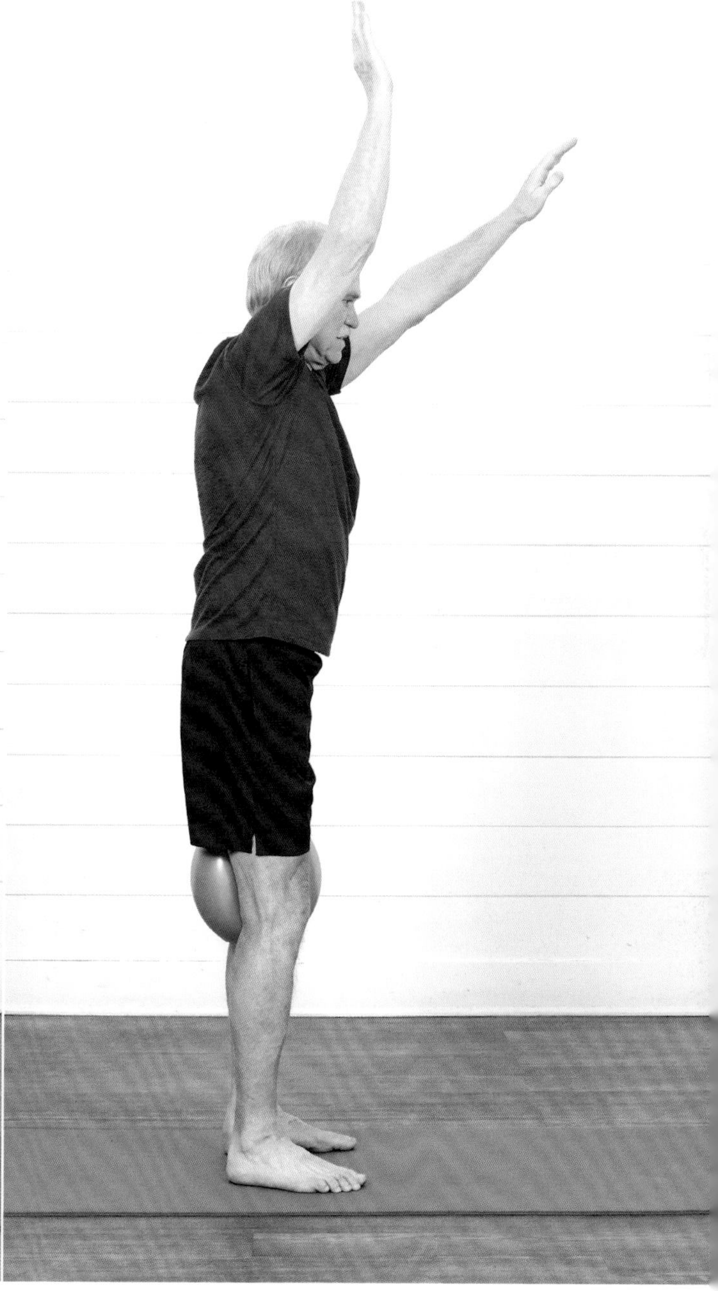

Standing Boxing

These movements will target your entire arm (especially your triceps), upper back, and chest muscles. Because this is a standing exercise, you'll strengthen your leg and gluteal muscles while also improving balance and coordination.

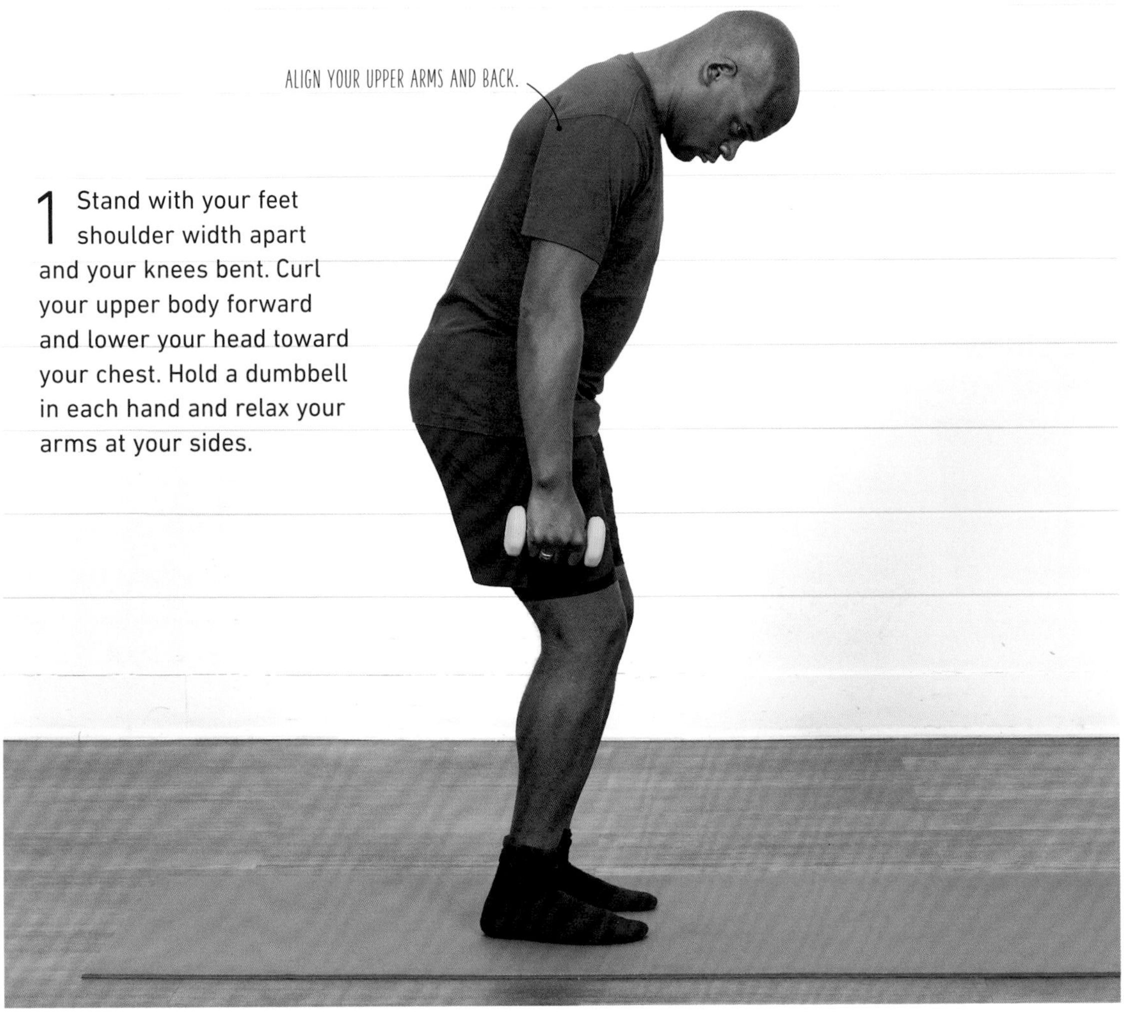
ALIGN YOUR UPPER ARMS AND BACK.

1 Stand with your feet shoulder width apart and your knees bent. Curl your upper body forward and lower your head toward your chest. Hold a dumbbell in each hand and relax your arms at your sides.

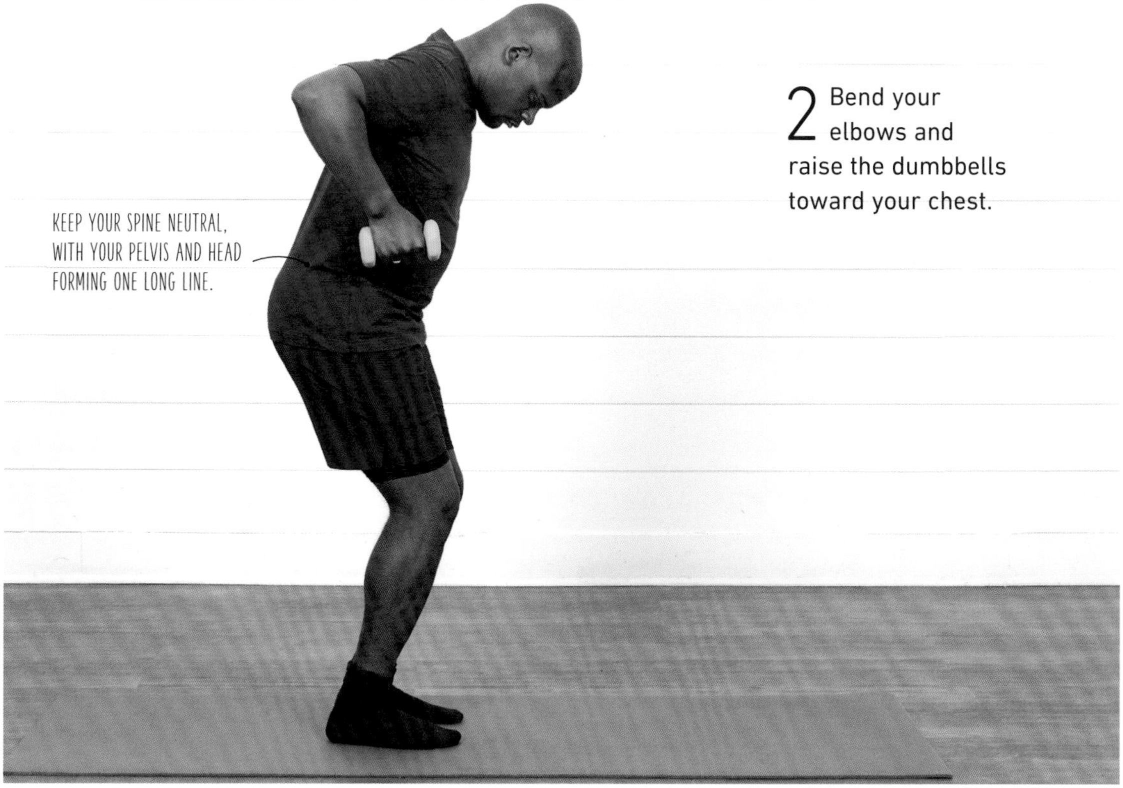

KEEP YOUR SPINE NEUTRAL, WITH YOUR PELVIS AND HEAD FORMING ONE LONG LINE.

2 Bend your elbows and raise the dumbbells toward your chest.

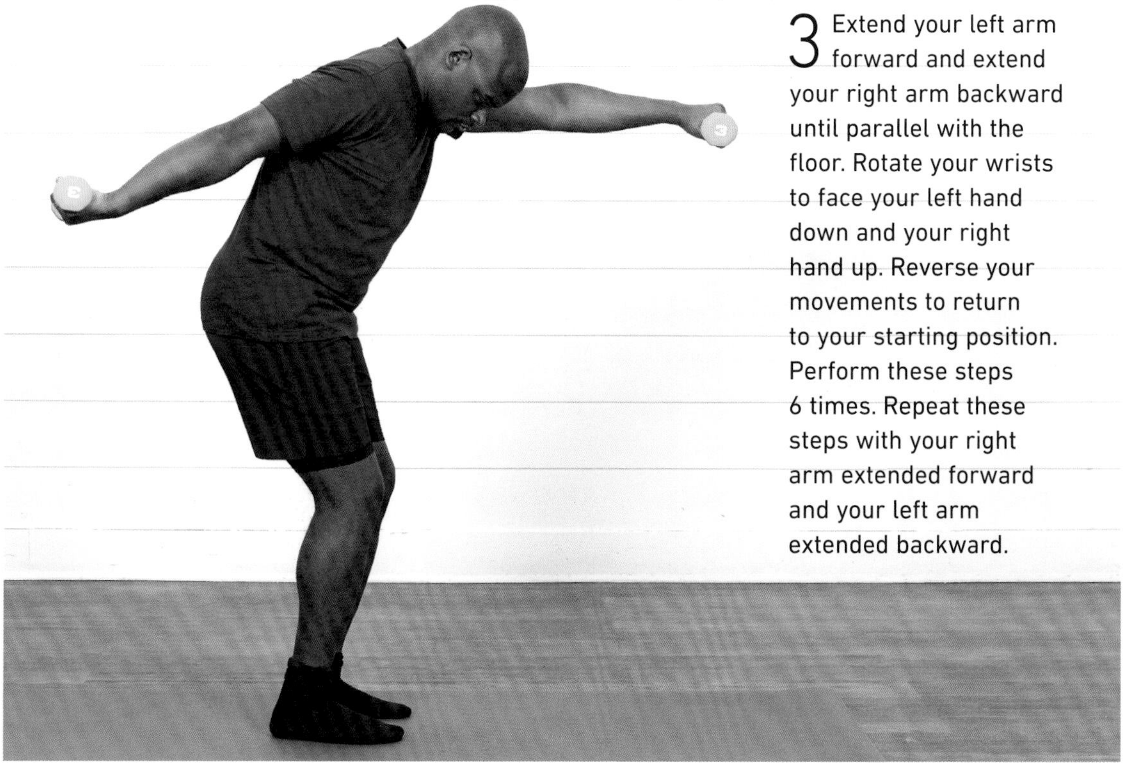

3 Extend your left arm forward and extend your right arm backward until parallel with the floor. Rotate your wrists to face your left hand down and your right hand up. Reverse your movements to return to your starting position. Perform these steps 6 times. Repeat these steps with your right arm extended forward and your left arm extended backward.

WITHOUT WEIGHTS >>>

In step 1, relax your arms and your empty hands at your sides. Continue with the remaining text.

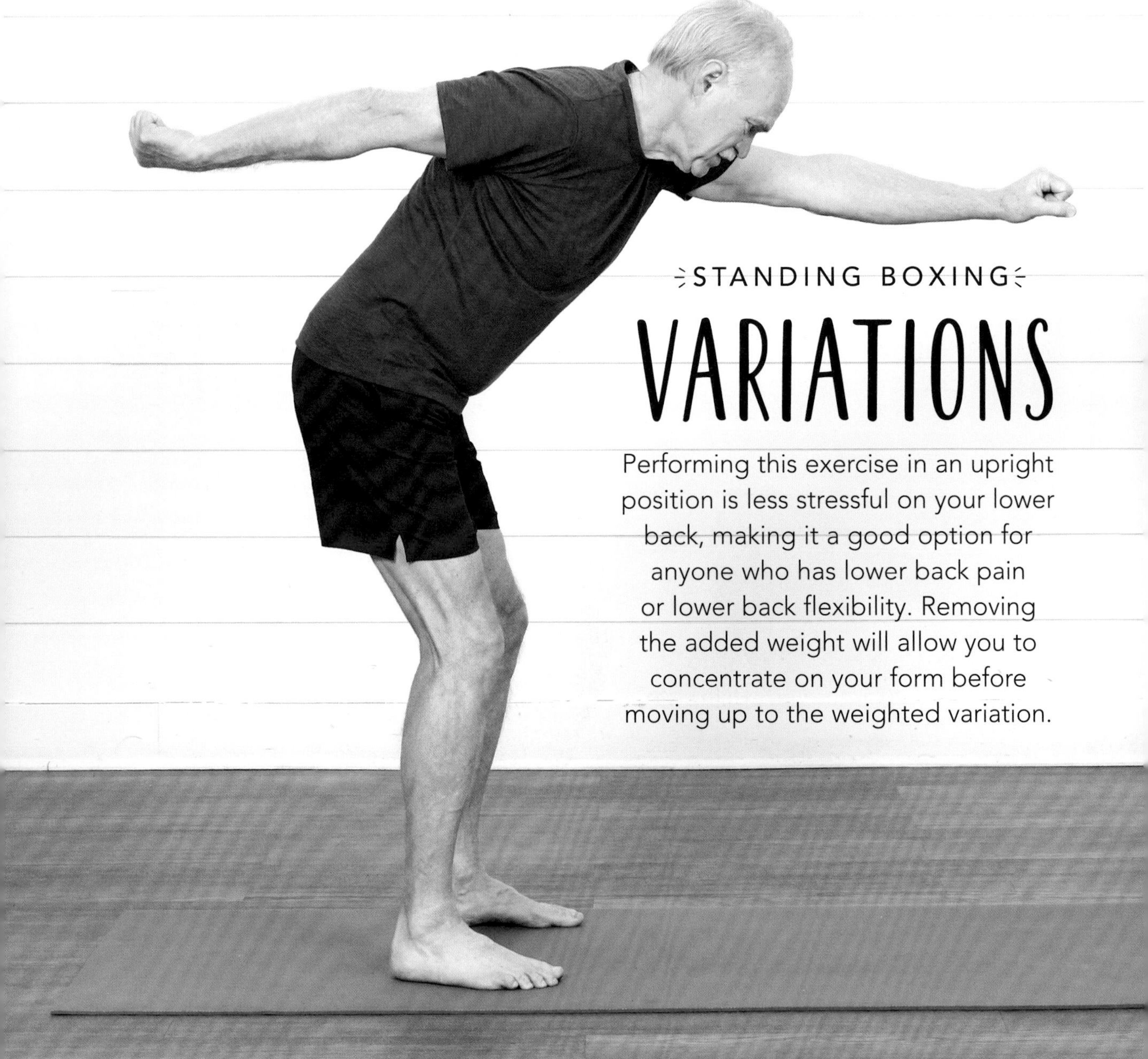

STANDING BOXING

VARIATIONS

Performing this exercise in an upright position is less stressful on your lower back, making it a good option for anyone who has lower back pain or lower back flexibility. Removing the added weight will allow you to concentrate on your form before moving up to the weighted variation.

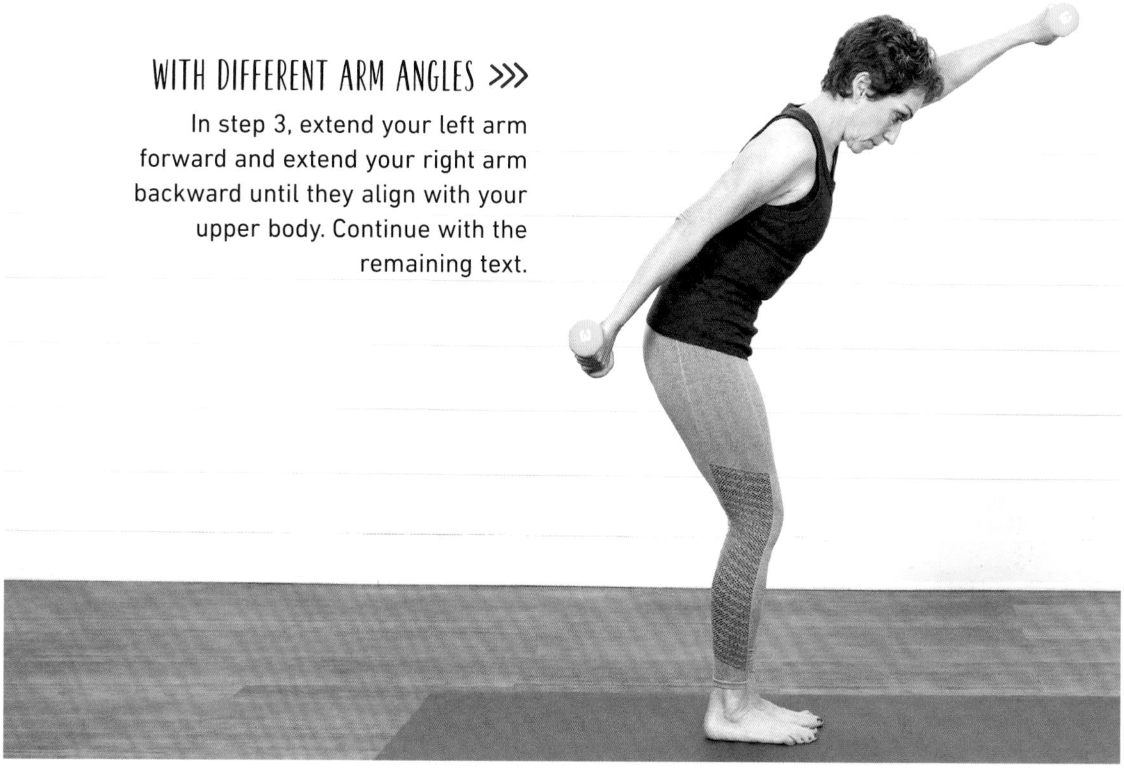

WITH DIFFERENT ARM ANGLES >>>

In step 3, extend your left arm forward and extend your right arm backward until they align with your upper body. Continue with the remaining text.

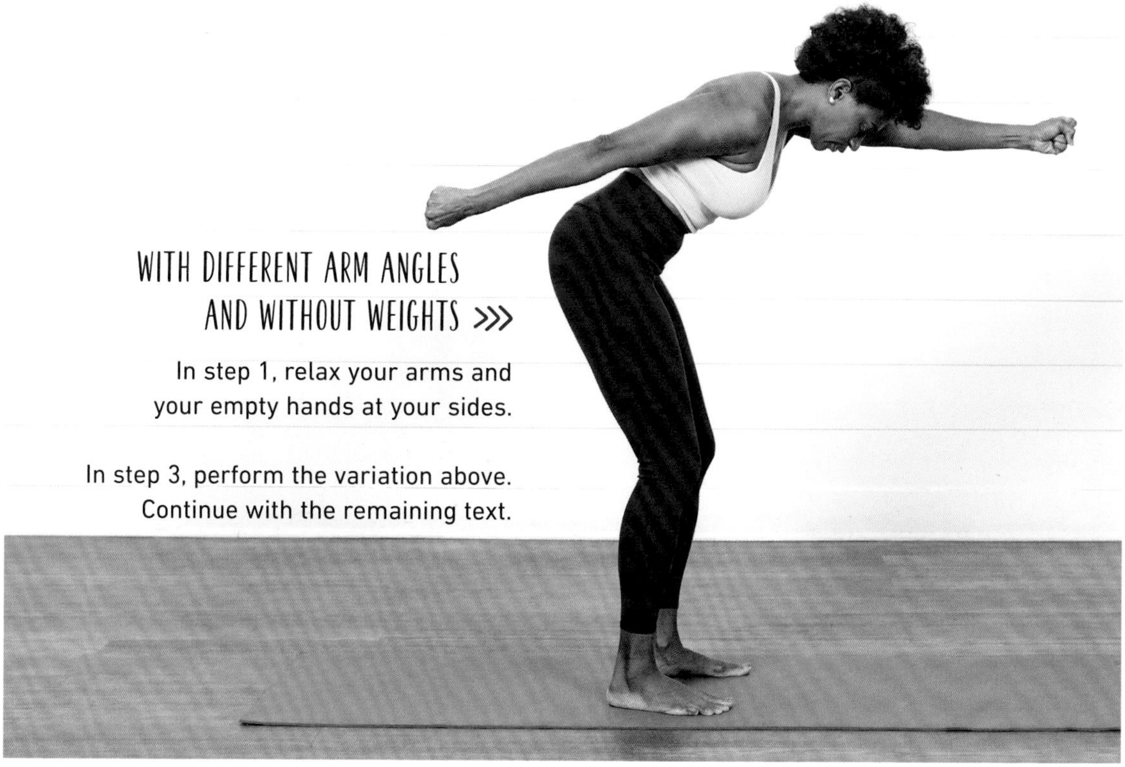

WITH DIFFERENT ARM ANGLES AND WITHOUT WEIGHTS >>>

In step 1, relax your arms and your empty hands at your sides.

In step 3, perform the variation above. Continue with the remaining text.

Standing Arm Circles

Arm circles are useful as a dynamic warm-up before performing an upper- or full-body workout. Performing these movements works the deltoids, trapezius, biceps, and triceps. They can also help improve balance, core strength, and coordination. Adding resistance or weight can make the exercise much more challenging.

1 Stand with your feet shoulder width apart. Hold a dumbbell in each hand and relax your arms in front of your thighs.

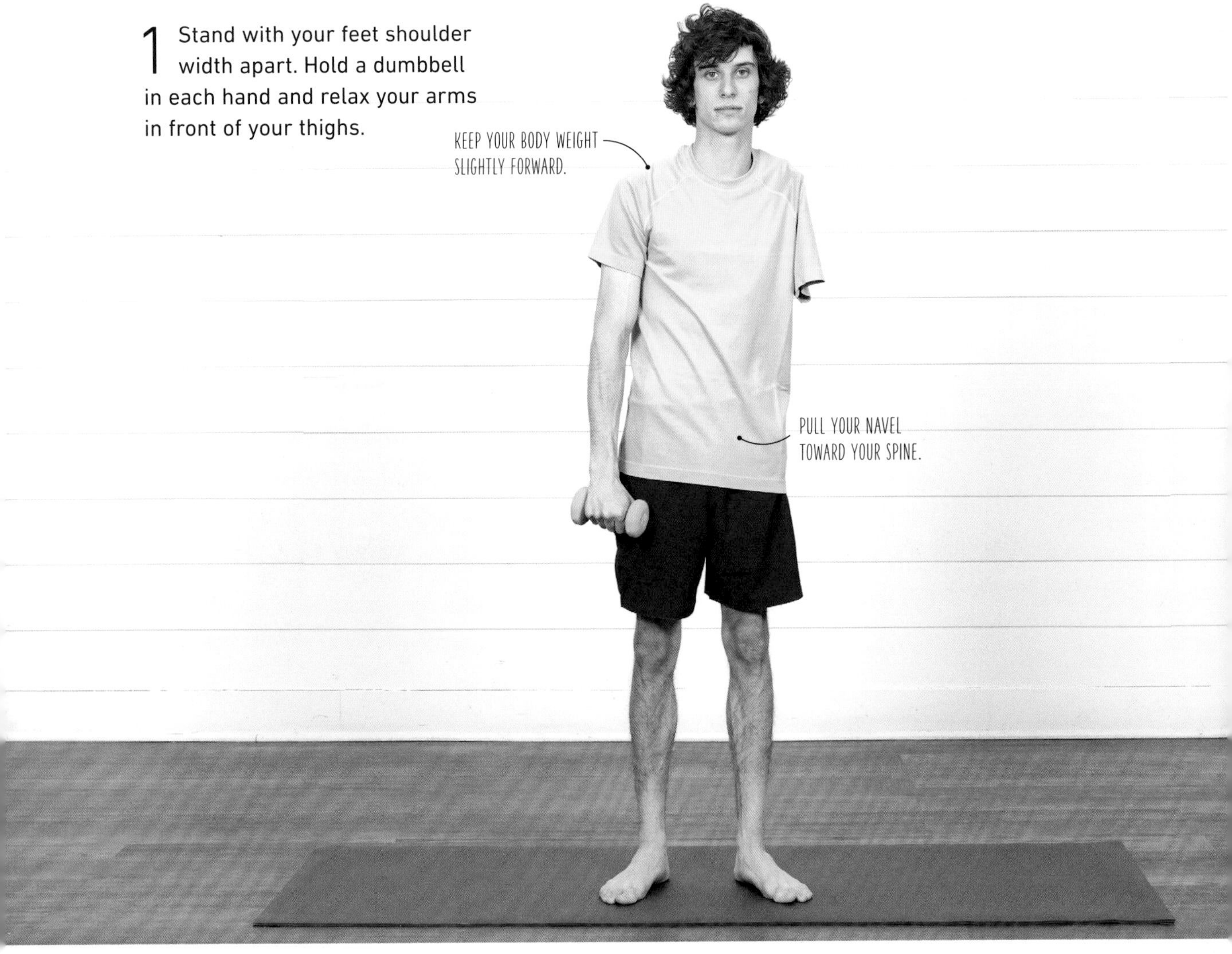
KEEP YOUR BODY WEIGHT SLIGHTLY FORWARD.
PULL YOUR NAVEL TOWARD YOUR SPINE.

2 Raise your arms and trace small clockwise circles, lifting your arms until they're just above your shoulders. Reverse your movements to trace small counterclockwise circles until your arms are lowered to your thighs. Perform these steps 5 times.

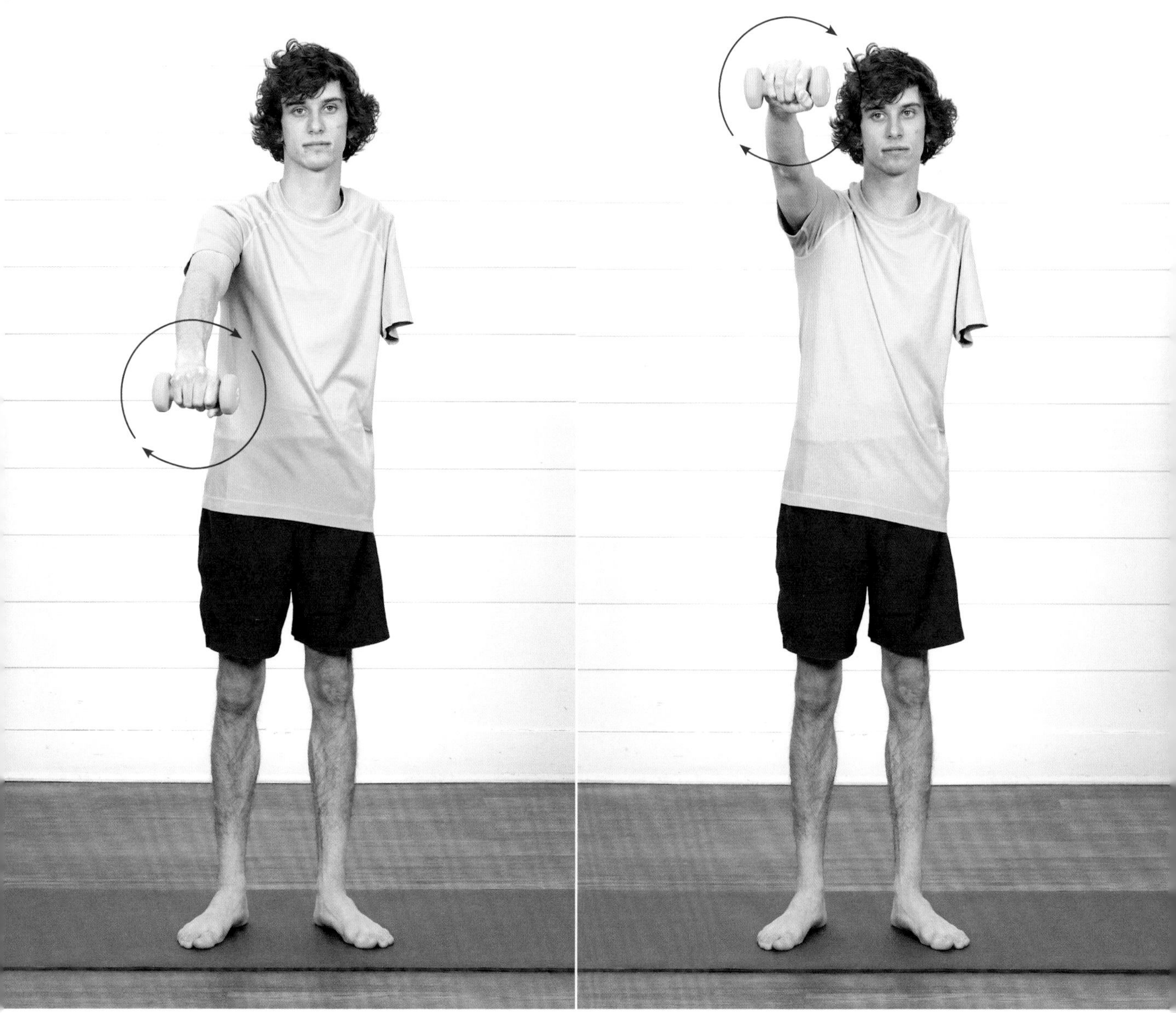

WITHOUT WEIGHTS >>>

In step 1, relax your arms and your empty hands at your sides. Continue with the remaining text.

STANDING ARM CIRCLES

VARIATIONS

If you experience shoulder pain or you've had a shoulder injury, performing this exercise without the weights or without raising your arms above your shoulders is a better alternative. If balance is a challenge, you might benefit from the seated variation.

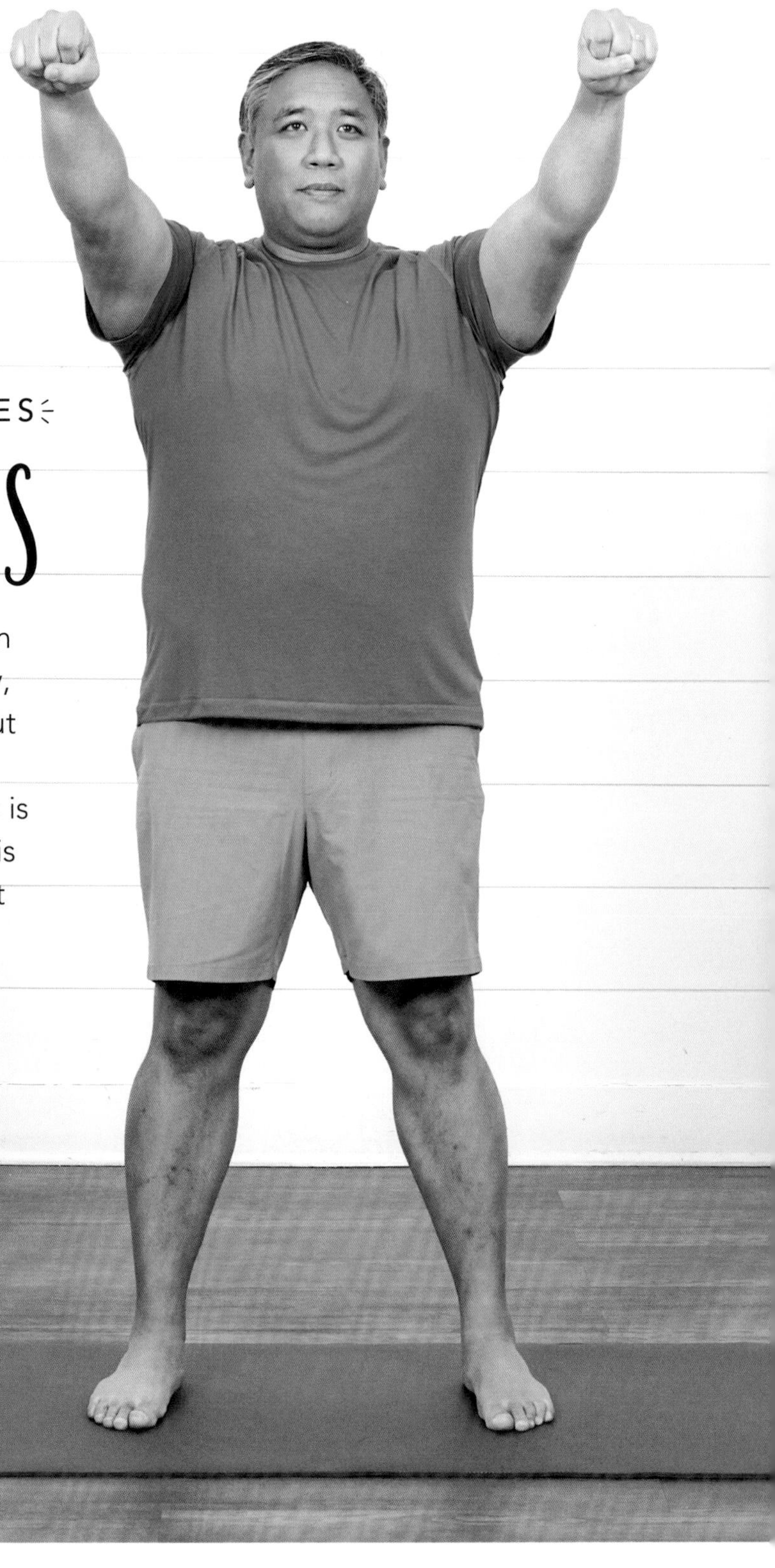

ARMS AT SHOULDER HEIGHT >>>

In step 2, raise your arms to shoulder height. Continue with the remaining text.

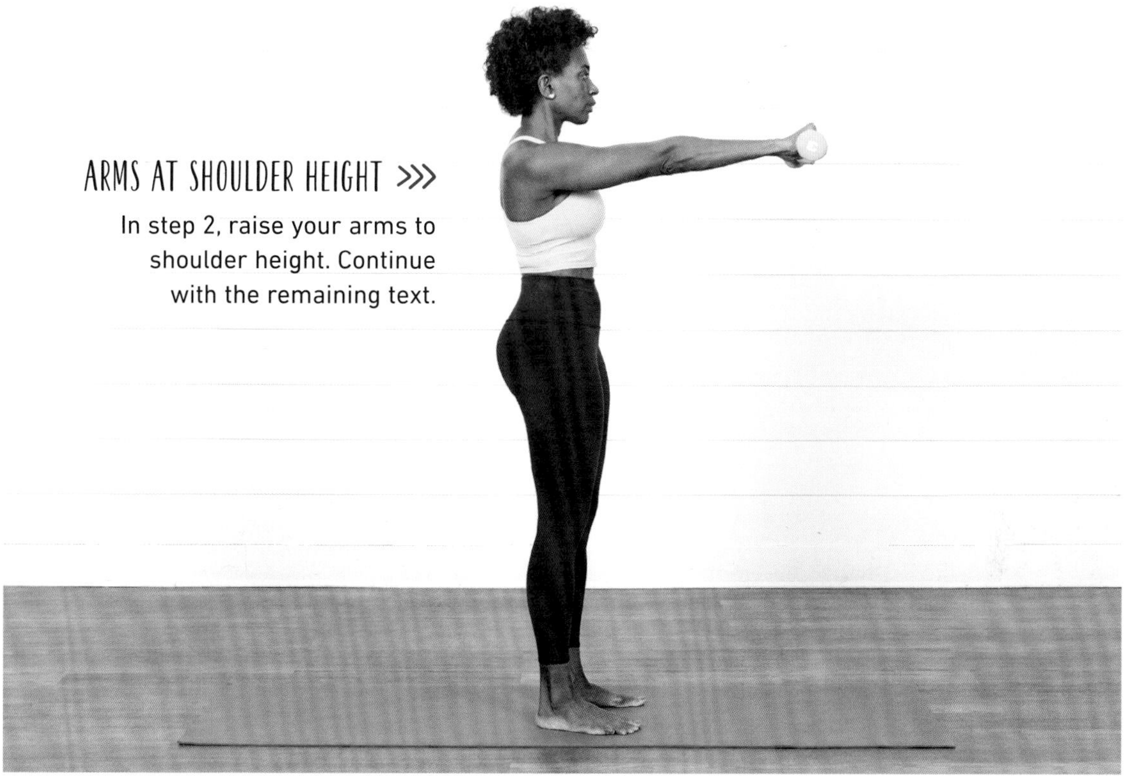

<<< SITTING IN A CHAIR

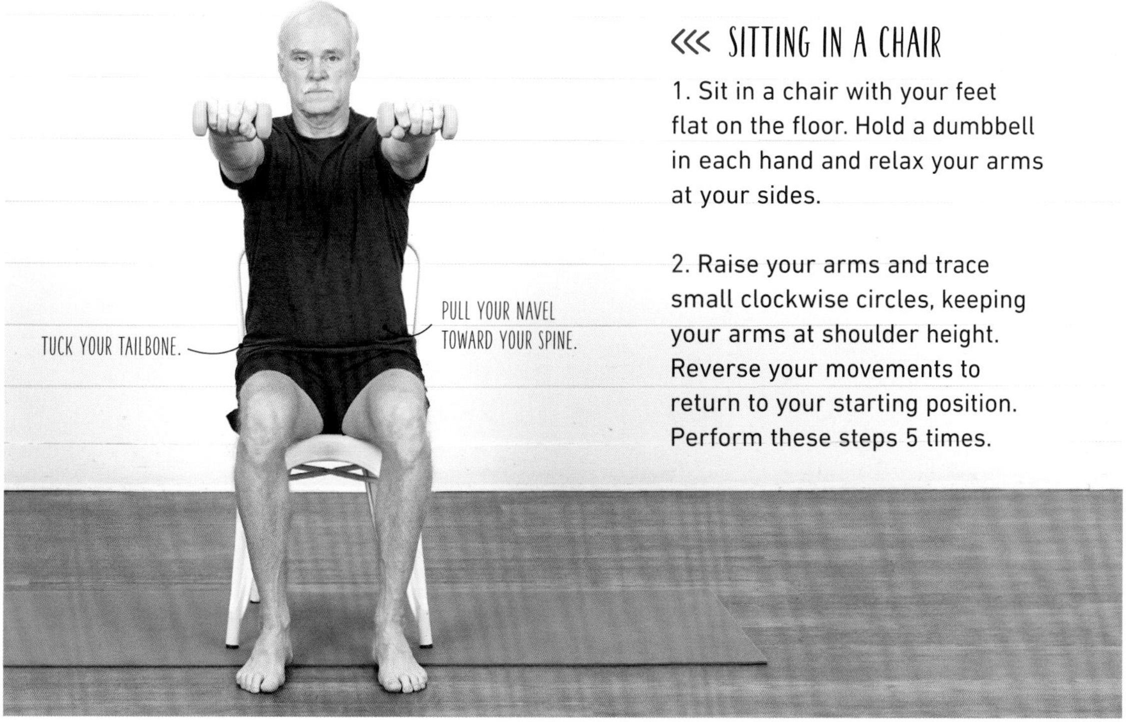
TUCK YOUR TAILBONE.
PULL YOUR NAVEL TOWARD YOUR SPINE.

1. Sit in a chair with your feet flat on the floor. Hold a dumbbell in each hand and relax your arms at your sides.

2. Raise your arms and trace small clockwise circles, keeping your arms at shoulder height. Reverse your movements to return to your starting position. Perform these steps 5 times.

Standing Biceps Curls

These curls target your biceps, your shoulders, and your deltoid muscles. This standing variation also works your abdominal muscles—they isometrically contract (shorten without changing length) to help stabilize your body.

1 Stand with your feet shoulder width apart. Hold a dumbbell in each hand. Relax your arms at your sides and face your hands toward your legs.

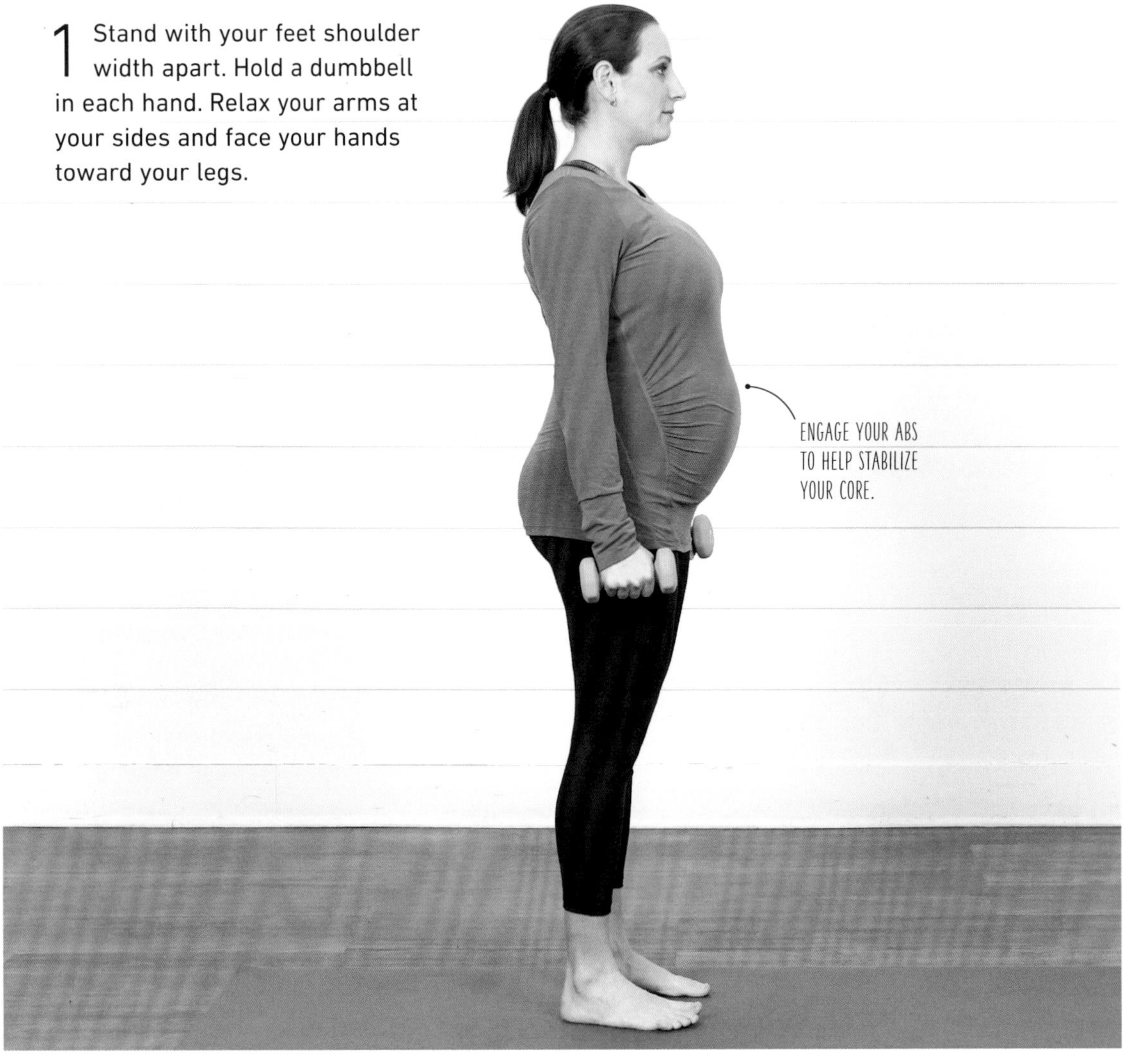
ENGAGE YOUR ABS TO HELP STABILIZE YOUR CORE.

2 Bend your elbows, and as you exhale, raise the weights to your chest and toward your shoulders. As you inhale, reverse your movements to return to your starting position. Perform these steps 8 times.

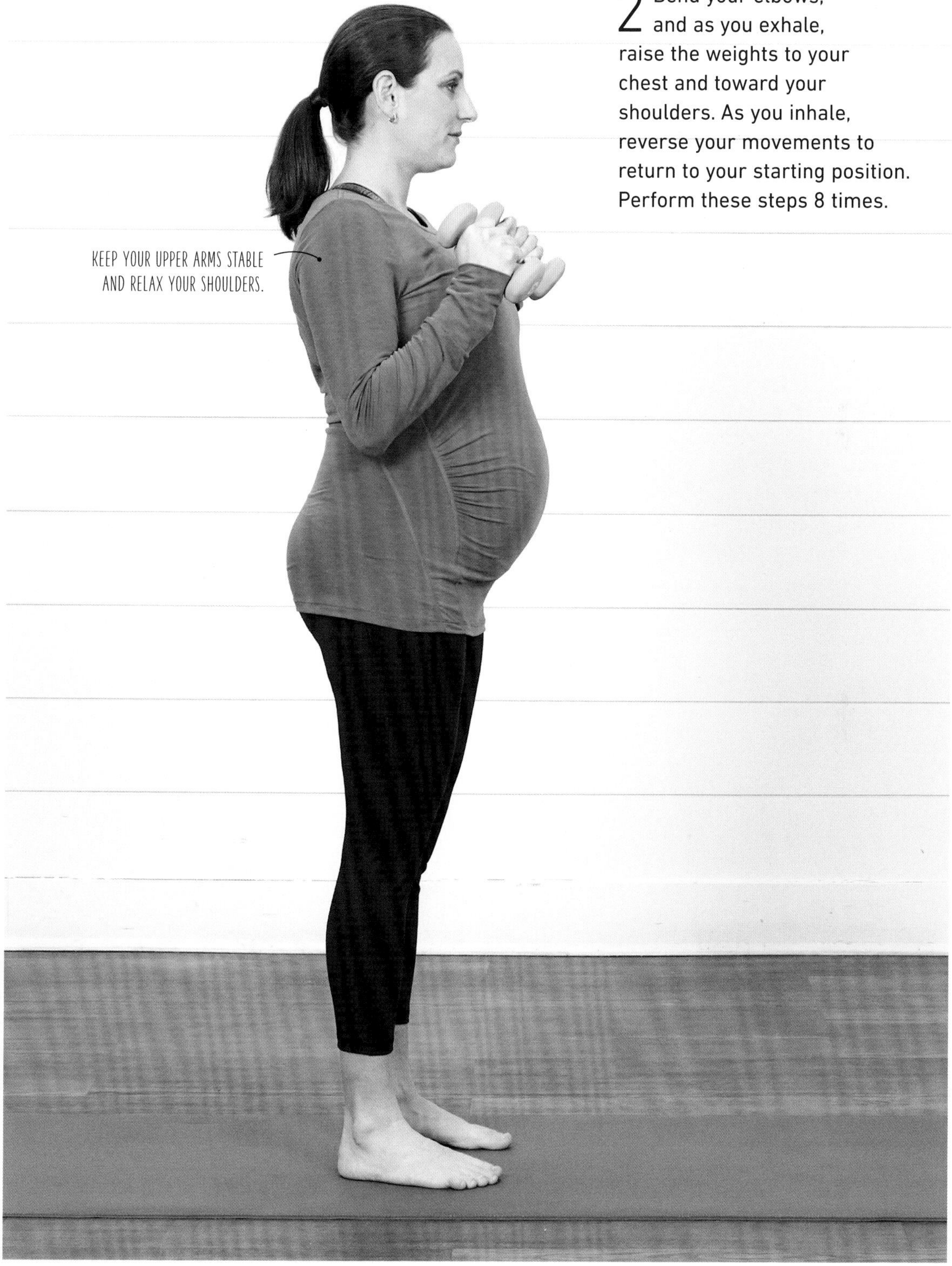

KEEP YOUR UPPER ARMS STABLE
AND RELAX YOUR SHOULDERS.

STANDING BICEPS CURLS

VARIATIONS

These variations allow you to not use weights or to use a resistance band while performing the movements. You can also perform this exercise while sitting in a chair.

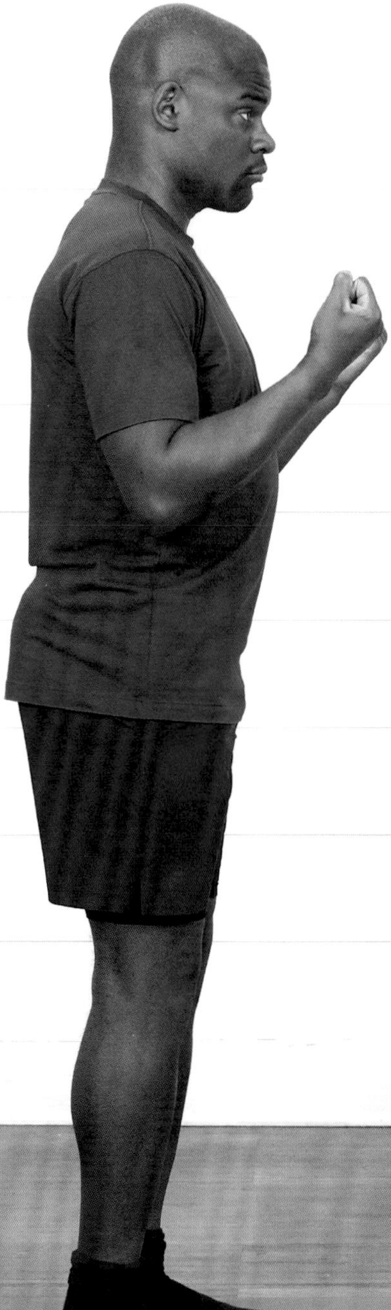

WITHOUT WEIGHTS

In step 1, relax your arms and your empty hands at your sides. Continue with the remaining text.

<<< WITH A RESISTANCE BAND

1. Stand with your right foot slightly ahead of your left foot. Loop a resistance band under your right foot and hold the ends of the band in your right hand. Relax your arms at your sides.

2. Bend your right elbow and raise the band until it's at shoulder height. Reverse your movements to return to your starting position. Perform these steps 6 times. Repeat these steps with the band under your right foot.

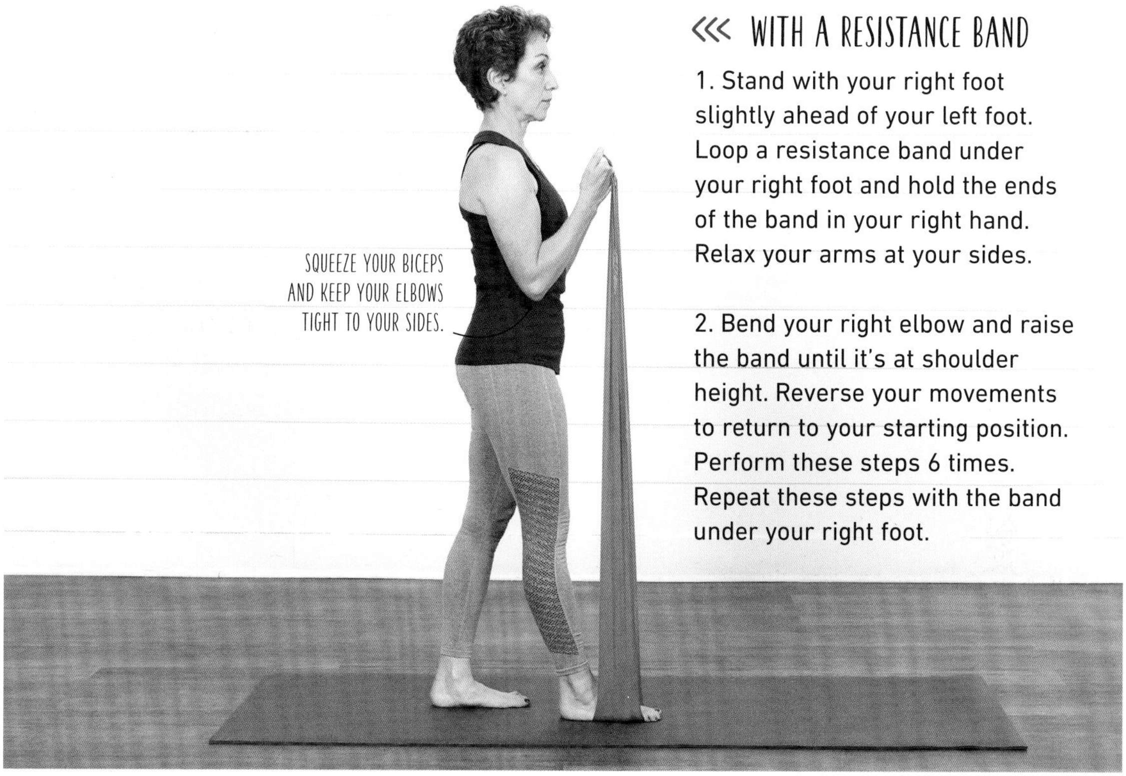

SQUEEZE YOUR BICEPS AND KEEP YOUR ELBOWS TIGHT TO YOUR SIDES.

<<< SITTING IN A CHAIR

1. Sit in a chair with a resistance band looped under your right foot. Hold the ends of the band in your right hand. Relax your arms at your sides or on your thighs.

2. Bend your right elbow and raise your right hand toward your right shoulder. Slowly reverse your movements to return to your starting position. Perform these steps 5 times. Repeat these steps with your left arm.

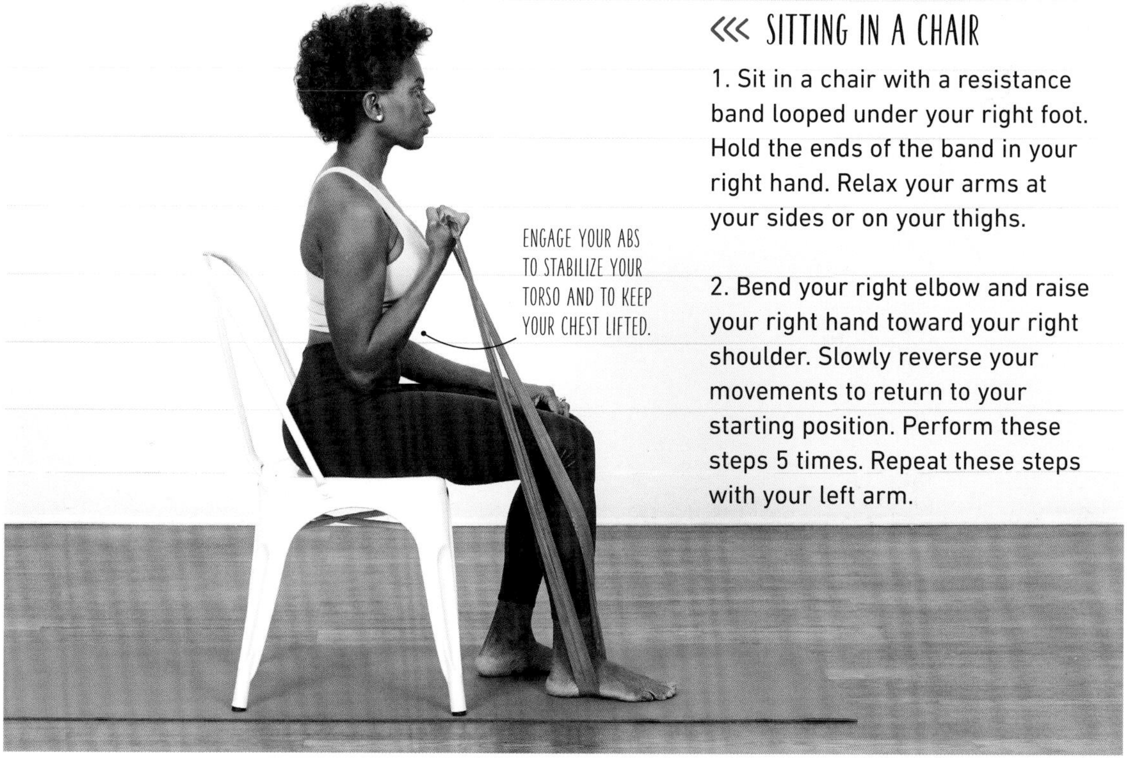

ENGAGE YOUR ABS TO STABILIZE YOUR TORSO AND TO KEEP YOUR CHEST LIFTED.

Standing Oblique Crunches

This exercise is great for working the muscles of your entire core, especially your obliques. Performing these movements can help you develop core strength, trunk mobility, lower-body stability, body awareness, and balance.

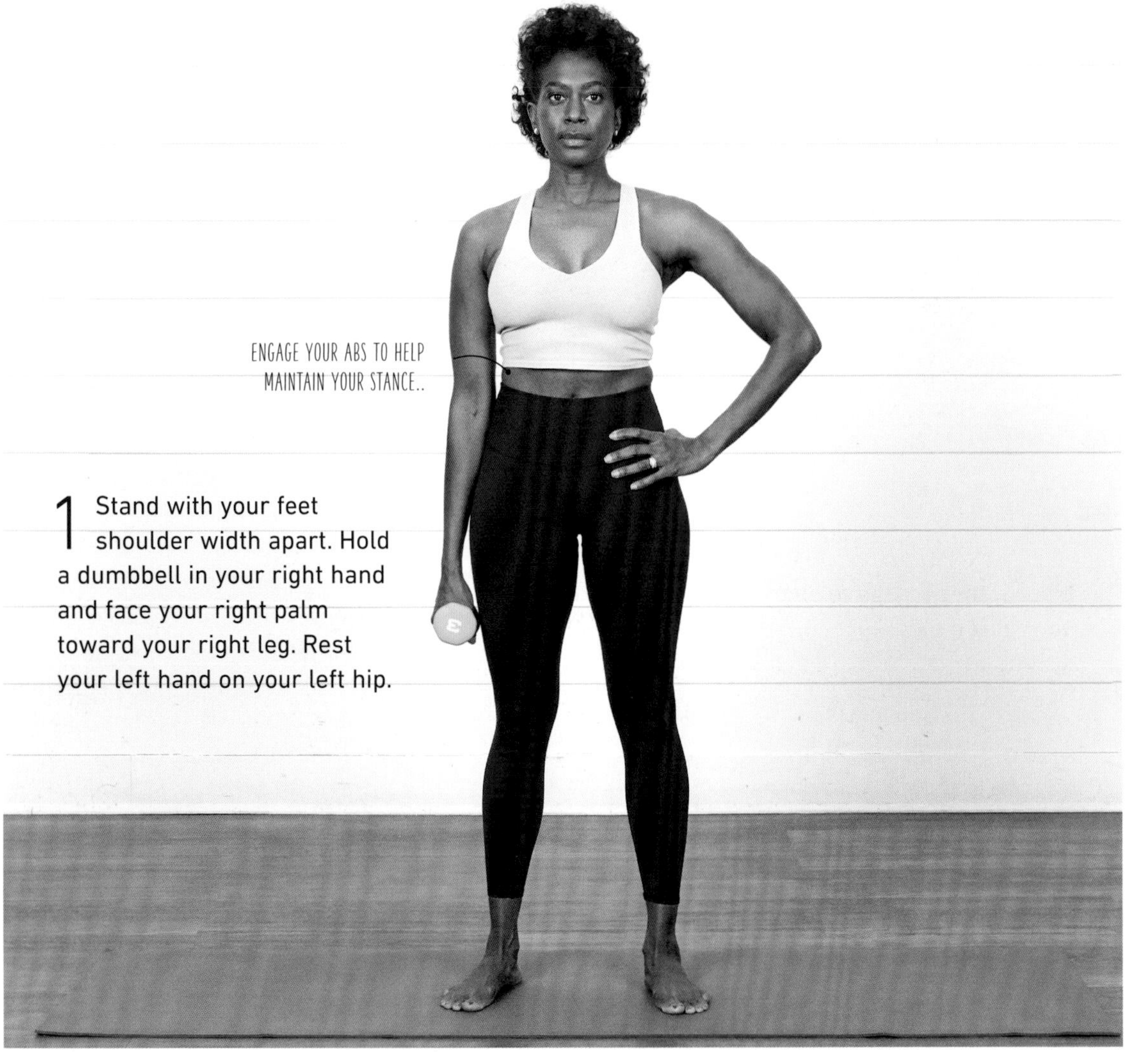

ENGAGE YOUR ABS TO HELP MAINTAIN YOUR STANCE..

1 Stand with your feet shoulder width apart. Hold a dumbbell in your right hand and face your right palm toward your right leg. Rest your left hand on your left hip.

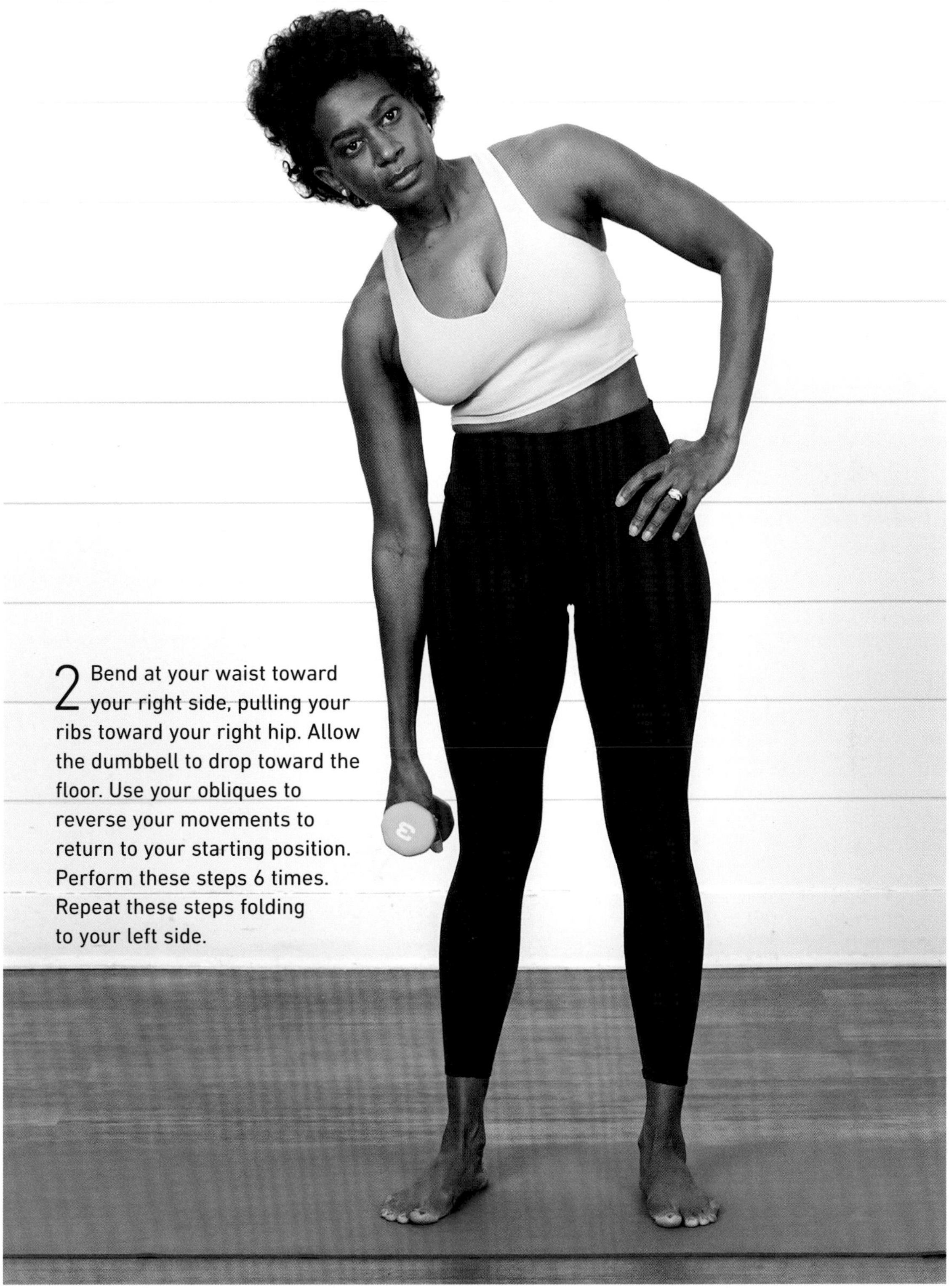

2 Bend at your waist toward your right side, pulling your ribs toward your right hip. Allow the dumbbell to drop toward the floor. Use your obliques to reverse your movements to return to your starting position. Perform these steps 6 times. Repeat these steps folding to your left side.

STANDING OBLIQUE CRUNCHES

VARIATIONS

If balance is a challenge for you, the seated variation is a good option. Performing this exercise without weights can help you learn the proper form. A resistance band is an affordable and portable option (if you don't have access to weights), with which you can progress as you get stronger.

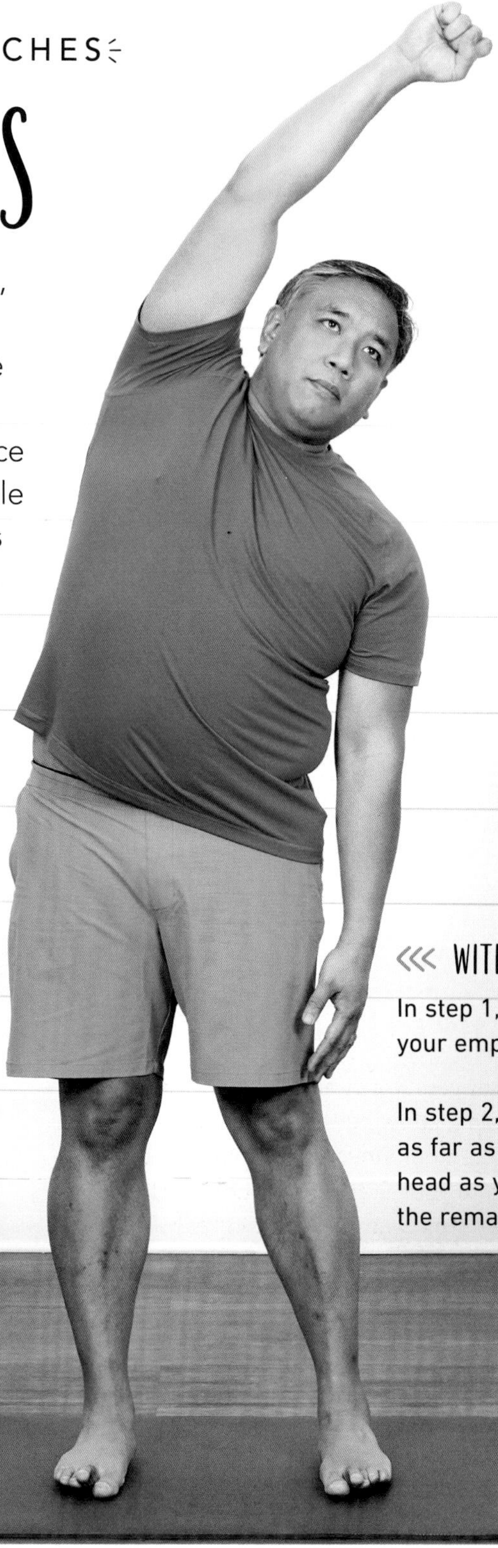

<<< WITHOUT WEIGHTS

In step 1, relax your arms and your empty hands at your sides

In step 2, extend your right arm as far as comfortable over your head as you bend. Continue with the remaining text.

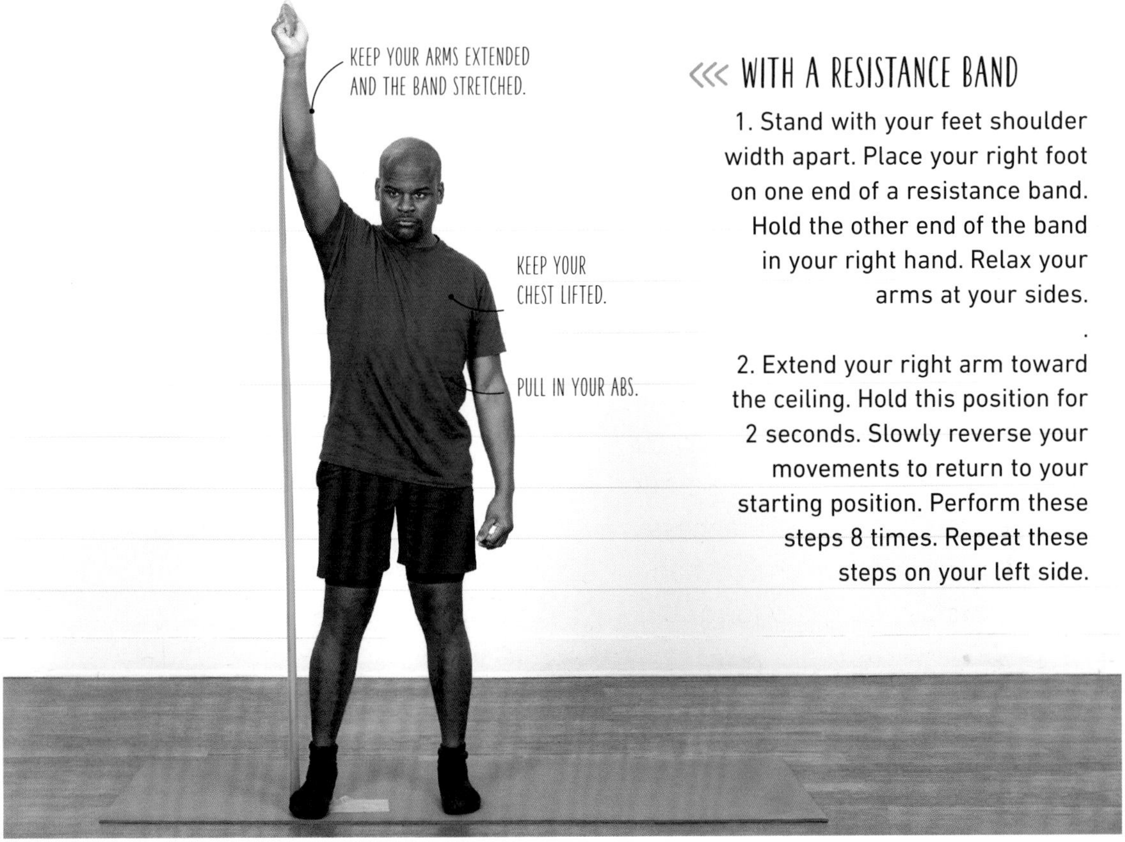

KEEP YOUR ARMS EXTENDED AND THE BAND STRETCHED.
KEEP YOUR CHEST LIFTED.
PULL IN YOUR ABS.

WITH A RESISTANCE BAND

1. Stand with your feet shoulder width apart. Place your right foot on one end of a resistance band. Hold the other end of the band in your right hand. Relax your arms at your sides.

2. Extend your right arm toward the ceiling. Hold this position for 2 seconds. Slowly reverse your movements to return to your starting position. Perform these steps 8 times. Repeat these steps on your left side.

SITTING IN A CHAIR

1. Sit in a chair with your feet flat on the floor. Hold a dumbbell in your right hand and relax your arms at your sides.

2. Bend at your waist and fold toward your right side, allowing the dumbbell to drop toward the floor. Reverse your movements to return to your starting position. Perform these steps 6 times. Repeat these steps with the dumbbell in your left hand and your body folding to your left side.

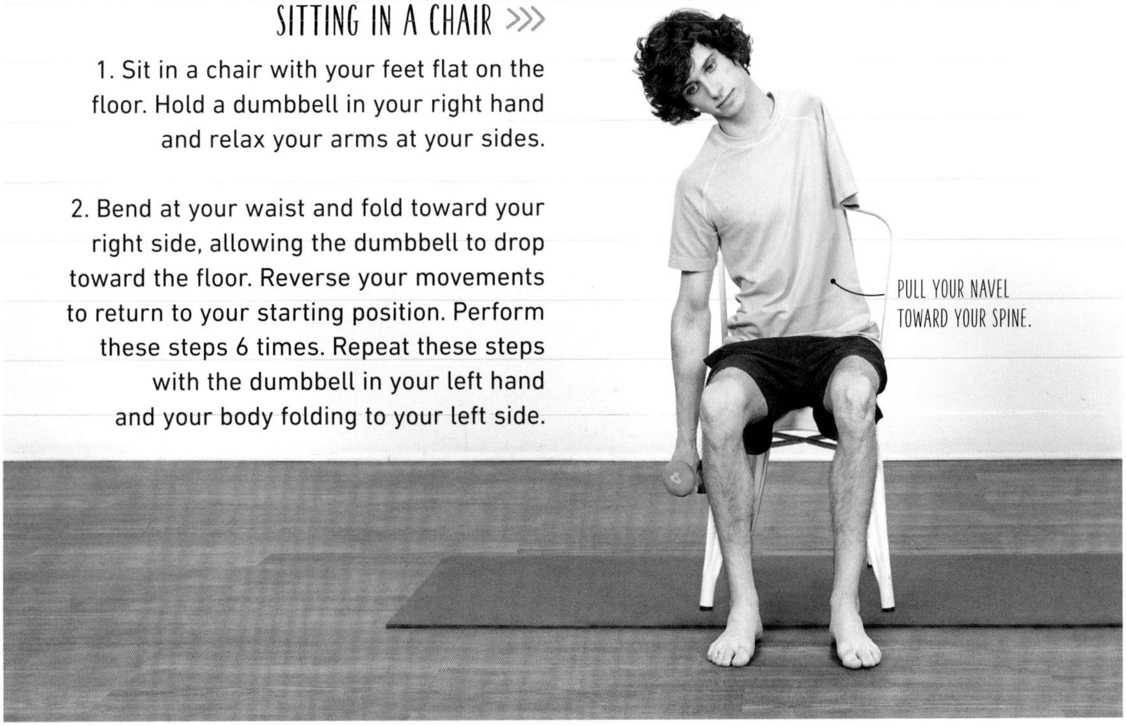

Standing Triceps Extensions

This is a push exercise that contracts your muscles when weight is pushed away from your body. It's also an isolation exercise that works your triceps, shoulders, chest, latissimus dorsi, and forearms, helping you become more functionally fit.

1 Stand with your feet shoulder width apart. Hold a dumbbell in each hand and relax your arms at your sides.

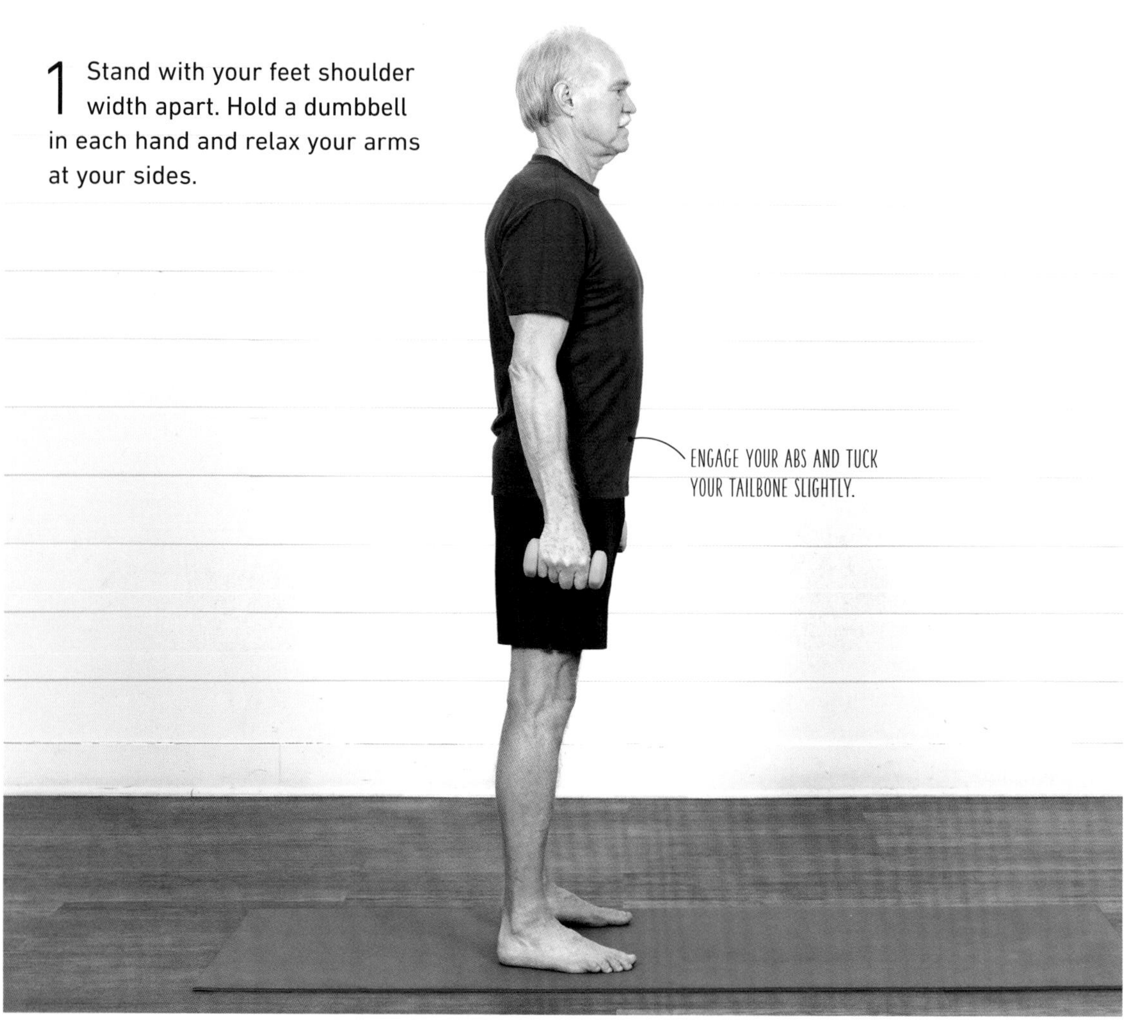

ENGAGE YOUR ABS AND TUCK YOUR TAILBONE SLIGHTLY.

2 Extend your arms toward the ceiling. Slowly bend your elbows and lower the dumbbells behind your head until your arms almost reach your neck. Reverse your movements to return to your starting position. Perform these steps 6 times.

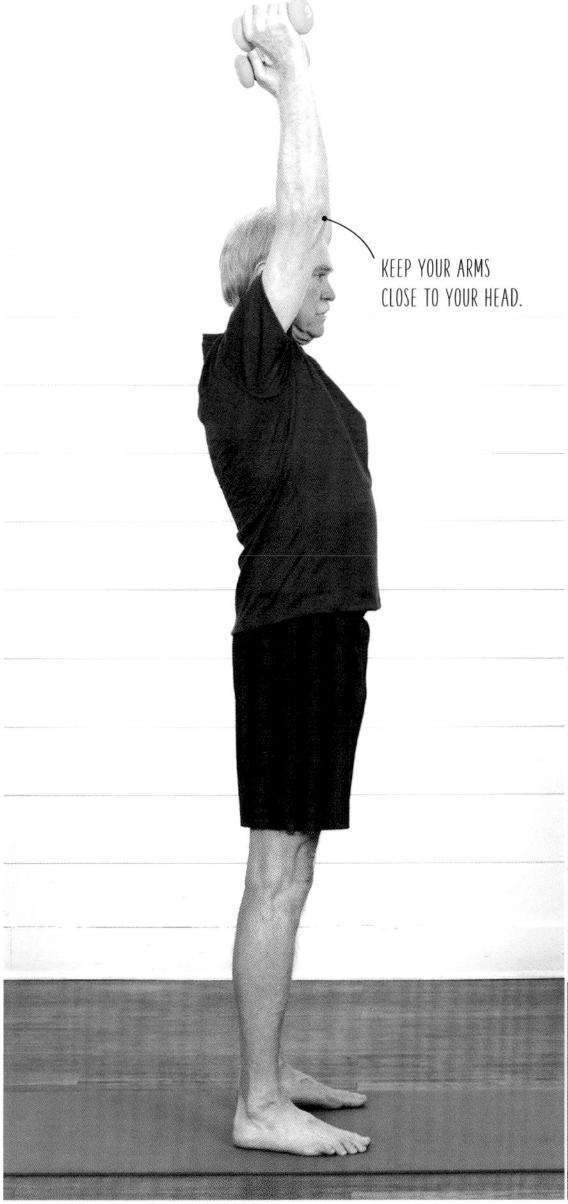

KEEP YOUR ARMS
CLOSE TO YOUR HEAD.

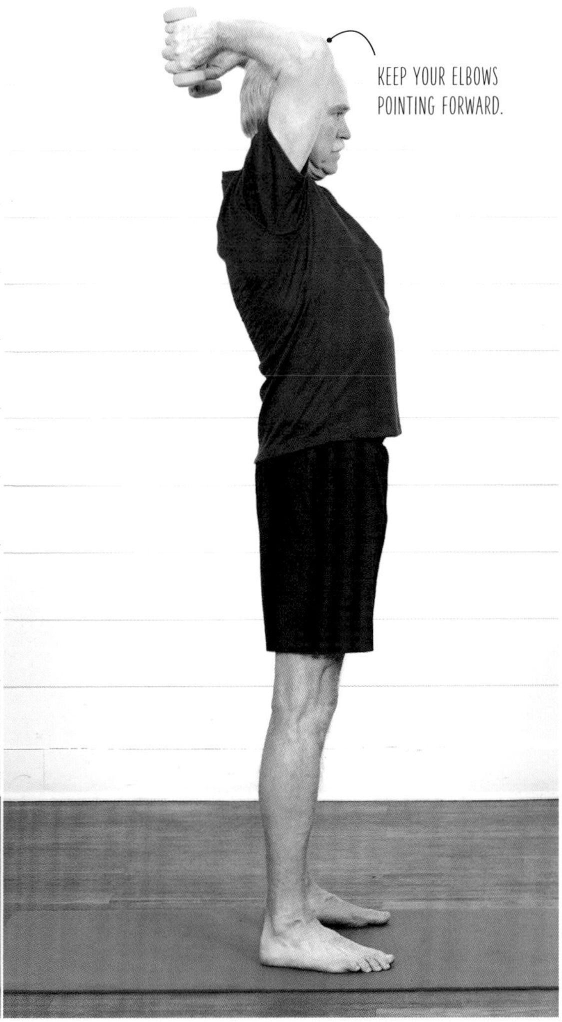

KEEP YOUR ELBOWS
POINTING FORWARD.

STANDING TRICEPS EXTENSIONS

VARIATIONS

Using less weight and/or changing your body position to engage your core less will make this exercise easier. Performing this exercise while seated makes it easier for you to maintain good posture and form.

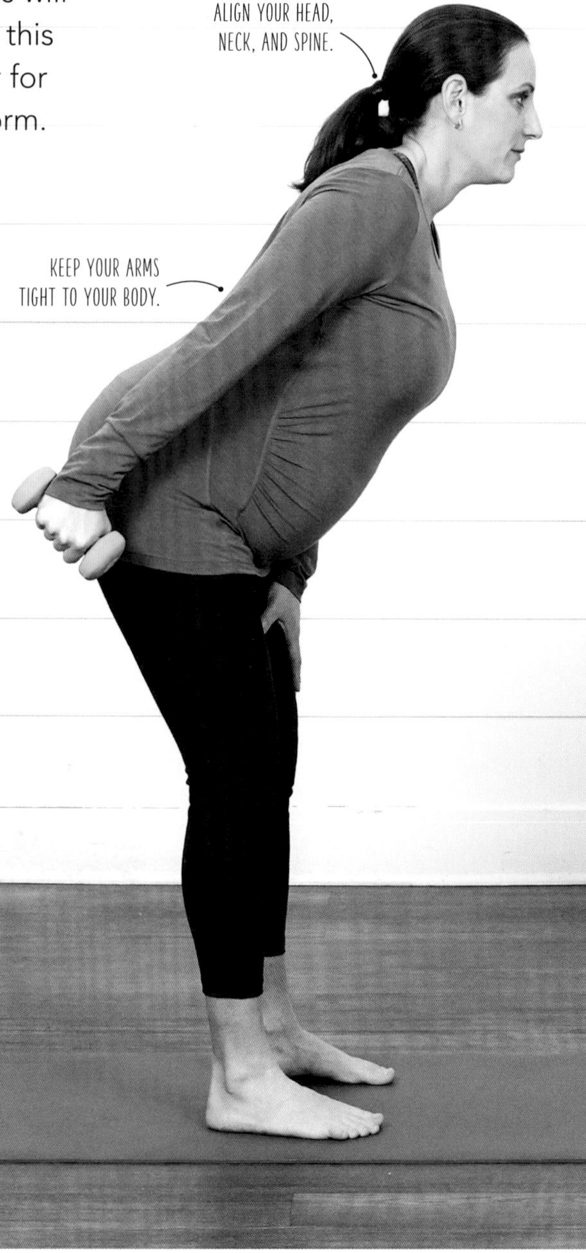

ALIGN YOUR HEAD, NECK, AND SPINE.
KEEP YOUR ARMS TIGHT TO YOUR BODY.

HINGED AT THE WAIST >>>

1. Stand with your feet shoulder width apart. Hold a dumbbell in your right hand and relax your right arm at your right side. Place your left hand on your left thigh.

2. Bend at your waist and fold forward to a comfortable position. As you exhale, slowly extend your right arm backward as far as you can. Reverse your movements to return to your starting position. Perform these steps 6 times. Repeat these steps with your left arm extended backward.

WITHOUT WEIGHTS >>>

In step 1 of the variation on page 198, relax your right arm and your empty right hand at your right side.

In step 2, extend your right arm backward until parallel with the floor. Continue with the remaining text.

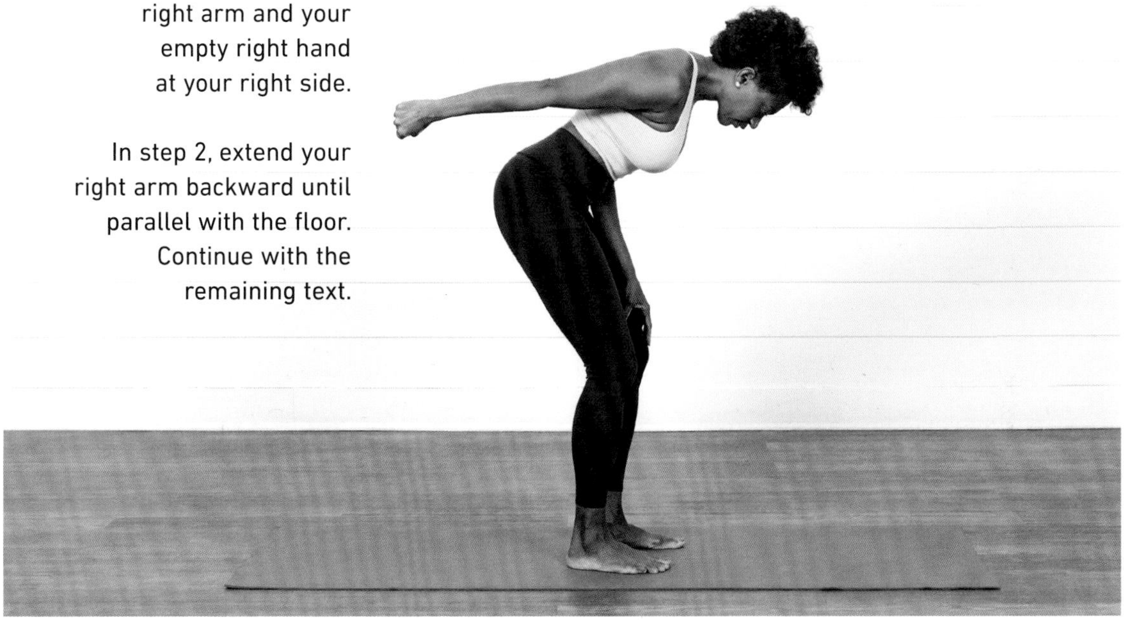

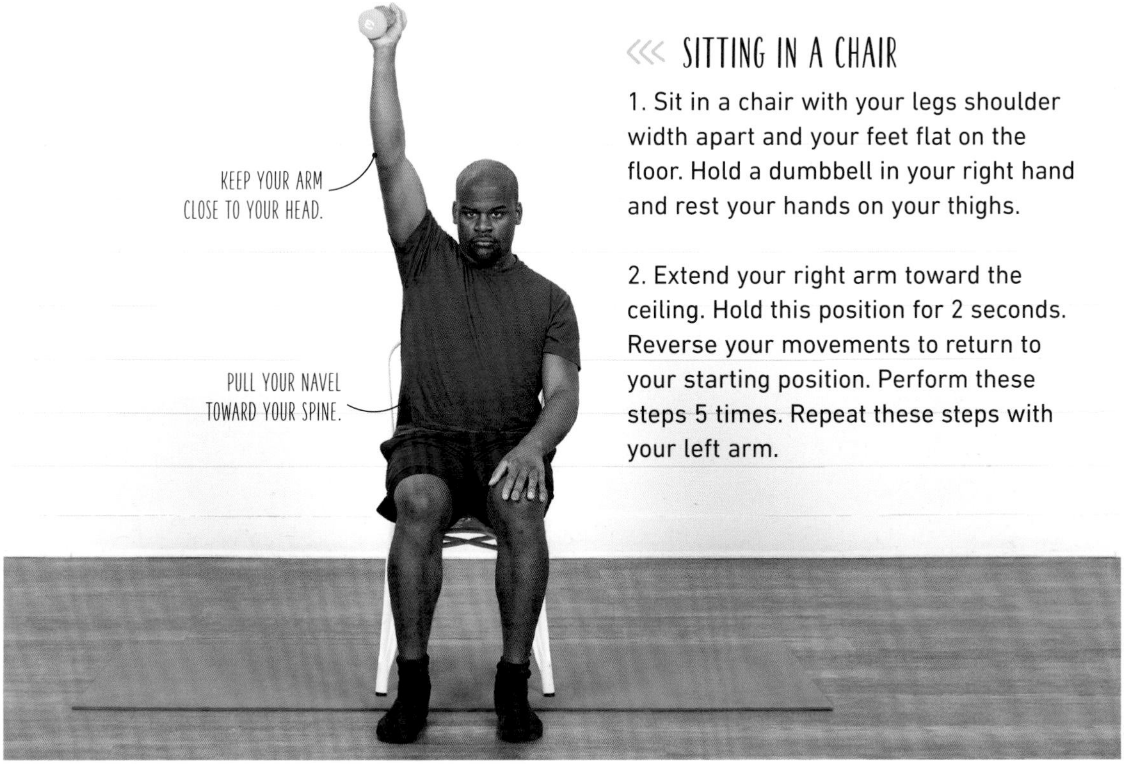
KEEP YOUR ARM CLOSE TO YOUR HEAD.
PULL YOUR NAVEL TOWARD YOUR SPINE.

<<< SITTING IN A CHAIR

1. Sit in a chair with your legs shoulder width apart and your feet flat on the floor. Hold a dumbbell in your right hand and rest your hands on your thighs.

2. Extend your right arm toward the ceiling. Hold this position for 2 seconds. Reverse your movements to return to your starting position. Perform these steps 5 times. Repeat these steps with your left arm.

ANDREW BLUM

I'm an actor, dreamer, and full-time procrastinator. The number of times I've said "I'll get in shape next year" is quite high but ironic to say the least because ever since I started a new job, I've been walking about six miles a day while working.

While I love walking, I want to talk about how I first learned to ride a bicycle. As a young child, I never really cared about learning to ride a bike because I simply assumed I couldn't do it at all because I thought it would be too difficult for me to balance. As a kid, I was never too bothered about not knowing how to ride a bike because none of my friends really rode bikes for fun anyway.

When I was 14 years old, after putting this off for so long, my dad had finally had enough and decided today was going to be the day I learned. He got one of the old bikes out of the garage and told me to get on it and ride down the hill in our yard. I reluctantly agreed and barely made it a few feet before I fell off. Attempt after attempt, I felt like I was only making a fool of myself until something started to catch on. I noticed I was actually balancing a little longer each time. Before I knew it, I was fully balancing this old bike by myself without even falling off. I was appalled it took me this long to even attempt to learn.

Shortly after I learned to ride a bike, I absolutely fell in love with it. I rode every chance I could get and started getting quite good at it. If I wanted to get in shape fast, I just had to ride my bike on the hilly back roads near my house every day and I was set for the summer. Thanks, Dad!

The photo shoot for this project was so much fun. Everyone was so kind, energetic, and super easy to work with while also introducing me to the amazing world of Indian food. The laughs and stories we shared are something I'll always keep close to my heart. To everyone involved with *Pilates for Everyone*, thank you!

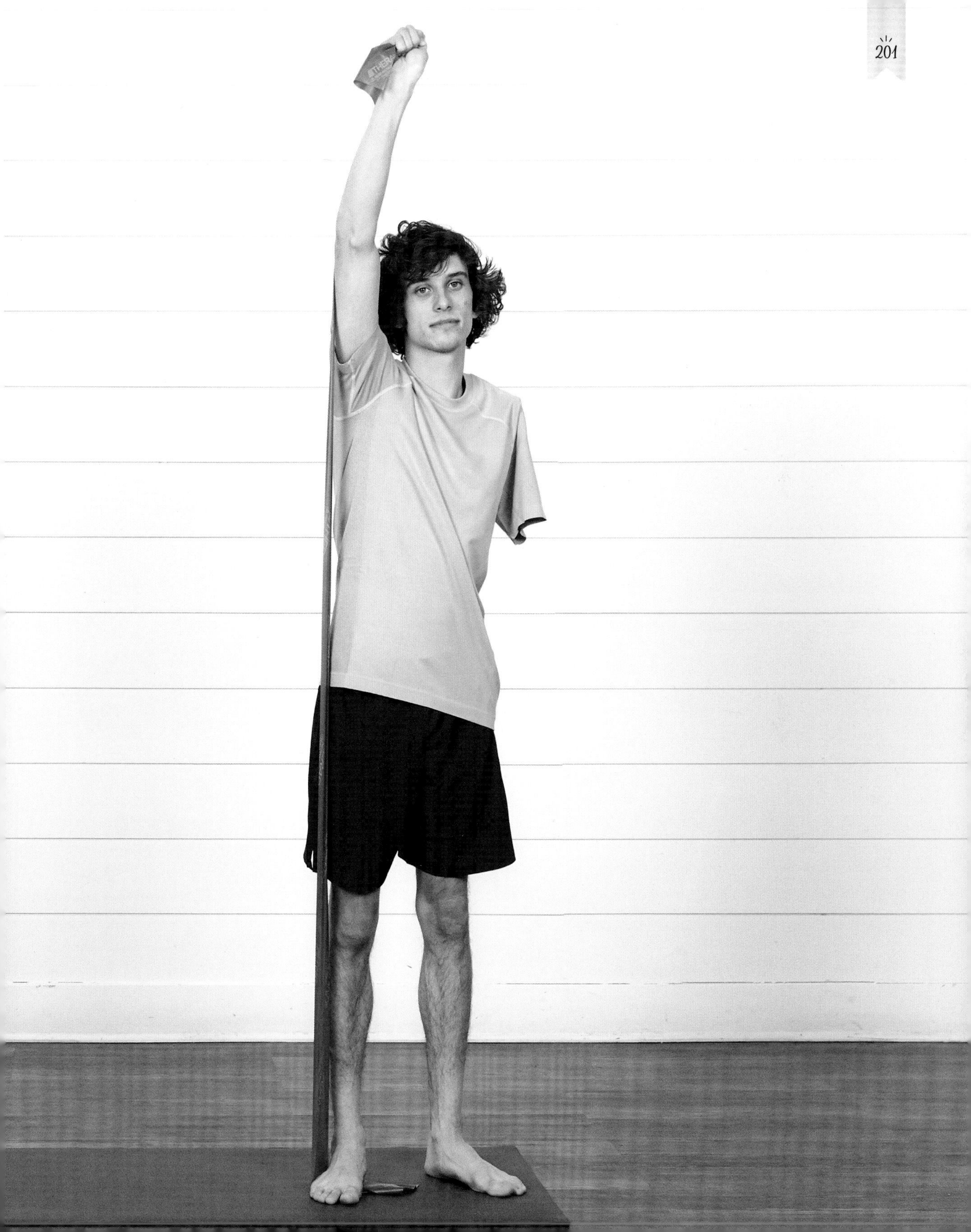

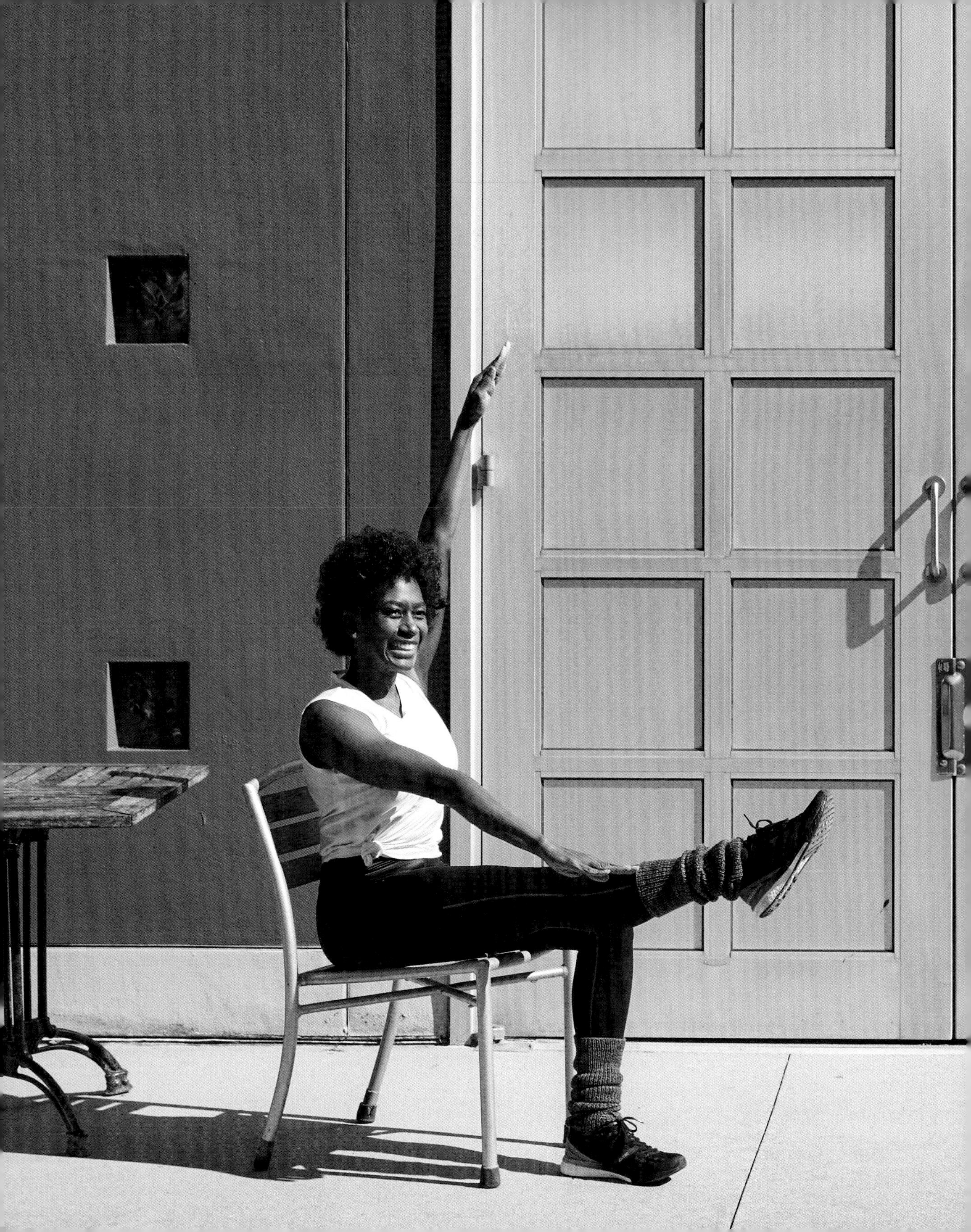

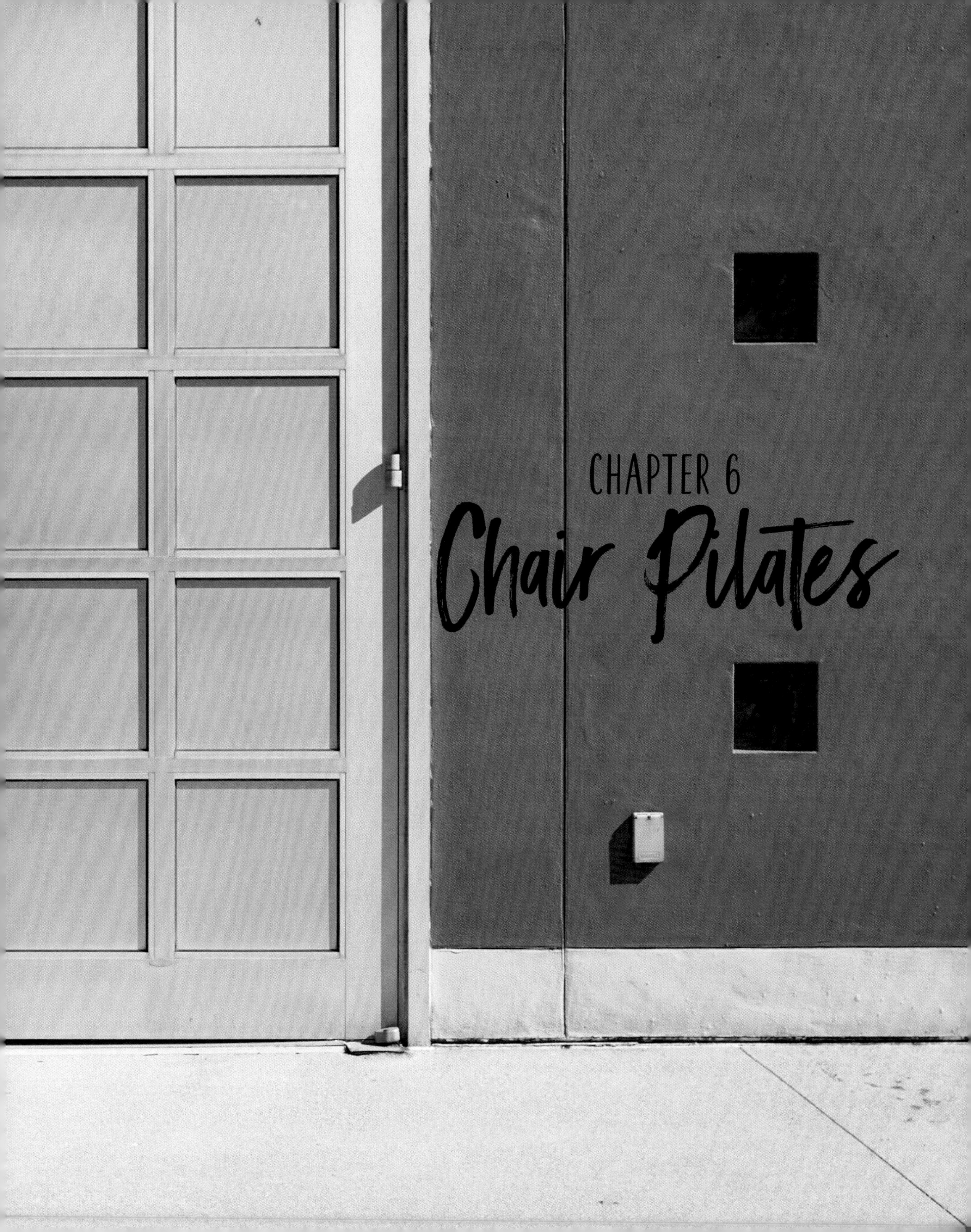

CHAPTER 6
Chair Pilates

Seated Biceps Curls

Performing this exercise works the biceps muscles as well as muscles of the lower arm. Biceps curls can increase your biceps and deltoid strength as well as increase your wrist stability. You use these muscles anytime you pick something up, making this biceps curl a great functional exercise.

1 Sit on the front edge of a chair with your feet flat on the floor. Hold a dumbbell in each hand and relax your arms at your sides, with your palms facing up.

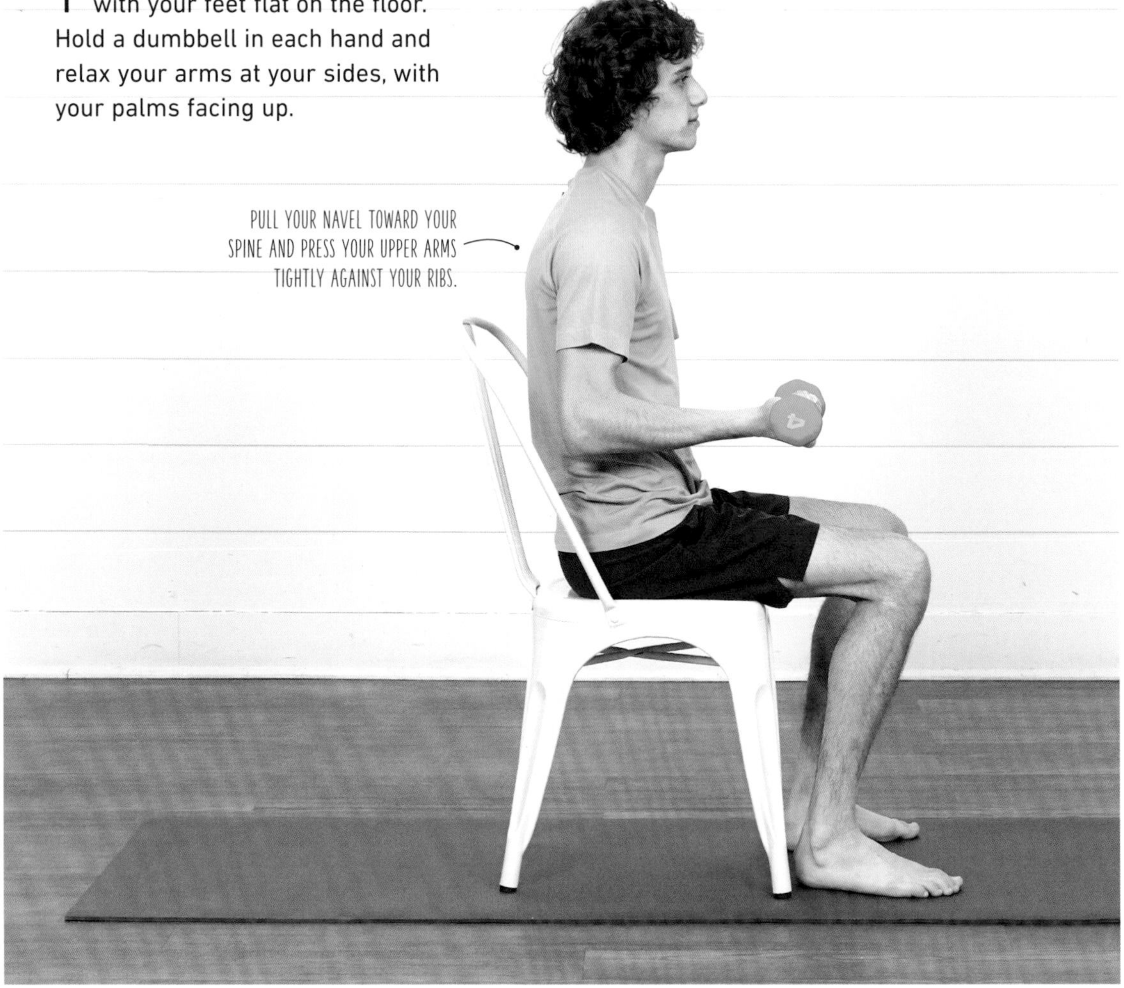

PULL YOUR NAVEL TOWARD YOUR SPINE AND PRESS YOUR UPPER ARMS TIGHTLY AGAINST YOUR RIBS.

2 Bend your elbows and raise the weights toward your shoulders. Reverse your movements to return to your starting position. Perform these steps 5 times.

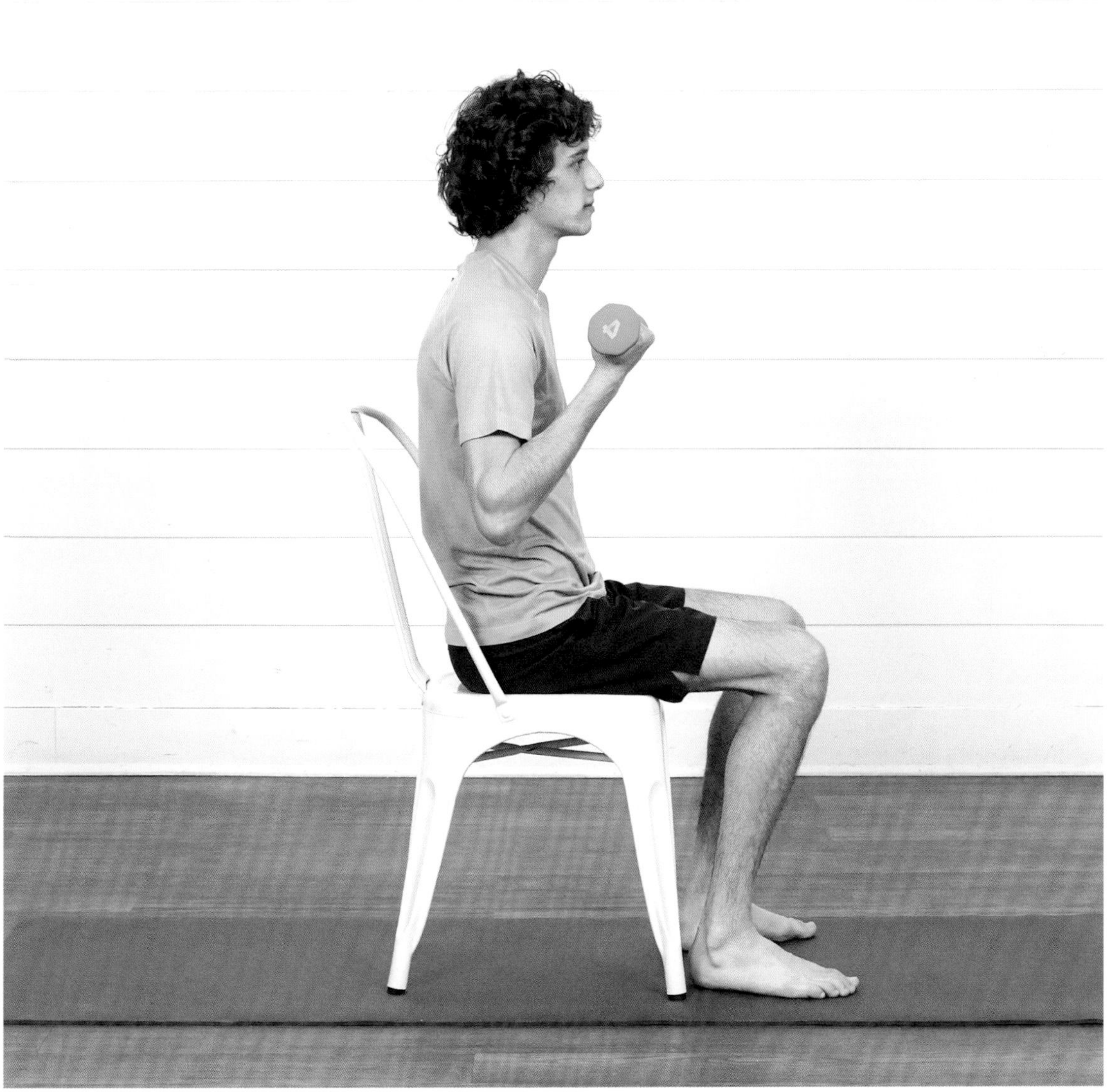

SEATED BICEPS CURLS

VARIATIONS

Facing your palms sideways or using a resistance band requires less muscle recruitment and makes for an excellent modification to help build the strength to perform the traditional exercise. Performing these movements without weights is also less strenuous on the arms.

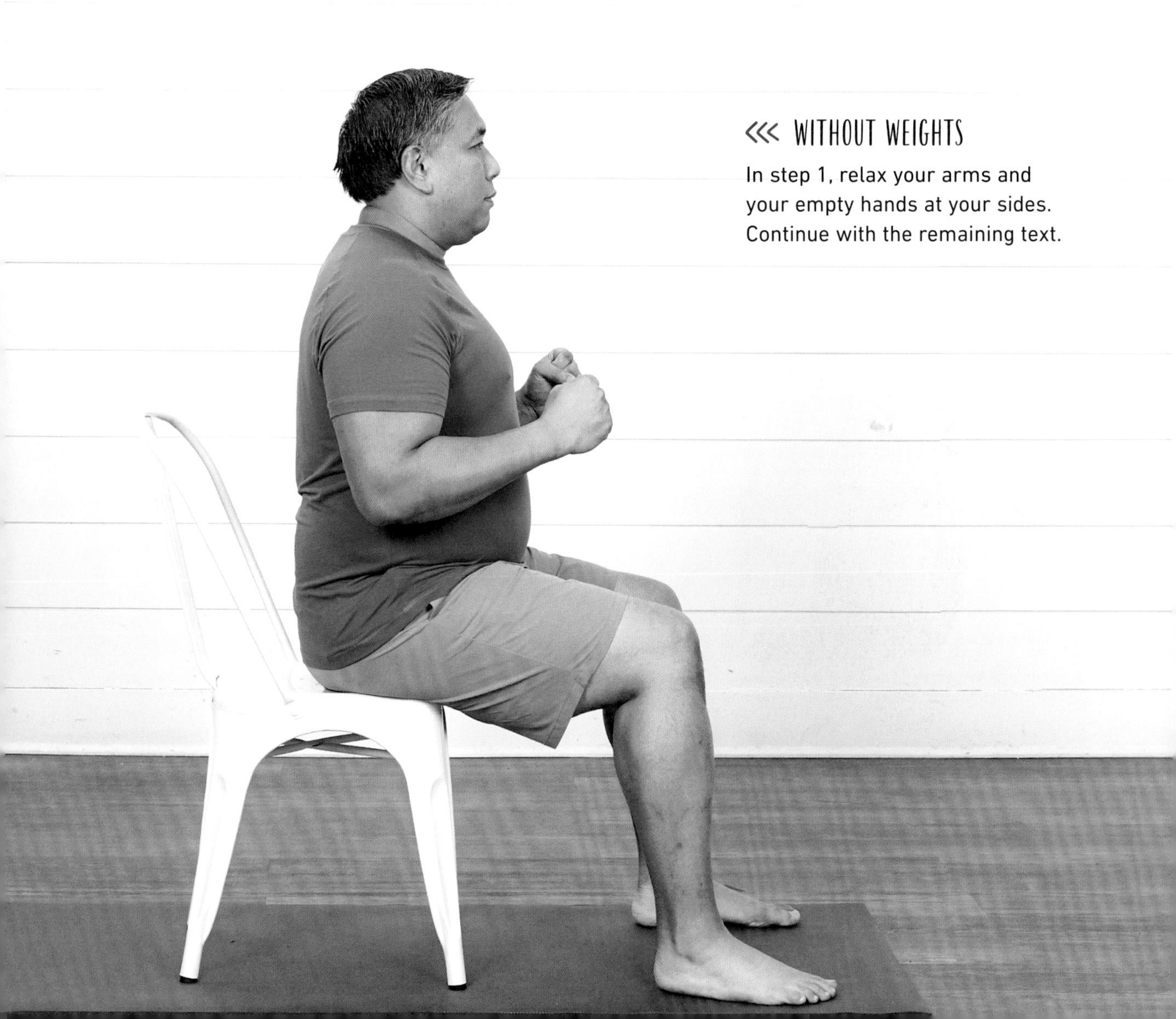

WITHOUT WEIGHTS

In step 1, relax your arms and your empty hands at your sides. Continue with the remaining text.

PALMS FACING IN >>>

In step 1, face your palms toward your legs. Continue with the remaining text.

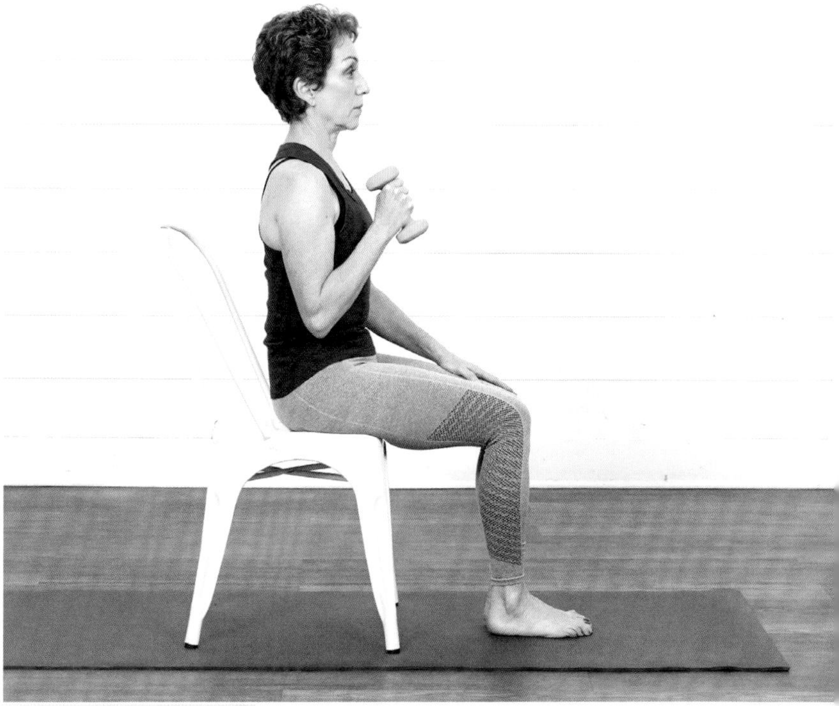

<<< WITH A RESISTANCE BAND

1. Sit in a chair with your legs shoulder width apart. Loop a resistance band under your feet. Hold one end of the band in each hand and face your palms toward your body.

2. Bend your elbows and raise your hands toward your shoulders. Reverse your movements to return to your starting position. Perform these steps 6 times.

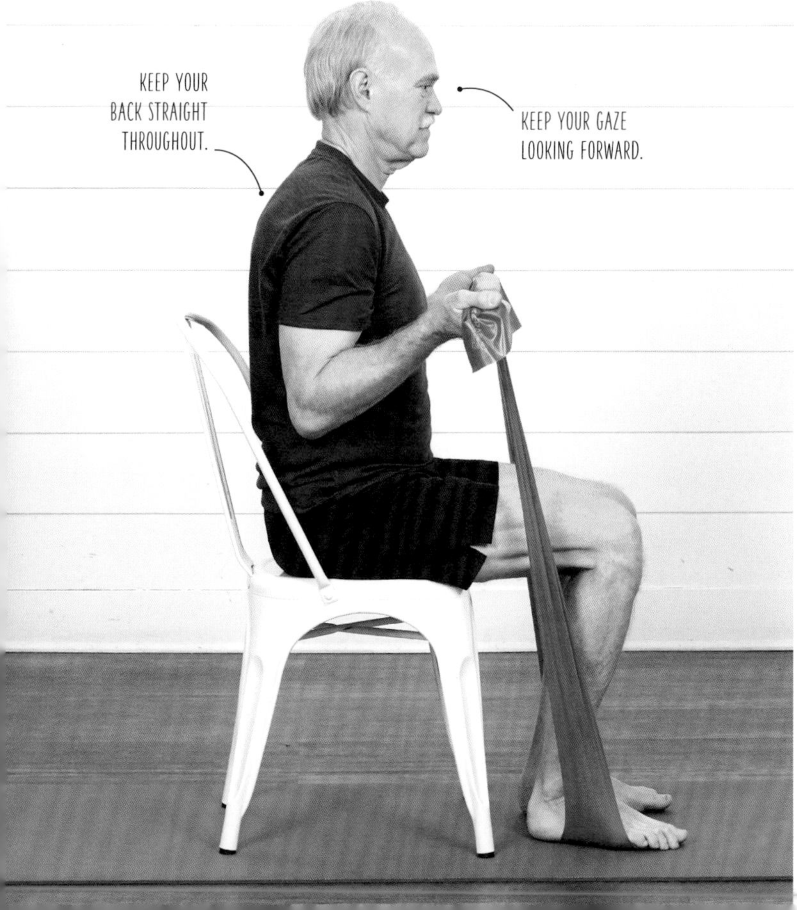

KEEP YOUR BACK STRAIGHT THROUGHOUT.
KEEP YOUR GAZE LOOKING FORWARD.

Seated Push-Ups

Push-ups are great for building upper-body and core strength. Performing push-up movements while sitting can help develop your chest, shoulder, triceps, back, and abdominal muscles as well as offer spinal compression relief.

1 Sit in a chair with your feet flat on the floor and shoulder width apart. Bend your elbows and place your hands on the front edge of the chair. (You can also place your hands on the sides of the chair.)

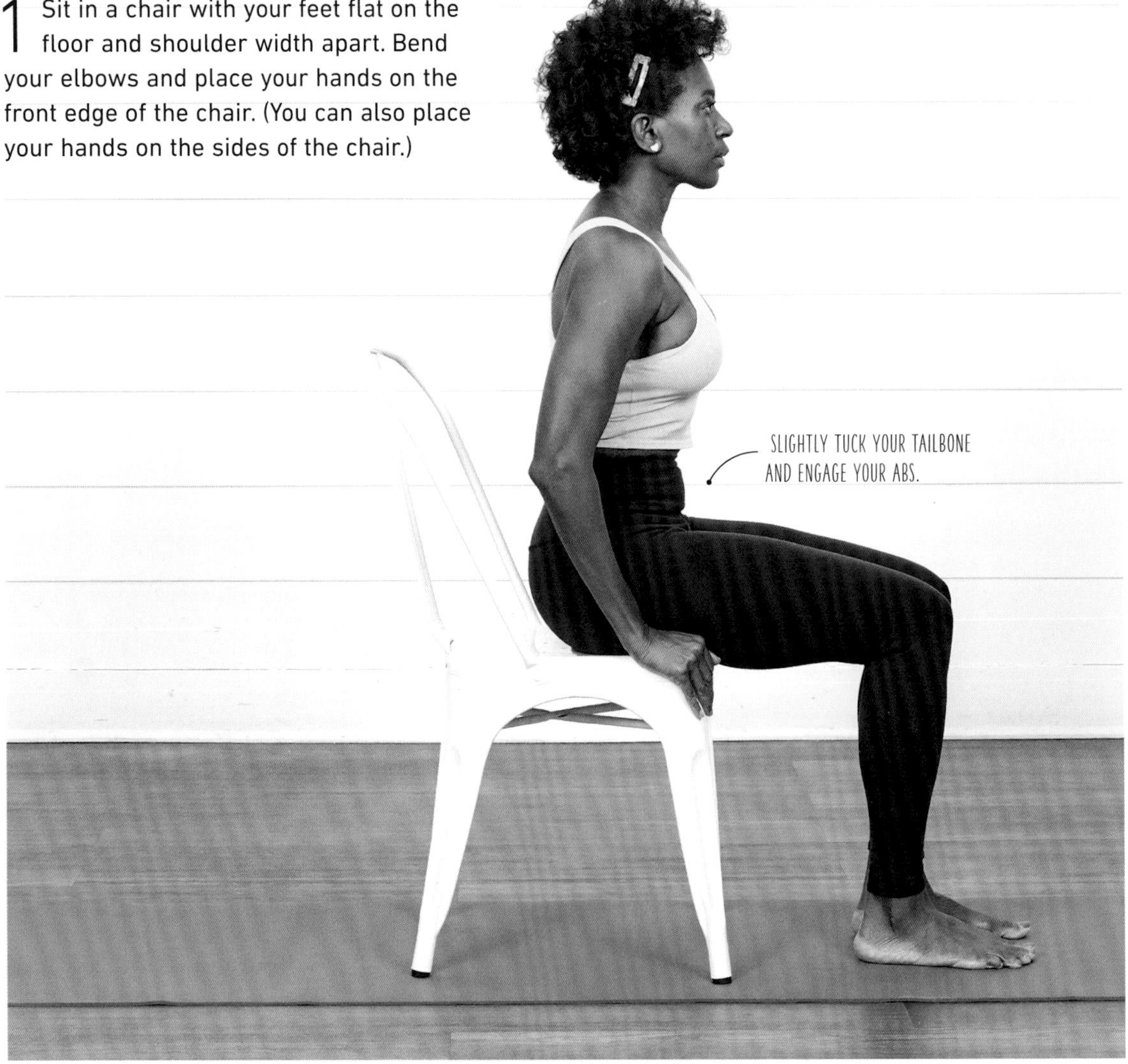
SLIGHTLY TUCK YOUR TAILBONE AND ENGAGE YOUR ABS.

2 Press your hands into the chair, straighten your arms, and raise your glutes off the chair. Reverse your movements to return to your starting position. Perform these steps 6 times.

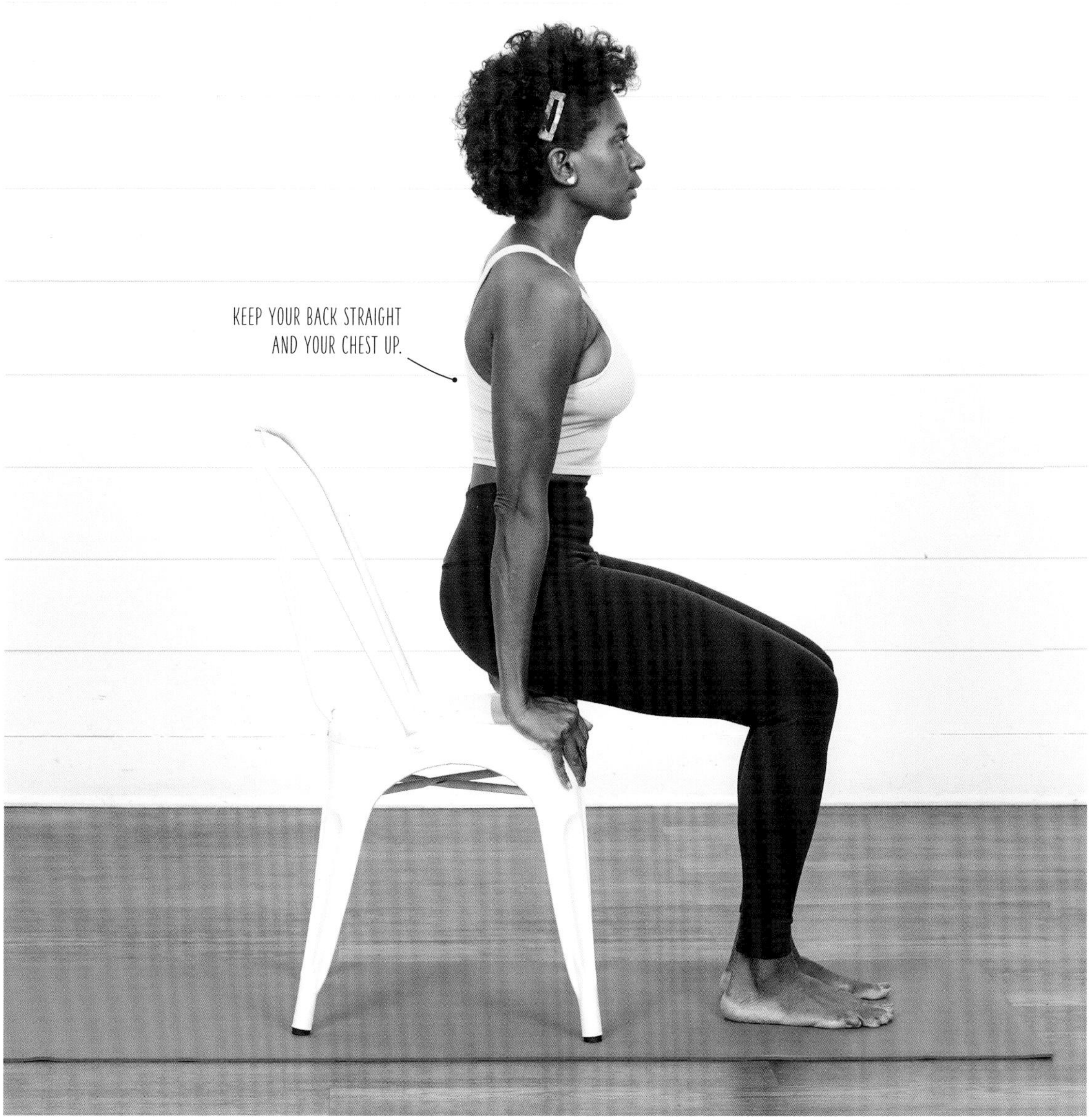

KEEP YOUR BACK STRAIGHT
AND YOUR CHEST UP.

SEATED PUSH-UPS

VARIATIONS

Using a resistance band or a loop band can help you lift your glutes off the chair. Performing this exercise with an isometric hold—muscle engagement without movement—can also help you build strength. These modifications can help you gain the strength required to execute a classic push-up.

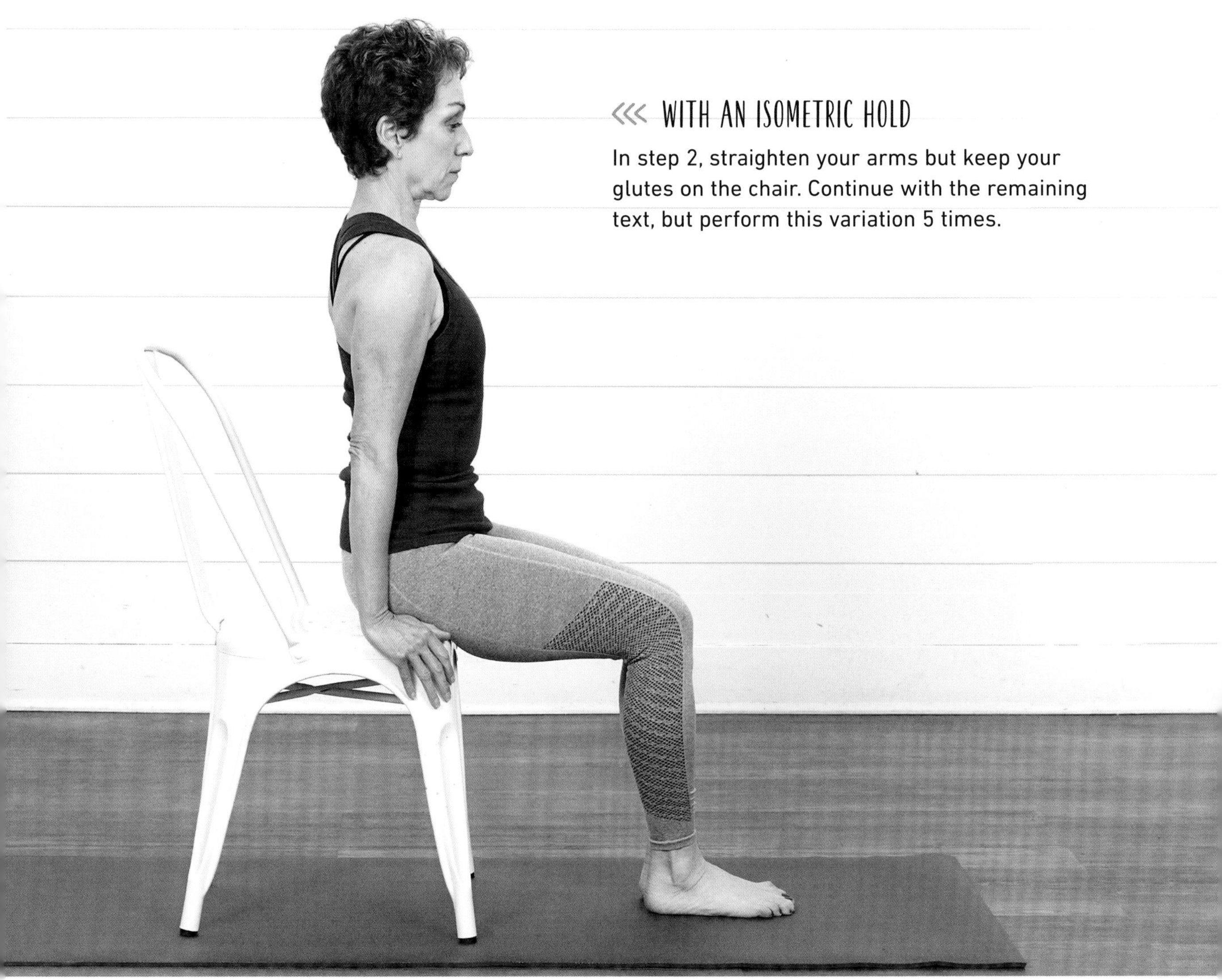

WITH AN ISOMETRIC HOLD

In step 2, straighten your arms but keep your glutes on the chair. Continue with the remaining text, but perform this variation 5 times.

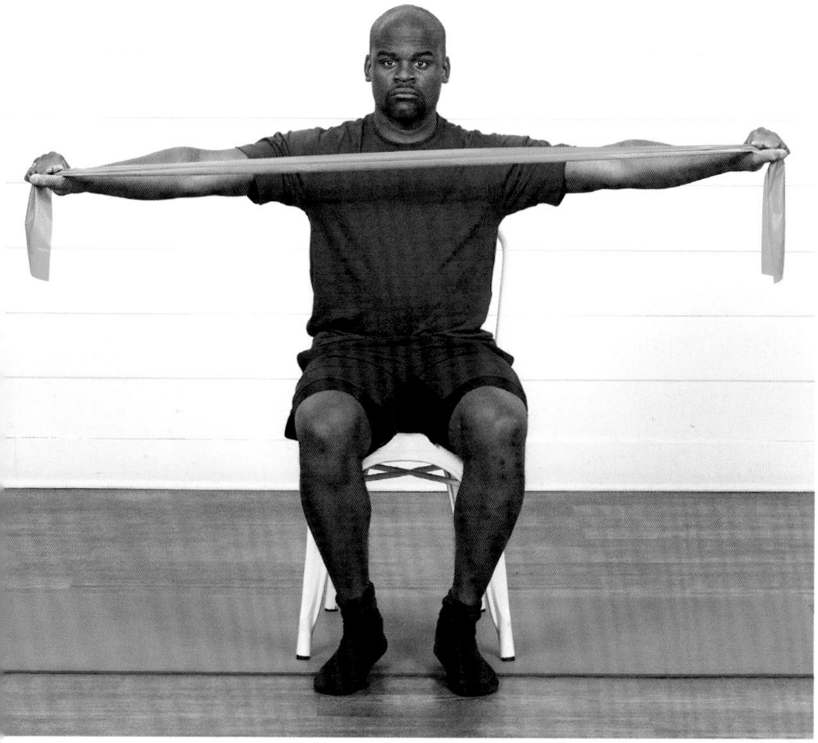

⋘ WITH A RESISTANCE BAND

1. Sit in a chair with your feet flat on the floor and shoulder width apart. Hold a resistance band in your hands at shoulder height.

2. Pull the band as you slowly squeeze your shoulder blades together. Hold for 1 second. Reverse your movements to return to your starting position. Perform these steps 5 times.

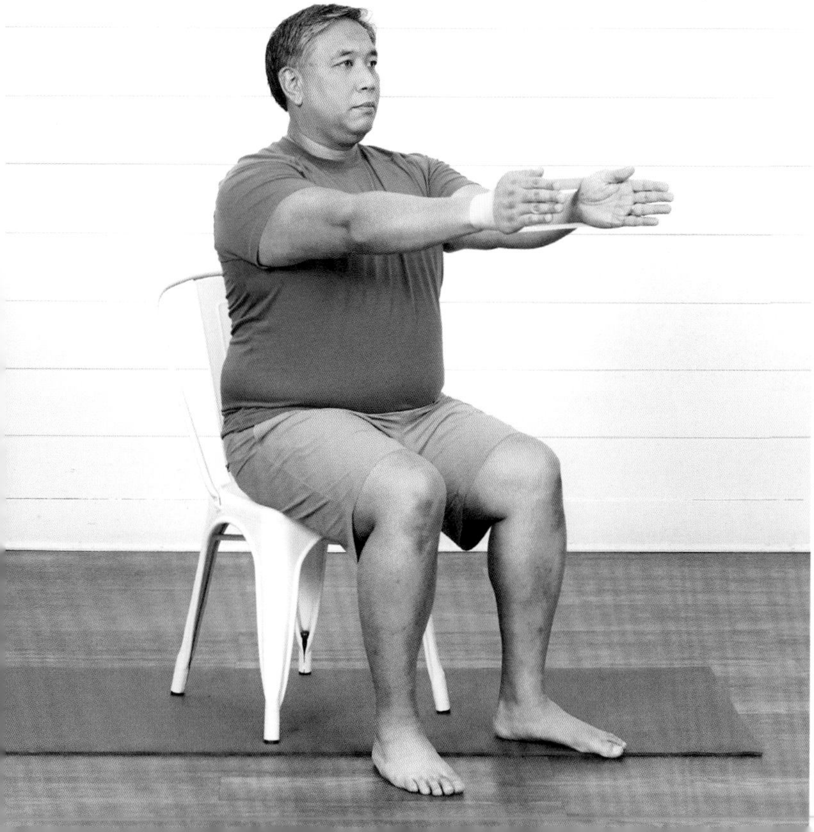

⋘ WITH A LOOP BAND

1. Sit in a chair with your feet flat on the floor and shoulder width apart. Place a loop band around your wrists and rest your arms on your thighs.

2. Extend your arms forward, keeping your glutes on the chair, and press your wrists against the band. Hold this position for 3 to 5 seconds. Reverse your movements to return to your starting position. Perform these steps 5 times.

Seated Swimming

Benefits of this exercise include increased body awareness as well as core, shoulder, back, and arm strength. You can also improve your coordination, posture, and spinal stability. This exercise is great as a warm-up before an upper-body workout.

1 Sit in a chair with your feet flat on the floor and shoulder width apart. Rest your hands on your thighs.

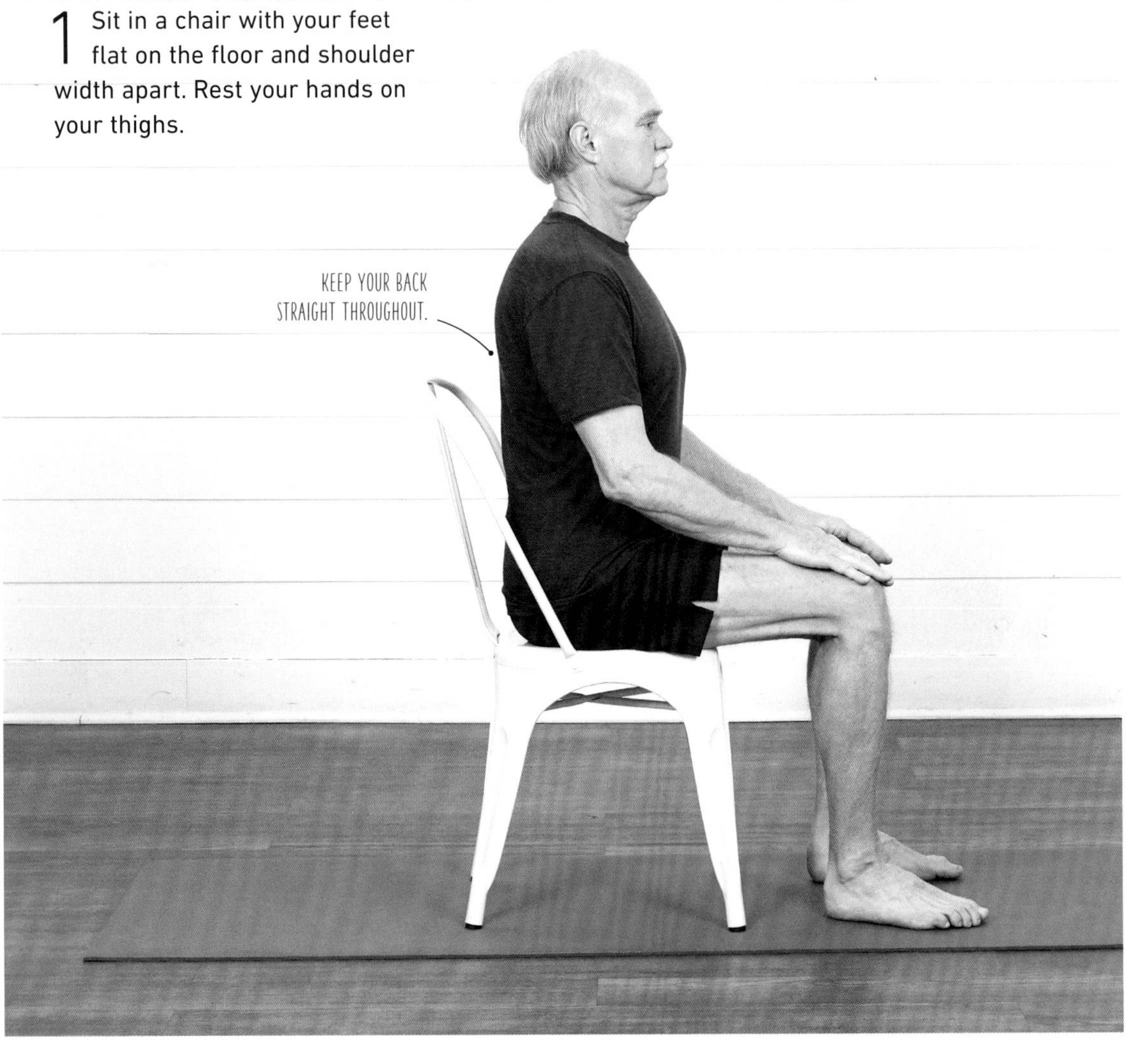
KEEP YOUR BACK STRAIGHT THROUGHOUT.

2 Raise your arms at the sides of your head and extend them toward the ceiling. Flutter your arms in a swimming motion for 10 seconds.

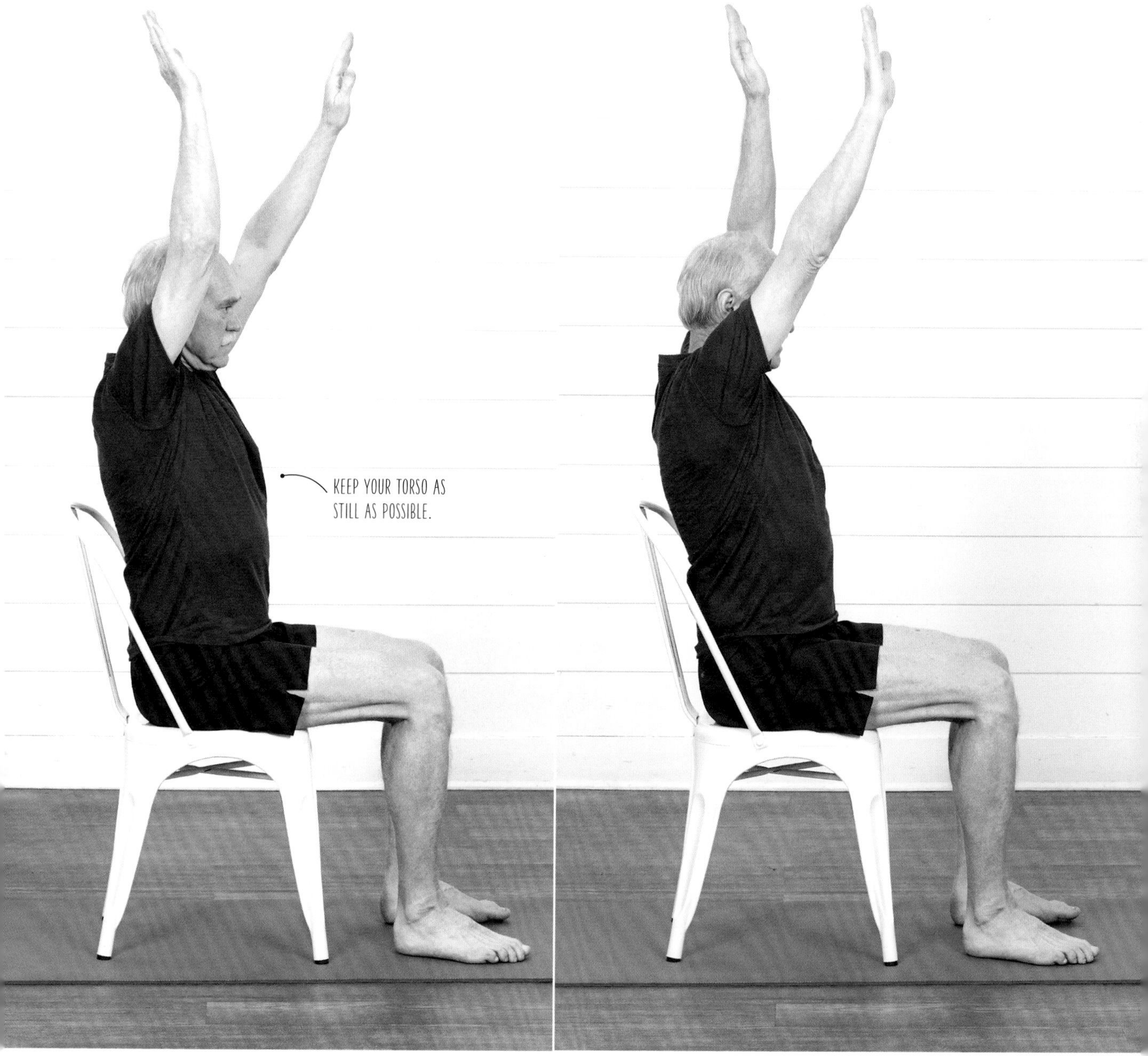
KEEP YOUR TORSO AS STILL AS POSSIBLE.

SEATED SWIMMING

VARIATIONS

Using the Magic Circle can help you engage your core: Squeezing the prop will aid in reducing the lumbar curve of your spine and tightening your abs. The moderate resistance of a loop band can help you develop muscle control and keep your legs and hips aligned properly. If your hamstrings or lower back is inflexible, sitting upright will ease the strain.

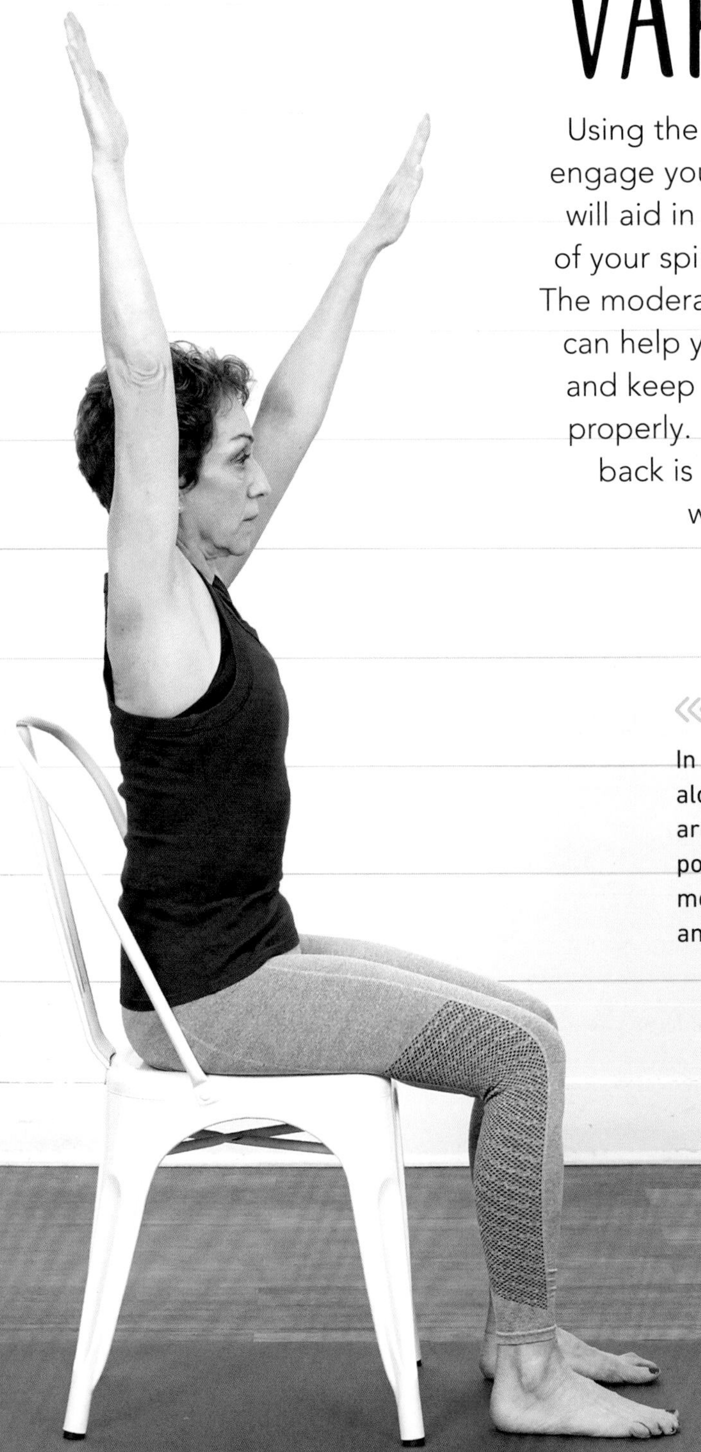

WITH ISOMETRIC HOLD

In step 2, extend your right arm alongside your right ear and your left arm slightly more forward. Hold this position for 3 seconds. Reverse your movements to switch arm positions and hold this position for 3 seconds.

WITH THE MAGIC CIRCLE >>>

In step 1, place the Magic Circle between your legs just above your ankles.

In step 2, squeeze the Magic Circle. Continue with the remaining text.

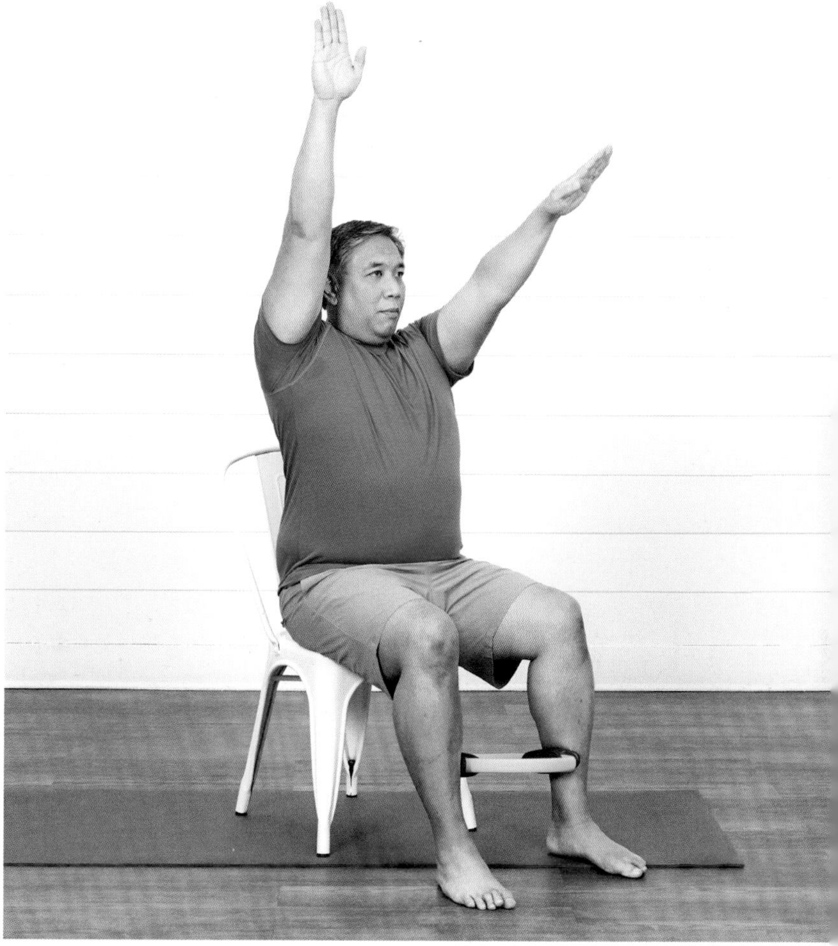

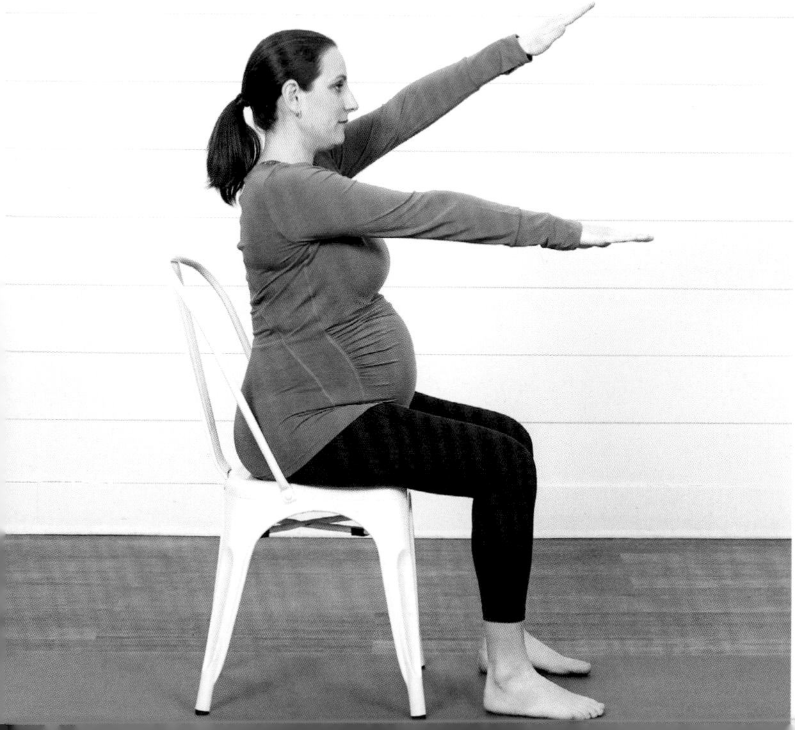

<<< ARMS AT SHOULDER HEIGHT

In step 2, raise your arms to shoulder height and parallel with the floor. Continue with the remaining text.

Seated Hundred

Performing these movements warms up the body, increases body awareness, and helps develop your ability to stabilize your core with added movement. This exercise can help strengthen your abdominal, back, arm, and shoulder muscles. Plus, it might help improve your posture, breath control, and spinal stability.

1 Sit in a chair with your legs shoulder width apart and your feet flat on the floor. Lean your upper body slightly forward and extend your arms forward at shoulder height, with your hands facing down.

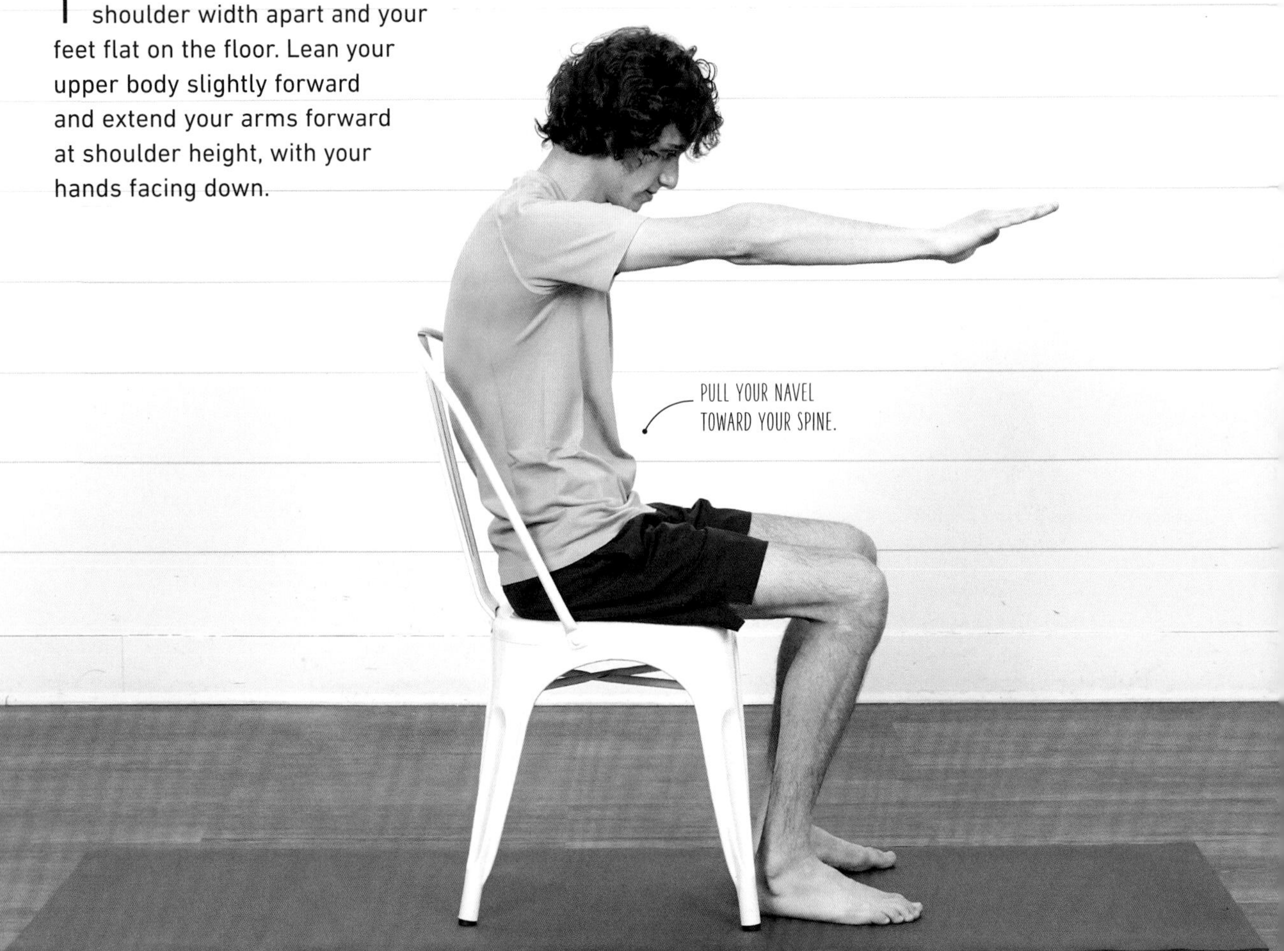
PULL YOUR NAVEL TOWARD YOUR SPINE.

2 Pulse your arms up and down as you inhale for 5 seconds and exhale for 5 seconds. Perform this step 5 times.

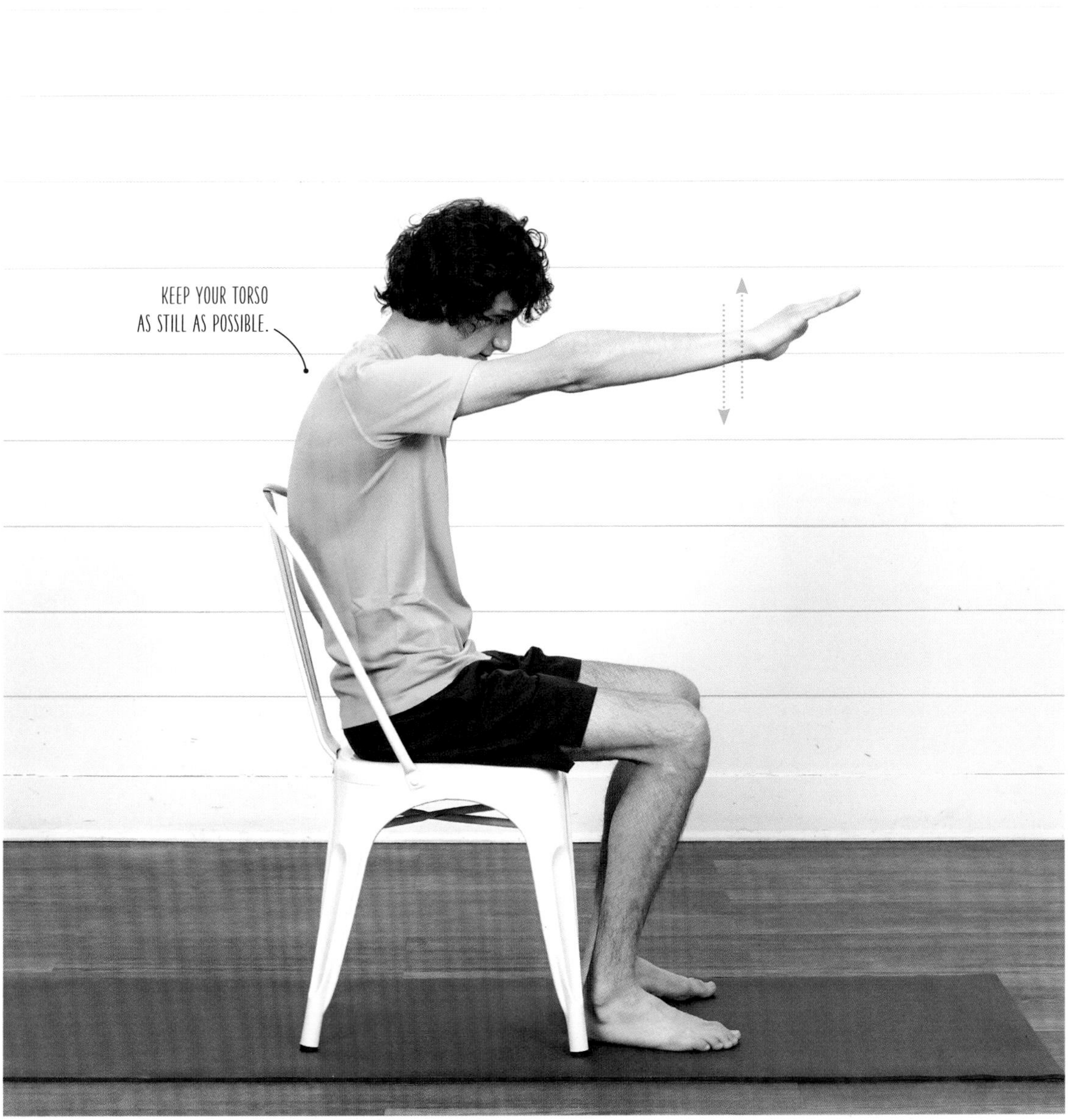
KEEP YOUR TORSO AS STILL AS POSSIBLE.

SEATED HUNDRED

VARIATIONS

Using the Magic Circle can help you engage your core as well as aid in reducing the lumbar curve of your spine and tighten your abs. The moderate resistance of a loop band can help you develop muscle control and keep your legs and hips aligned properly. If your hamstrings or lower back is inflexible, sitting upright will ease the strain.

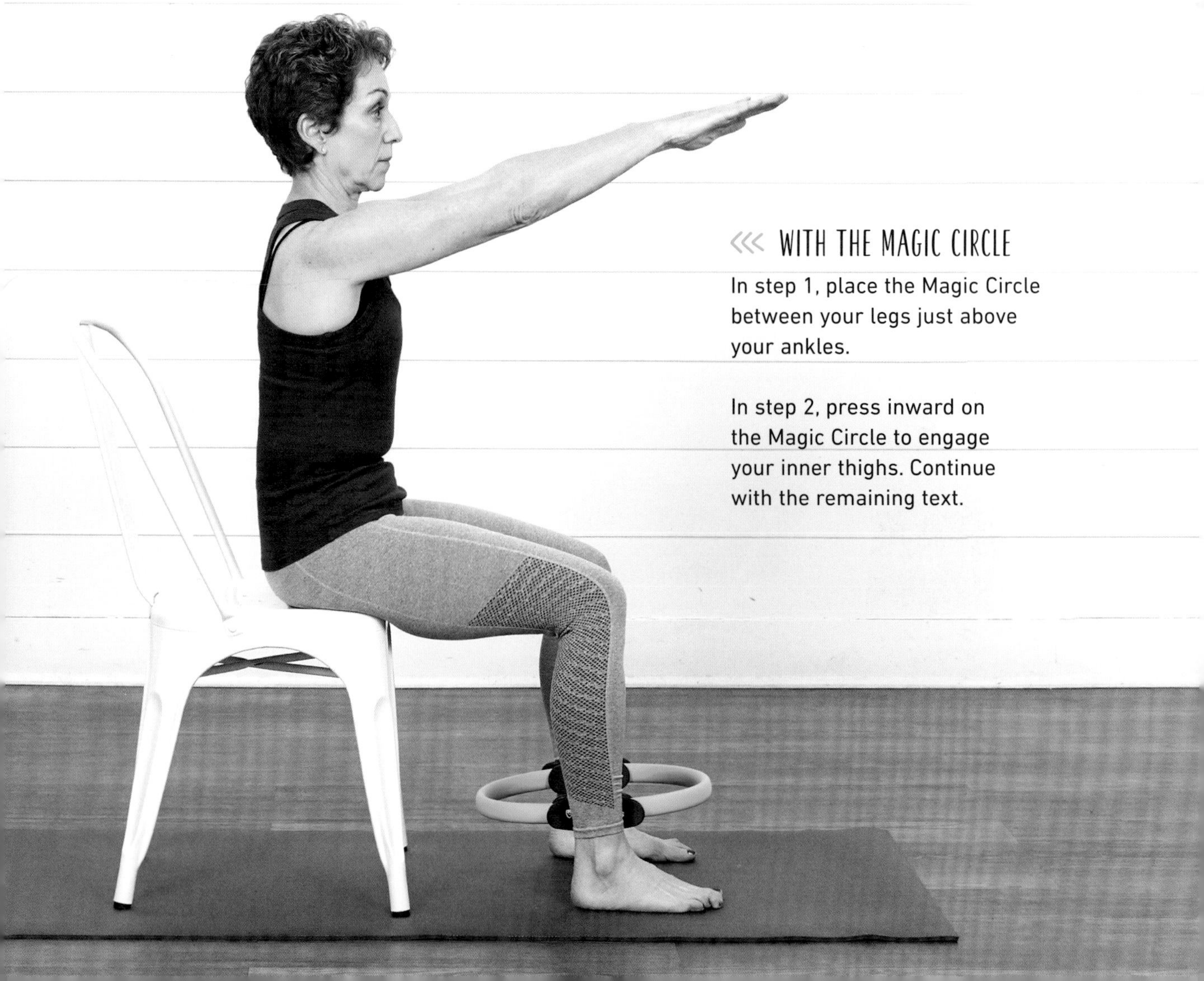

WITH THE MAGIC CIRCLE

In step 1, place the Magic Circle between your legs just above your ankles.

In step 2, press inward on the Magic Circle to engage your inner thighs. Continue with the remaining text.

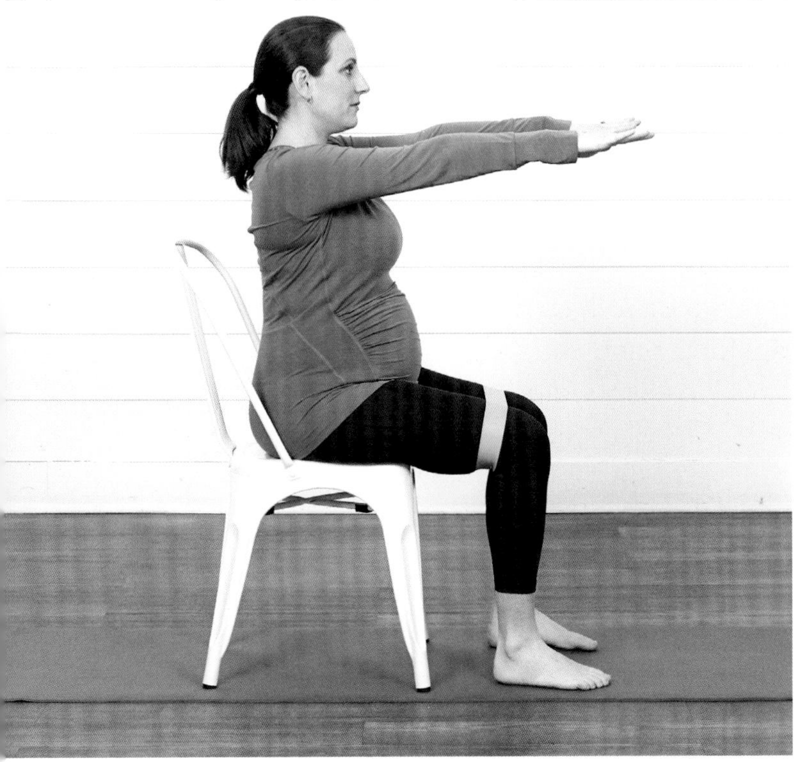

WITH A LOOP BAND

In step 1, place a loop band around your thighs just above your knees.

In step 2, press outward on the band to engage your outer thighs. Continue with the remaining text.

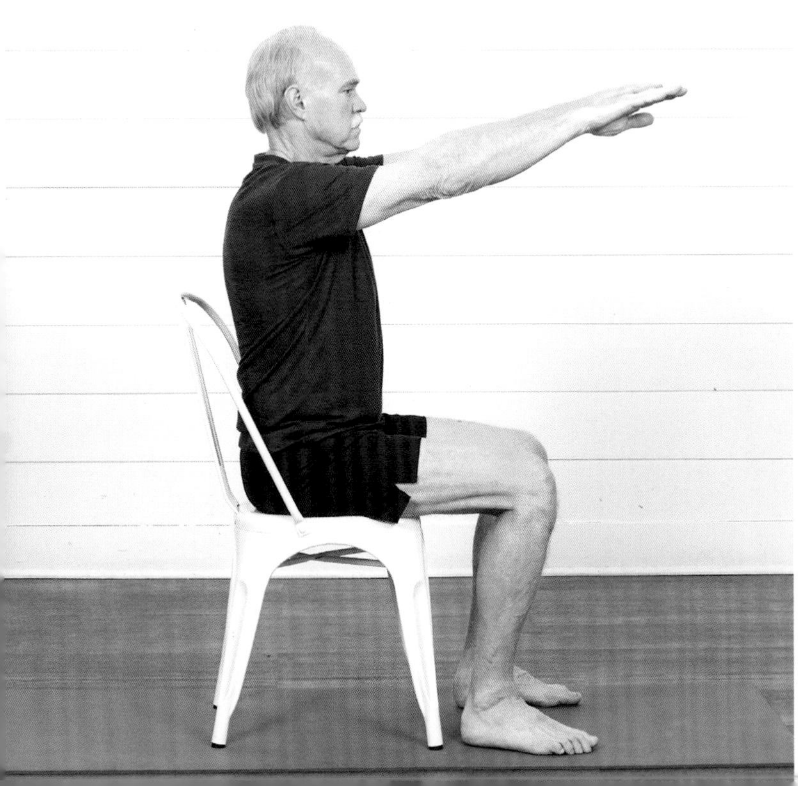

SITTING UPRIGHT

In step 1, keep your back straight. Continue with the remaining text.

Seated Criss-Cross

With a focus on your external obliques, this exercise works your entire abdominal wall. Your obliques play a major role in posture, trunk flexion (bending forward), and rotation (twisting to one side). Strengthening these muscles can help define your waistline and stabilize your spine.

1 Sit in a chair with your legs shoulder width apart and your feet flat on the floor. Place your hands behind your head, keeping your elbows slightly in front of your shoulders.

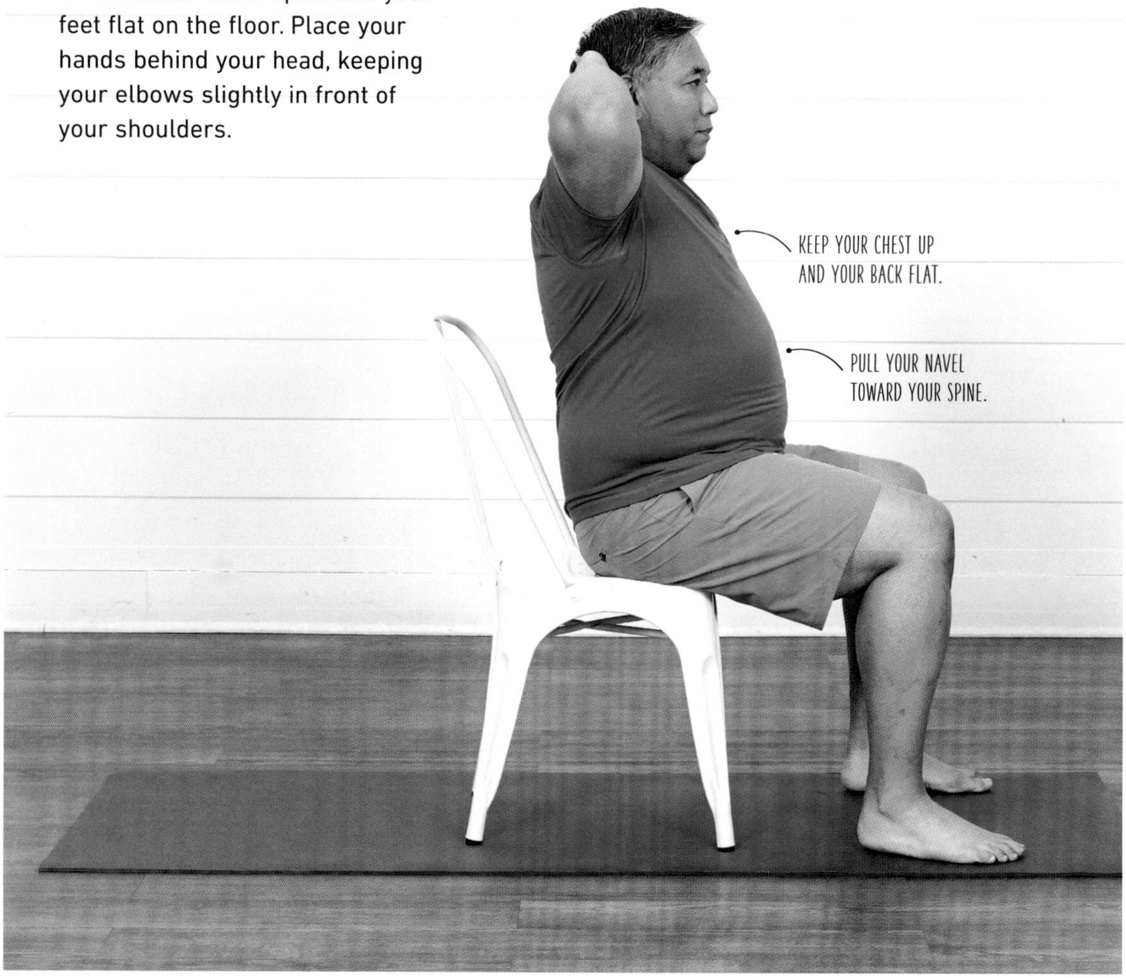
KEEP YOUR CHEST UP AND YOUR BACK FLAT.
PULL YOUR NAVEL TOWARD YOUR SPINE.

2 Raise your left foot and exhale as you simultaneously rotate your torso to your left. Inhale as you reverse your movements to return to your starting position.

3 Raise your right foot and exhale as you simultaneously rotate your torso to your right. Inhale as you reverse your movements to return to your starting position. Perform these steps 10 times.

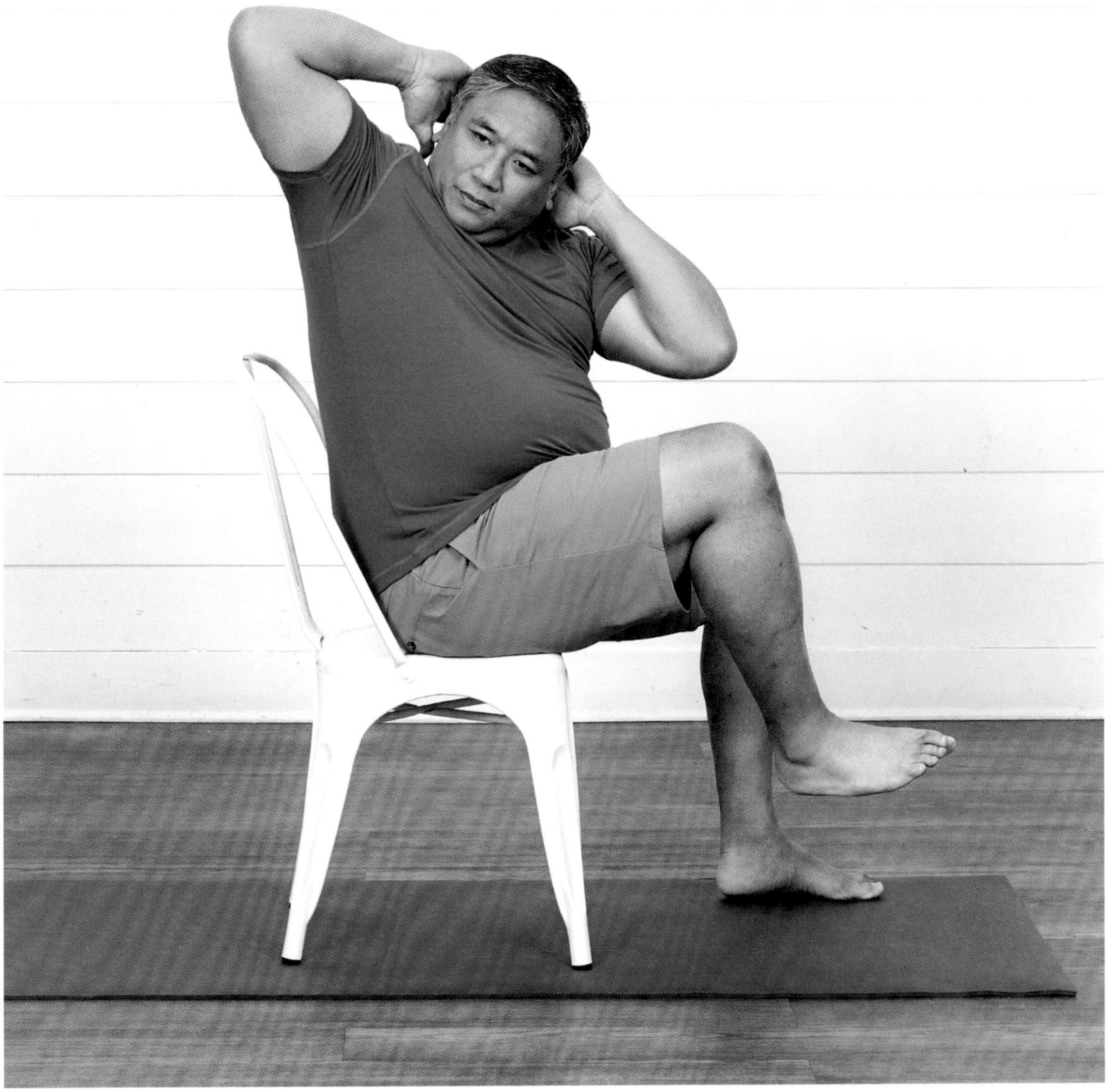

SEATED CRISS-CROSS

VARIATIONS

Keeping your feet on the floor when doing this exercise gives you lower body stability and requires less core activation. Sitting with your back against a wall can also provide upper body stability and back support.

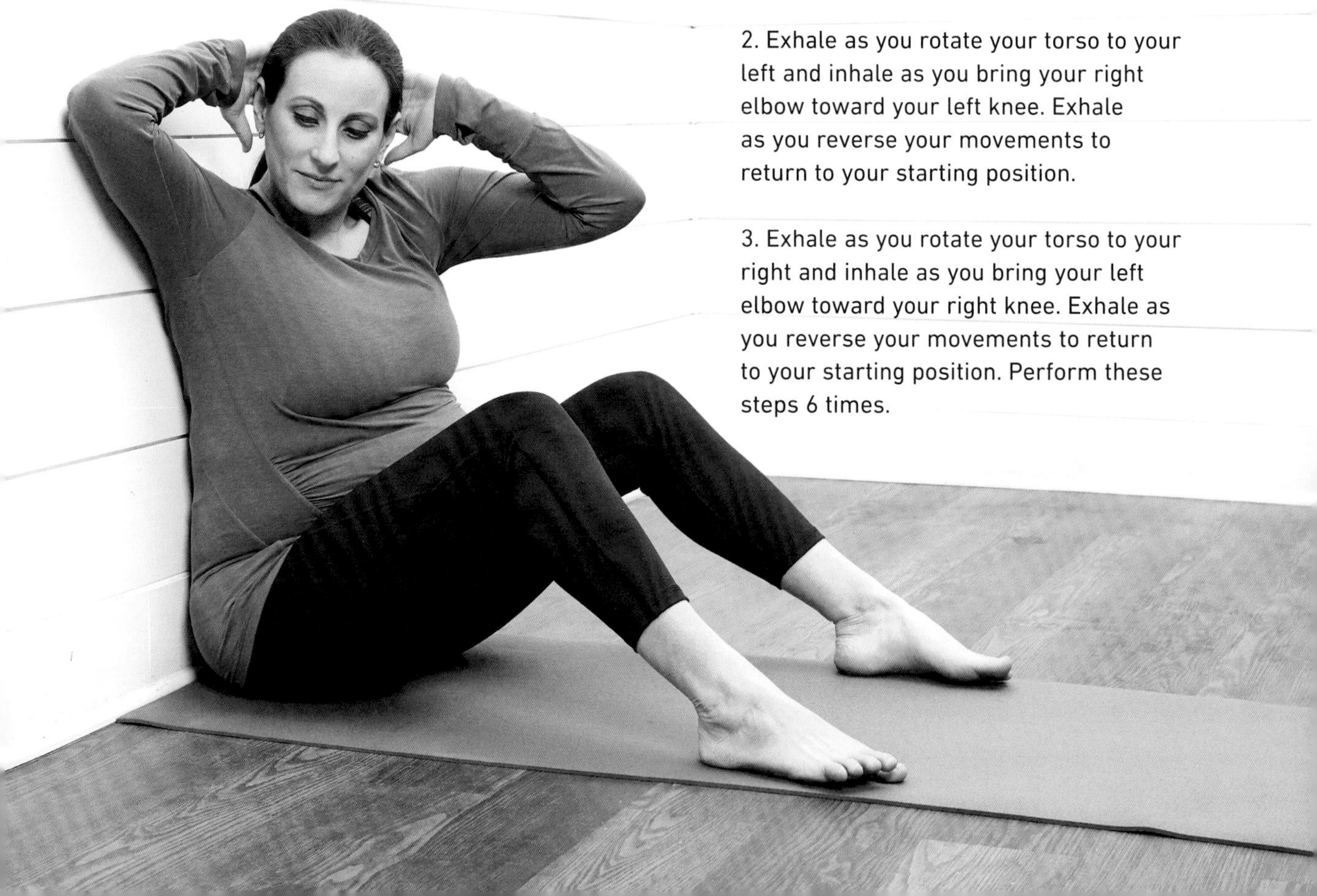

AGAINST THE WALL

1. Sit on the floor with your back against a wall. Bend your knees and place your feet flat on the floor and shoulder width apart. Place your hands behind your head, keeping your elbows slightly in front of your shoulders.

2. Exhale as you rotate your torso to your left and inhale as you bring your right elbow toward your left knee. Exhale as you reverse your movements to return to your starting position.

3. Exhale as you rotate your torso to your right and inhale as you bring your left elbow toward your right knee. Exhale as you reverse your movements to return to your starting position. Perform these steps 6 times.

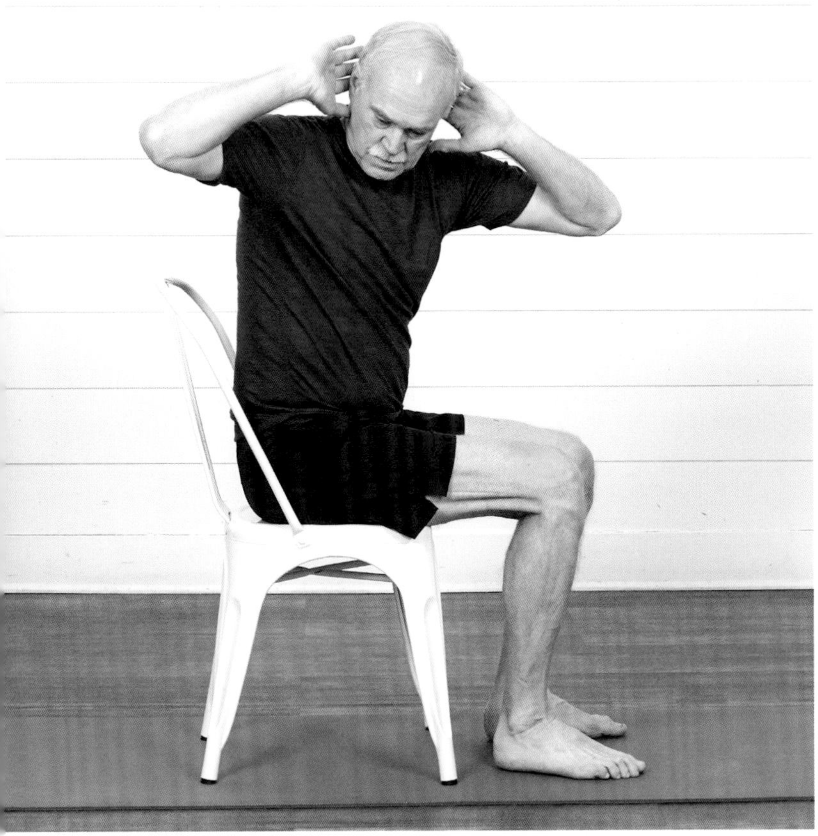

WITH FEET ON THE FLOOR

In steps 2 and 3, keep your feet flat on the floor. Continue with the remaining text.

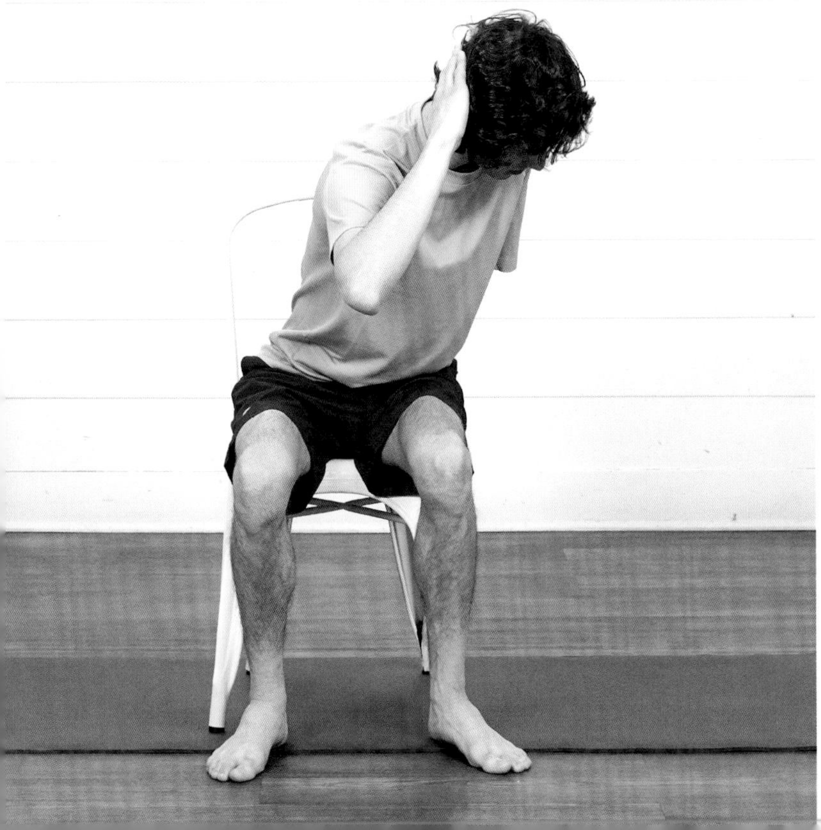

ONE ARM AT A TIME

In step 1, place your right hand behind your head with your elbow slightly in front of your shoulders.

In step 2, exhale as you rotate your right shoulder to your left side. Inhale as you bring your right elbow toward your left knee. Exhale as you reverse your movements to return to your starting position.

In step 3, exhale as you rotate your left shoulder to your right side. Inhale as you bring your left elbow toward your right knee. Exhale as you reverse your movements to return to your starting position. Perform these steps 3 times.

Seated Teaser

Fly like an arrow in this pose designed to strengthen your back muscles and stretch those muscles at the front of your body. These movements can also open the tight muscles of your quads and shoulders as well as stretch your abs.

1 Sit in a chair with your legs shoulder width apart and your feet flat on the floor. Extend your arms toward the ceiling.

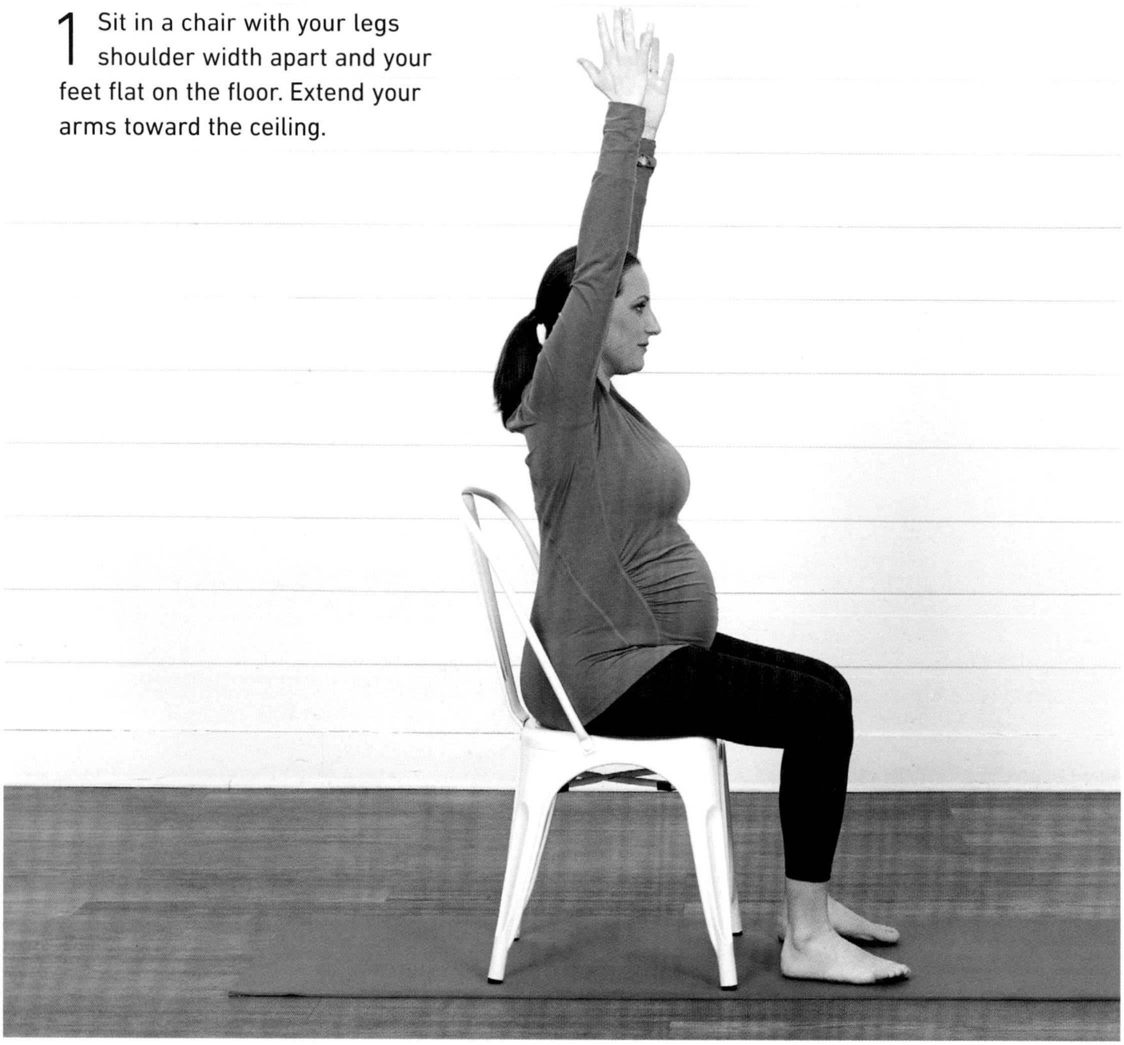

2 Raise your legs until they're parallel with the floor. Curl your chin toward your chest and round your back while lowering your arms to almost parallel with your legs. Reverse your movements to return to your starting position. Perform these steps 5 times.

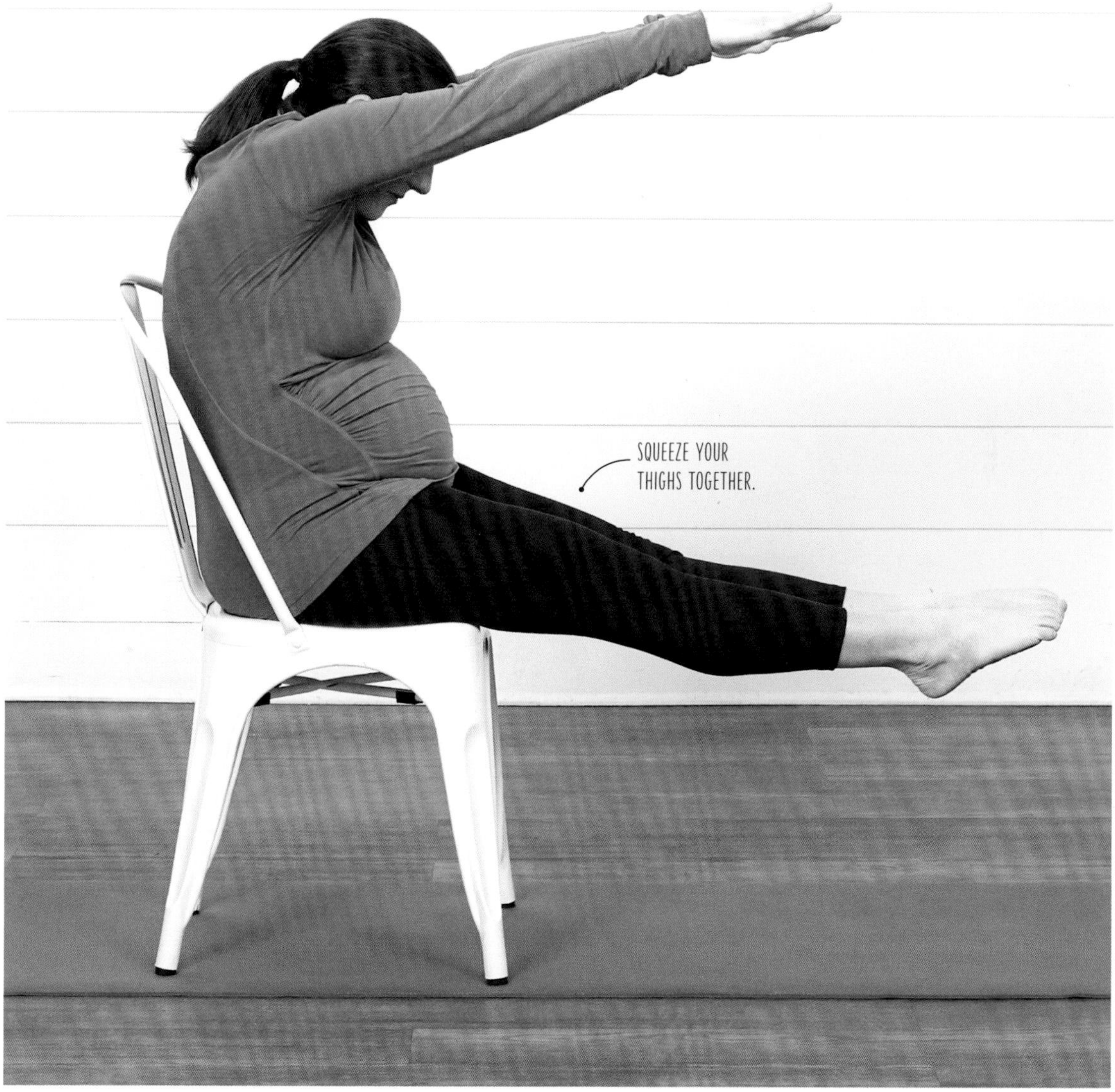
SQUEEZE YOUR
THIGHS TOGETHER.

SEATED TEASER

VARIATIONS

If you have trouble lifting both legs simultaneously, the single-leg or isometric variation is an effective modification. Using a small Pilates ball can also help you establish the core connection required to perform the movements.

WITH ONE LEG

1. Sit in a chair with your legs together and your feet flat on the floor. Extend your arms toward the ceiling.

2. Raise your right leg until parallel with the floor. Curl your chin toward your chest and round your back while you lower your right arm to parallel with your legs. Reverse your movements to return to your starting position.

3. Raise your left leg until parallel with the floor. Curl your chin toward your chest and round your back while you lower your left arm to parallel with your legs. Reverse your movements to return to your starting position. Perform these steps 6 times.

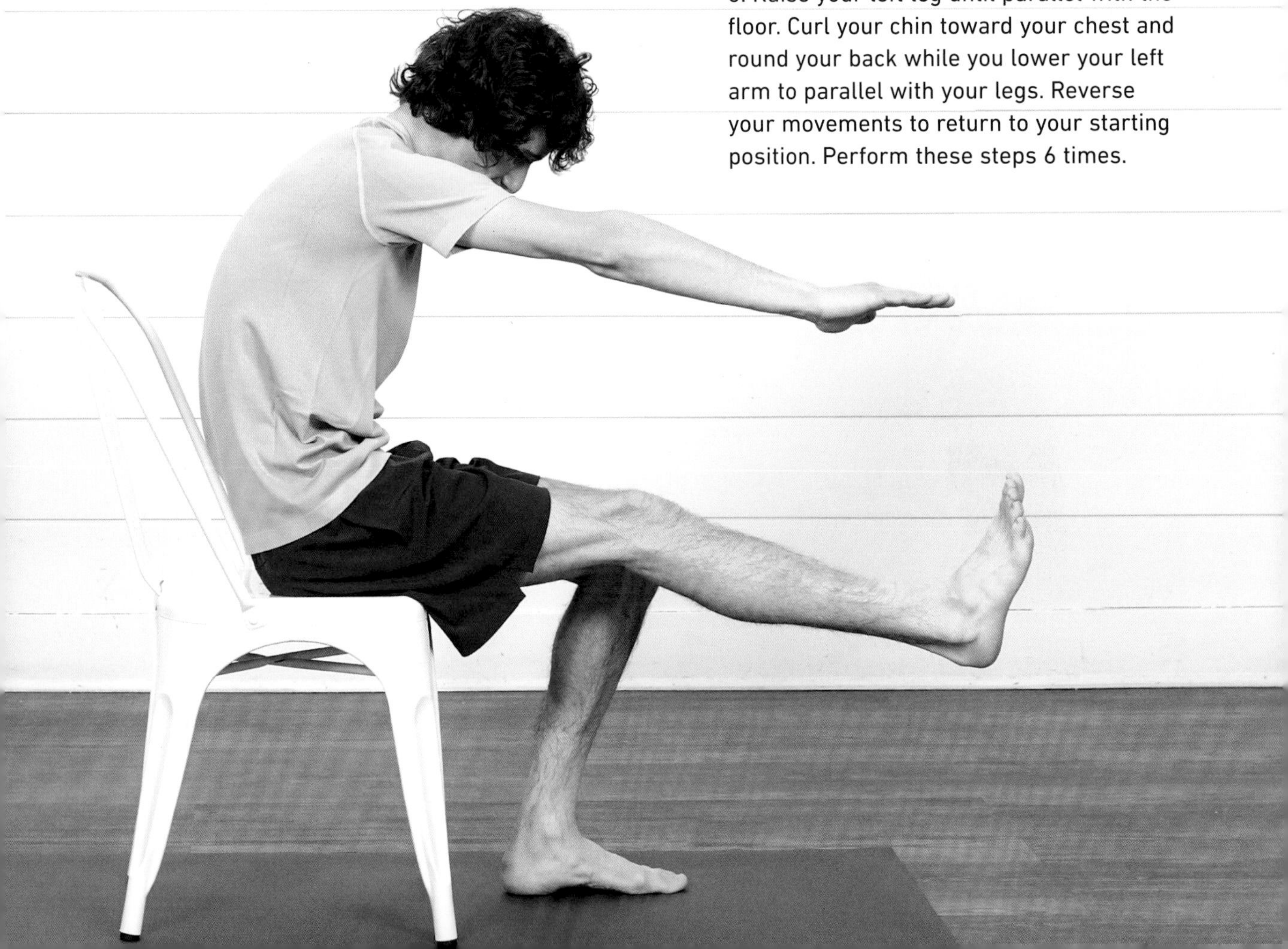

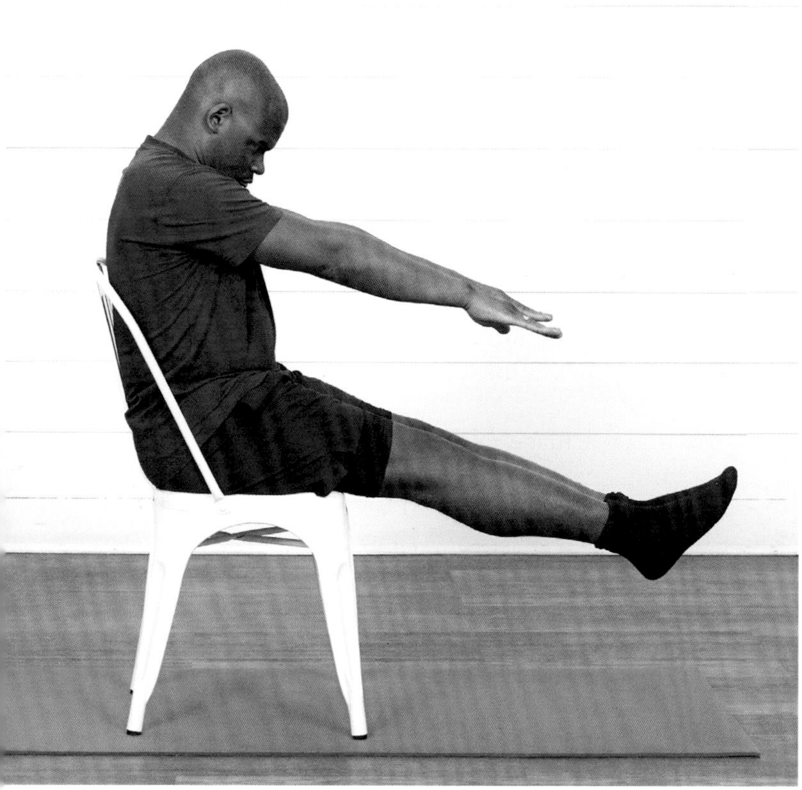

⋘ WITH AN ISOMETRIC HOLD

In steps 2 and 3 of the variation on page 226, raise one leg at a time and hold for 3 seconds. Continue with the remaining text.

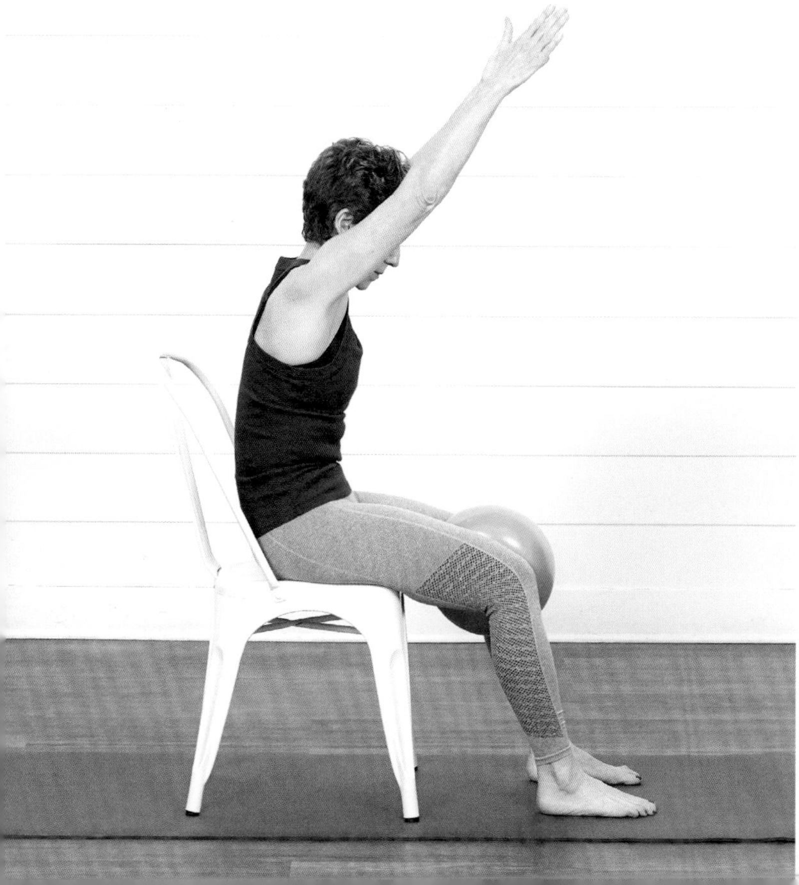

⋘ WITH A SMALL PILATES BALL

In step 1, place a small Pilates ball between your legs just above your knees.

In step 2, squeeze the ball as you bring your chin toward your chest and round your back. Continue with the remaining text.

Seated Leg Lifts

These movements will work your hip flexors, quadriceps, abs, and inner and outer thigh muscles. Performing this exercise while seated can help you strengthen your core as well as improve your spinal stability and posture. This exercise can also act as a warm-up for a lower-body workout.

1 Sit on the front edge of a chair with your legs shoulder width apart and your feet flat on the floor. Place your hands on the sides or the arms of the chair.

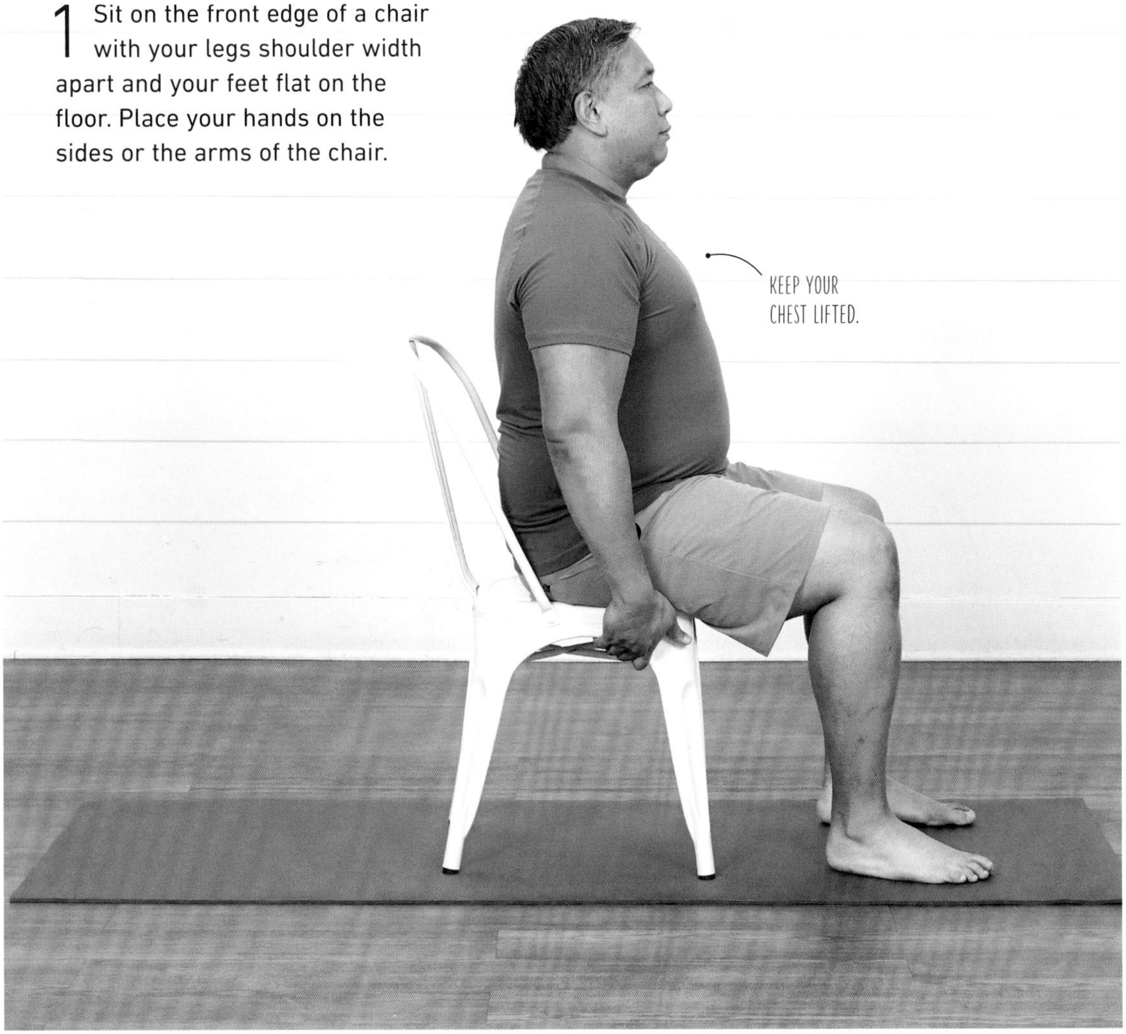

2 Extend your right leg forward until parallel with the floor and flex your right foot toward your body. Reverse your movements to lower your right foot toward the floor, but before your heel touches the floor, raise your right leg again. Perform this action 6 times. Repeat these steps with your left leg extended.

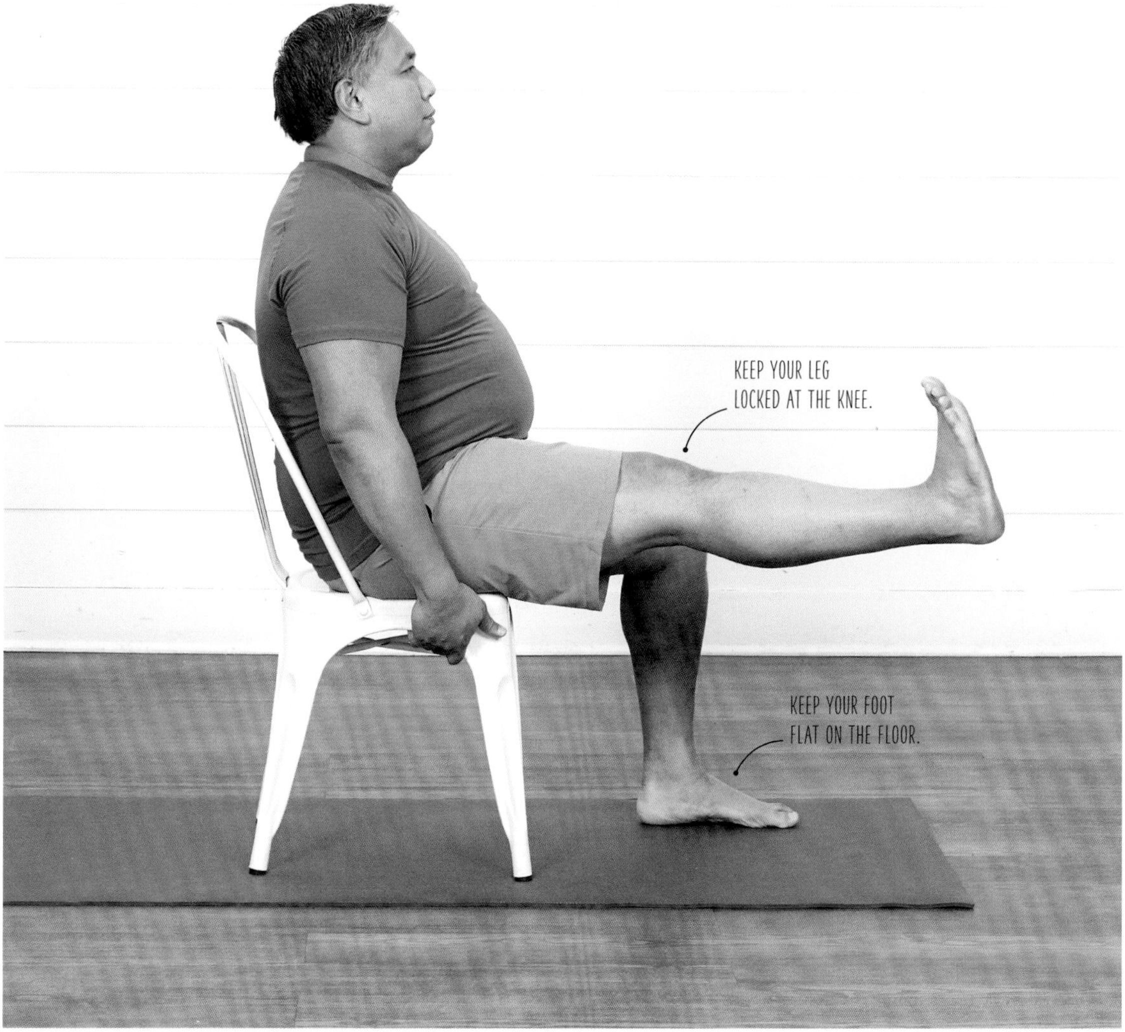
KEEP YOUR LEG
LOCKED AT THE KNEE.
KEEP YOUR FOOT
FLAT ON THE FLOOR.

SEATED LEG LIFTS

VARIATIONS

If you've had a knee injury or any kind of knee issue and you're unable to fully straighten either leg, keeping your knee bent while seated in a chair or against a wall might prove beneficial. Bending your knees can also help if you have weak hip flexors or quadriceps or you lack core strength.

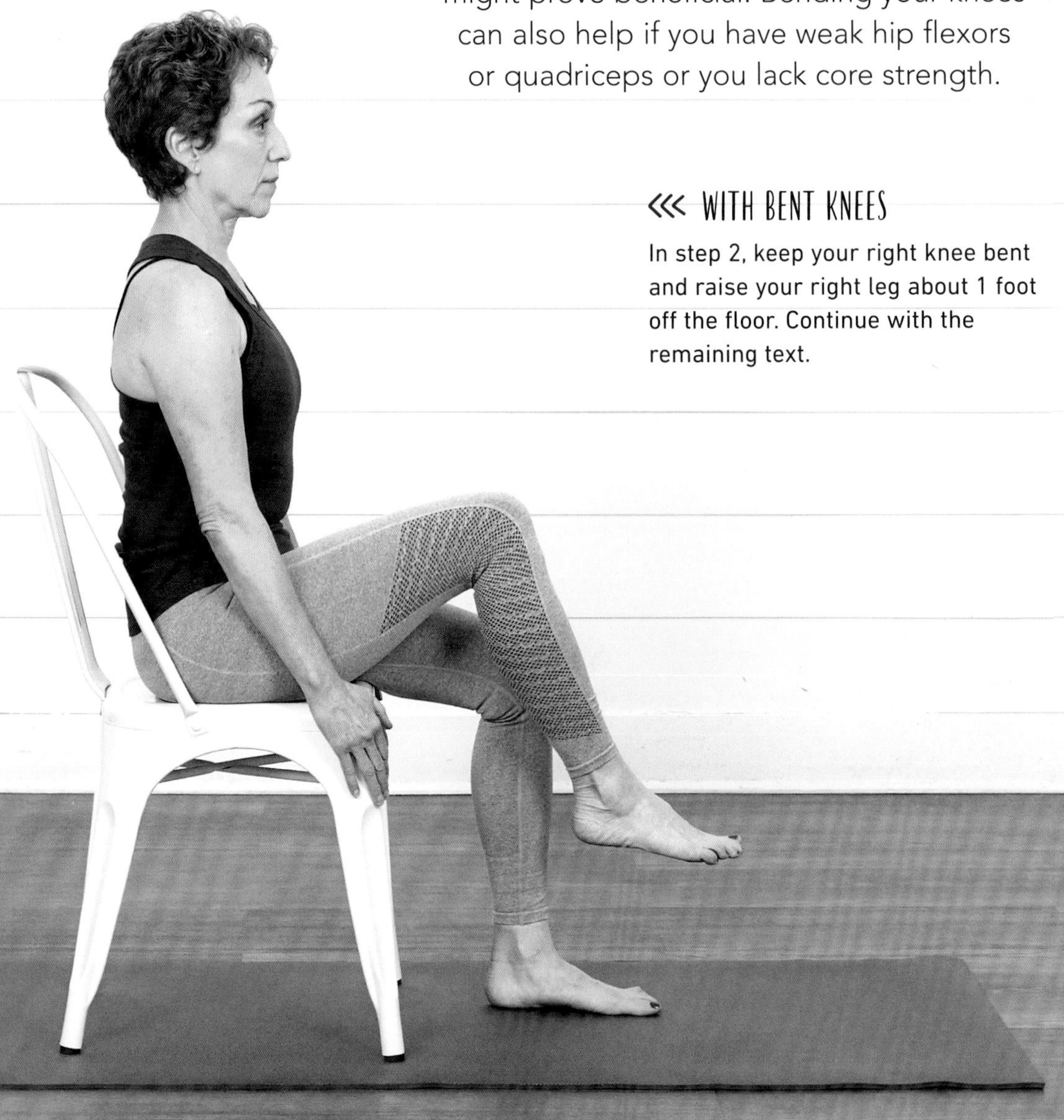

‹‹‹ WITH BENT KNEES

In step 2, keep your right knee bent and raise your right leg about 1 foot off the floor. Continue with the remaining text.

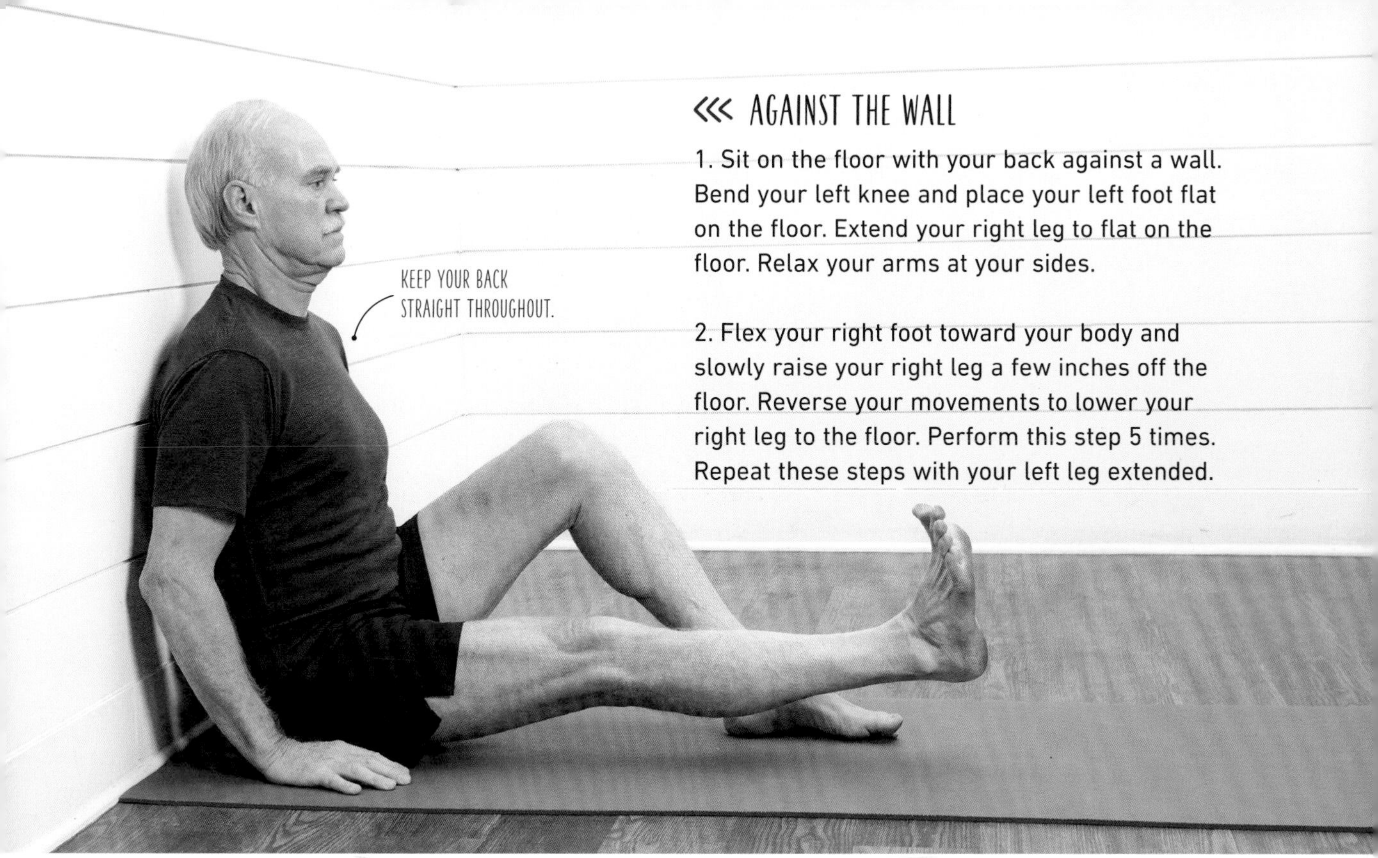
KEEP YOUR BACK STRAIGHT THROUGHOUT.

AGAINST THE WALL

1. Sit on the floor with your back against a wall. Bend your left knee and place your left foot flat on the floor. Extend your right leg to flat on the floor. Relax your arms at your sides.

2. Flex your right foot toward your body and slowly raise your right leg a few inches off the floor. Reverse your movements to lower your right leg to the floor. Perform this step 5 times. Repeat these steps with your left leg extended.

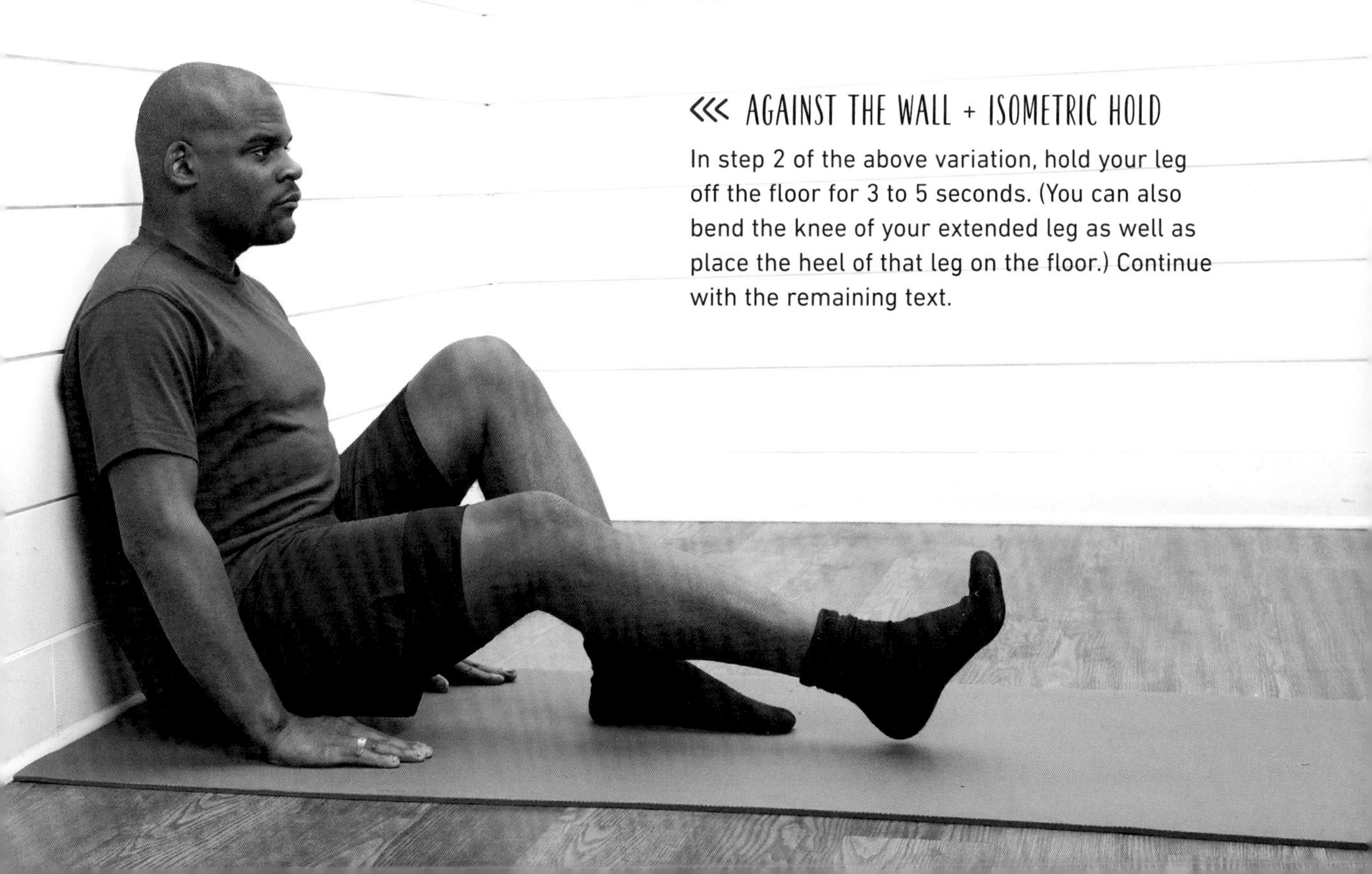

AGAINST THE WALL + ISOMETRIC HOLD

In step 2 of the above variation, hold your leg off the floor for 3 to 5 seconds. (You can also bend the knee of your extended leg as well as place the heel of that leg on the floor.) Continue with the remaining text.

Seated Spine Twists

If you're looking to strengthen your abs—especially your internal and external obliques, rectus abdominis, and transversus abdominis—this exercise is for you. Plus, not only can you increase flexibility in your lower back and hamstrings as well as your spinal rotation and mobility, but you can also improve your posture through these movements.

1 Sit in a chair with your arms extended to your sides at shoulder height. Extend your legs and place your heels flat on the floor.

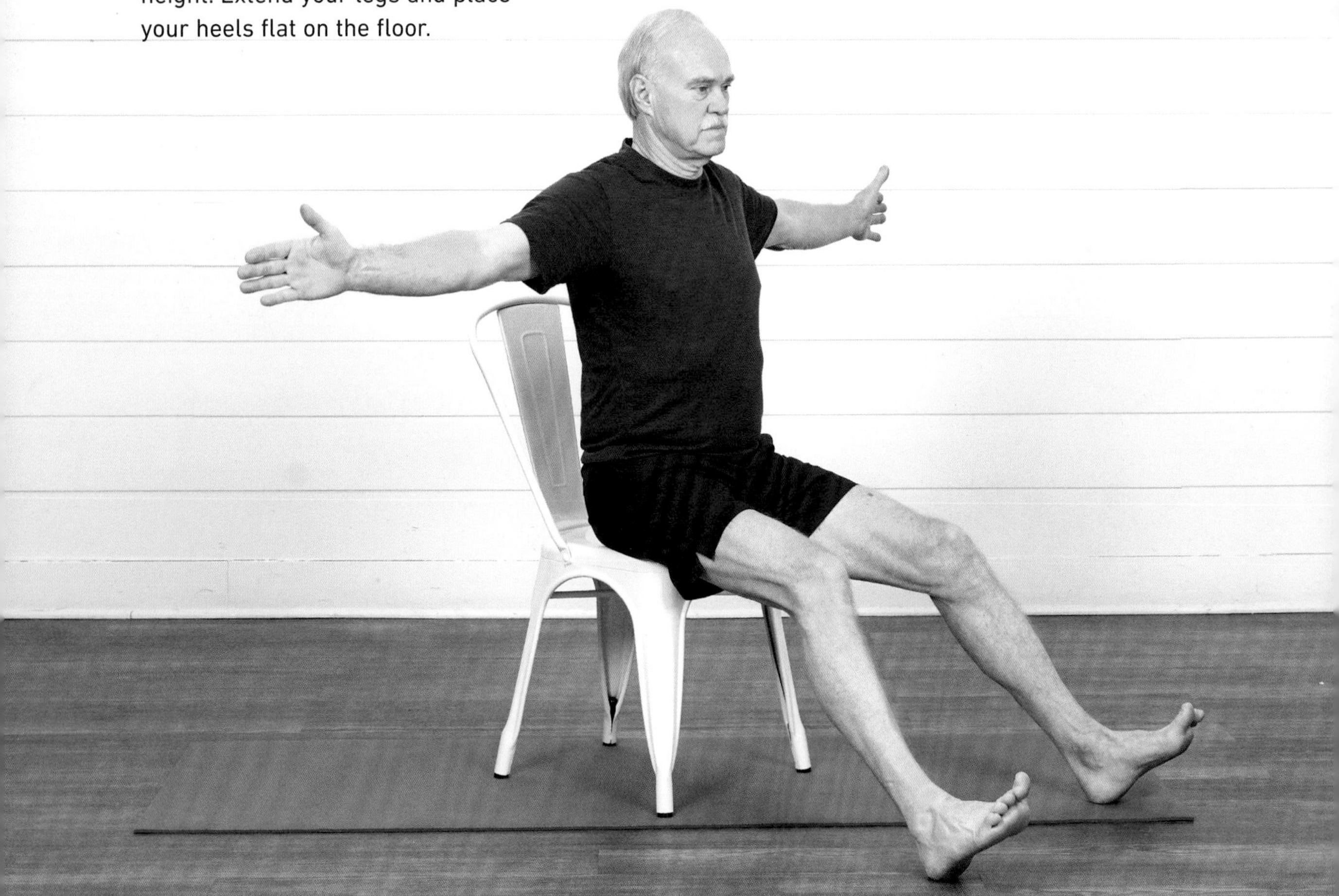

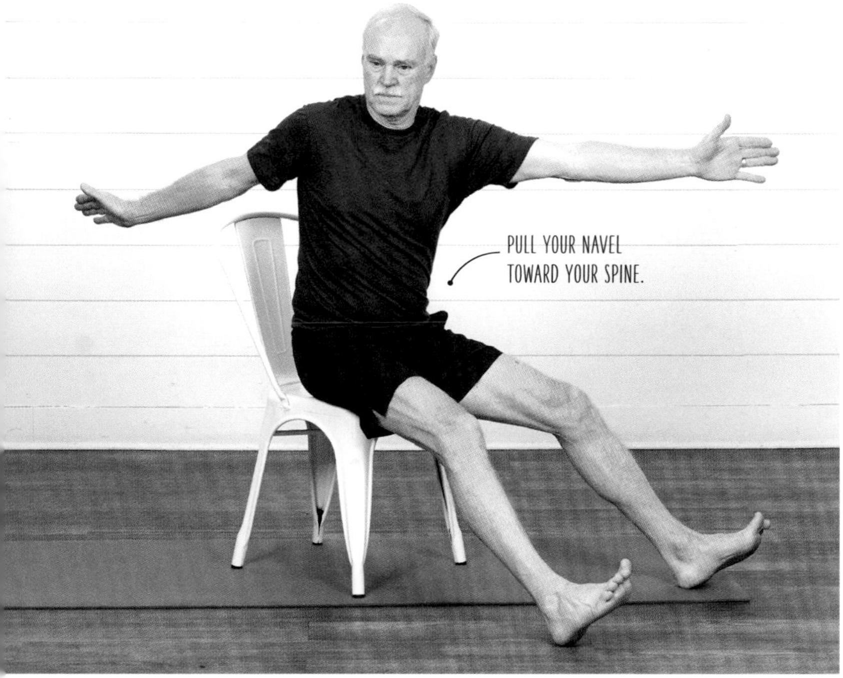
PULL YOUR NAVEL
TOWARD YOUR SPINE.

2 As you inhale, rotate your torso to your right.

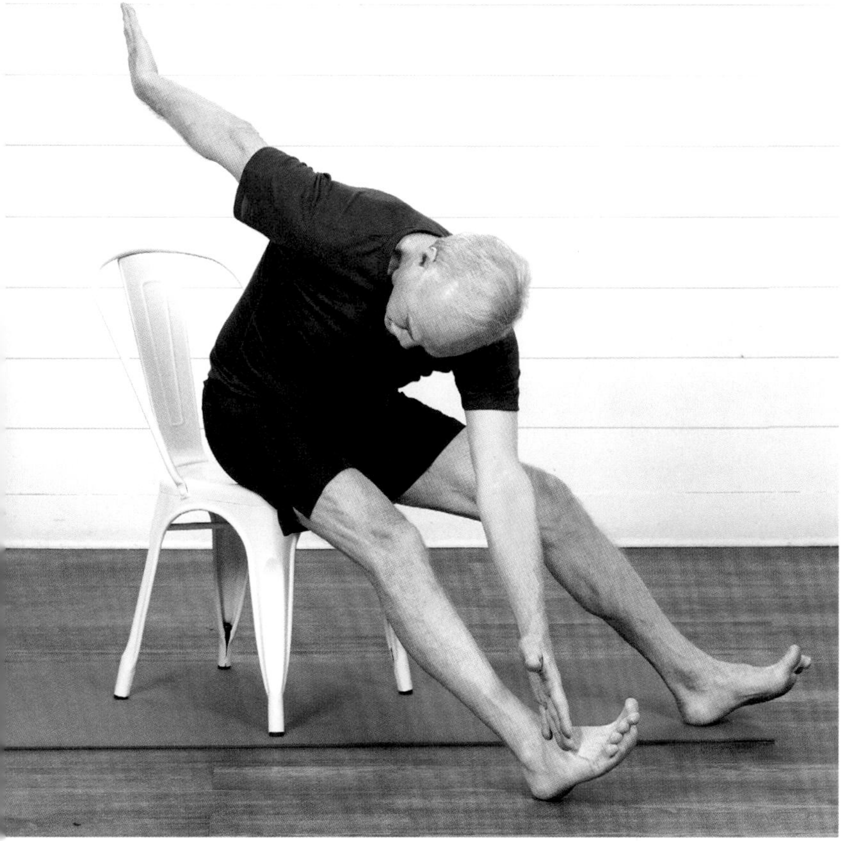

3 As you exhale, reach your left hand toward your right foot. Reverse your movements to return to your starting position. Perform these steps 6 times. Repeat these steps rotating to your left side.

SEATED SPINE TWISTS

VARIATIONS

If you lack flexibility in your hamstrings and lower back, placing your feet flat on the floor might help alleviate strain in these areas. Using the Magic Circle can give your muscles feedback, helping your body understand how to better direct your energy to improve your alignment and the elongation of your limbs.

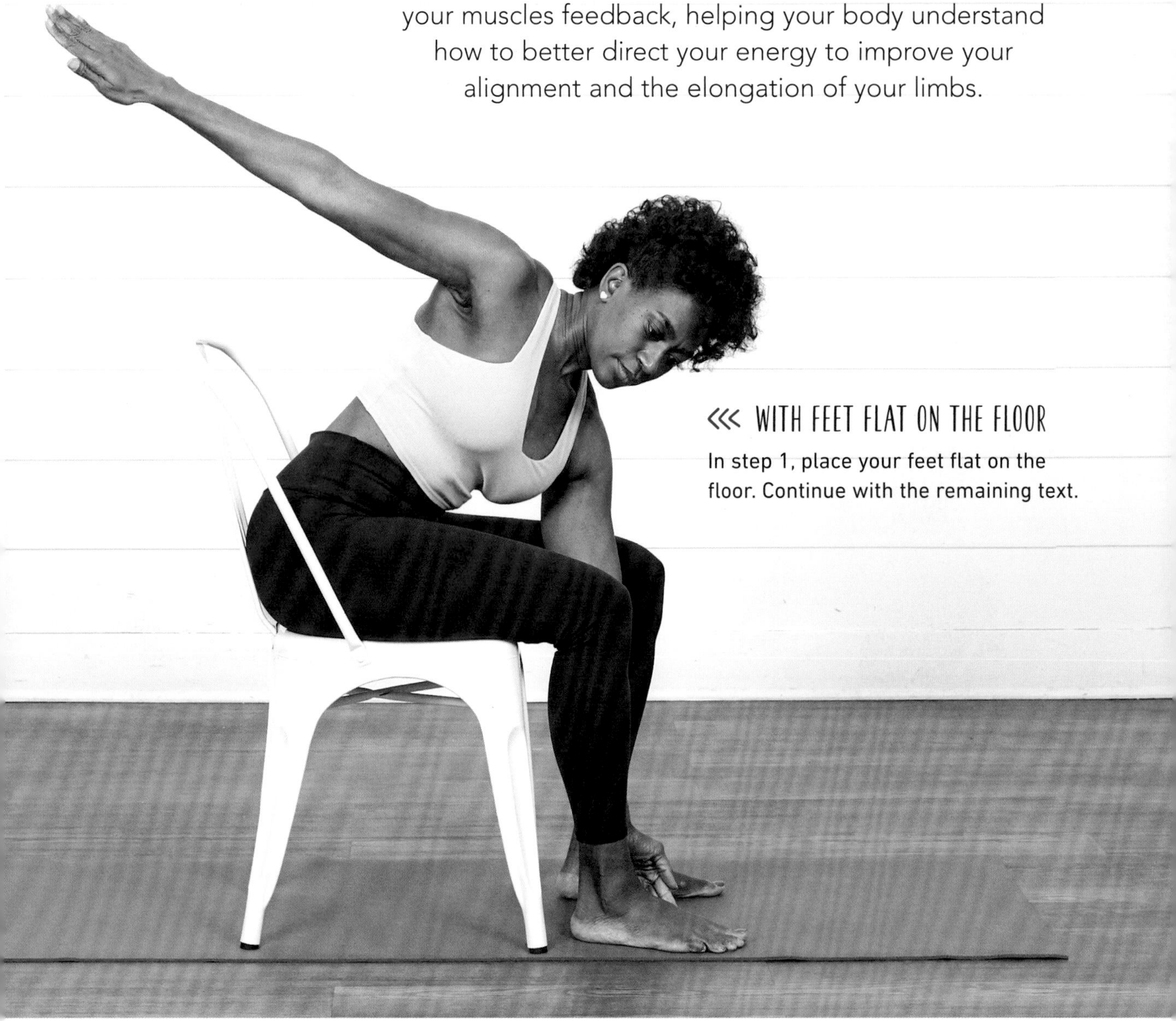

WITH FEET FLAT ON THE FLOOR

In step 1, place your feet flat on the floor. Continue with the remaining text.

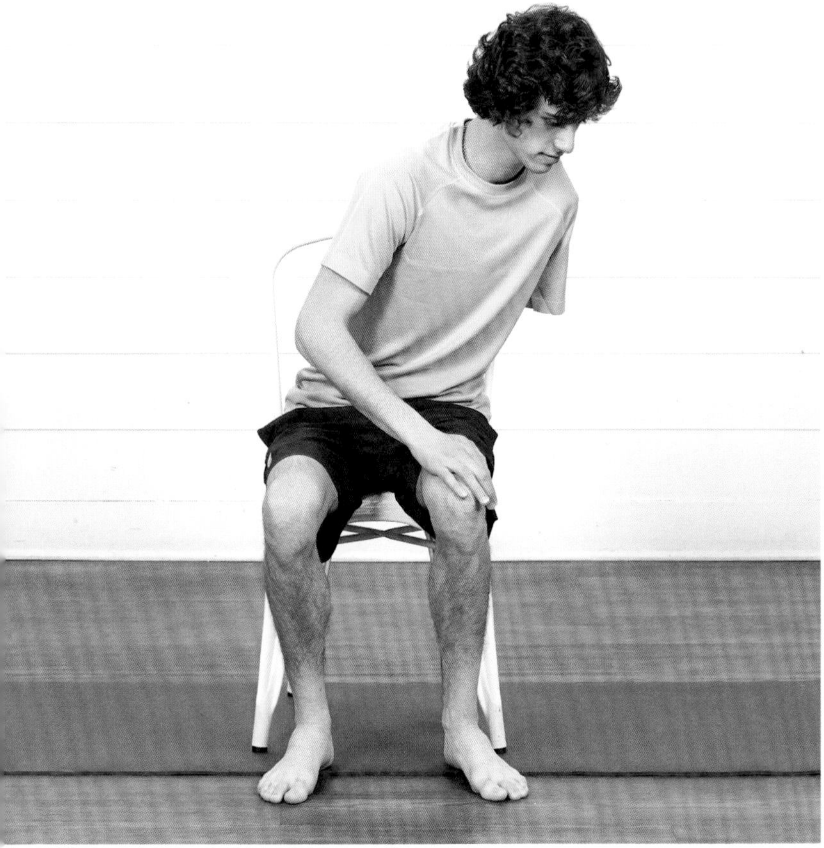

<<< WITH DIFFERENT HAND PLACEMENTS

In step 1, place your feet flat on the floor.

In step 3, reach your hand toward your opposite leg and place your hand on your knee. Continue with the remaining text.

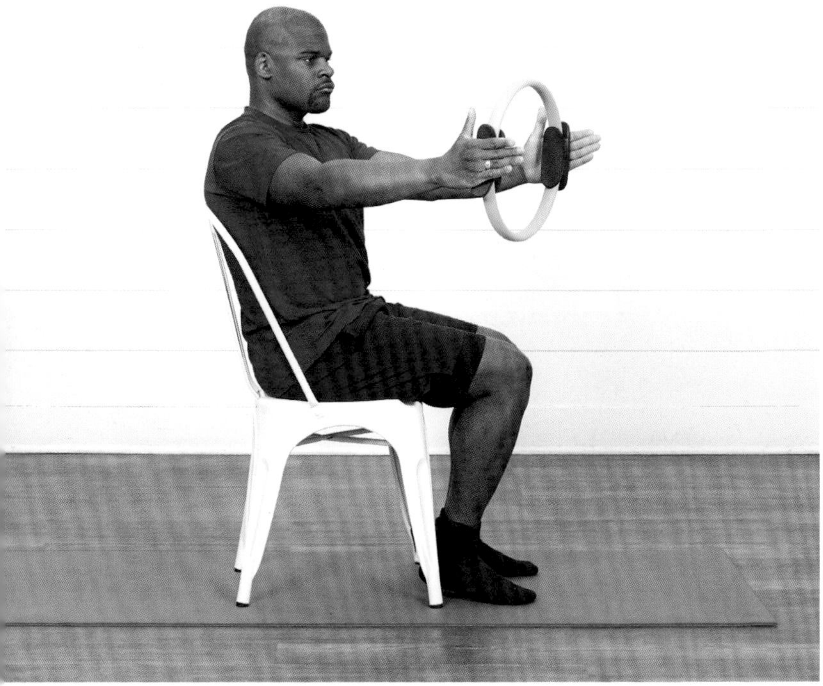

<<< WITH THE MAGIC CIRCLE

In step 1, hold the Magic Circle between the heels of your hands. Extend your arms forward until parallel with your shoulders.

In step 3, keep your arms extended. Continue with the remaining text.

Seated Figure Four Stretches

This is a popular backbending and heart-opening pose. Practicing these movements can also open your shoulders, lengthen the muscles of the front of your body, and strengthen the muscles of your back and upper body.

1 Sit on the front edge of a chair with your feet flat on the floor. Rest your hands on your thighs.

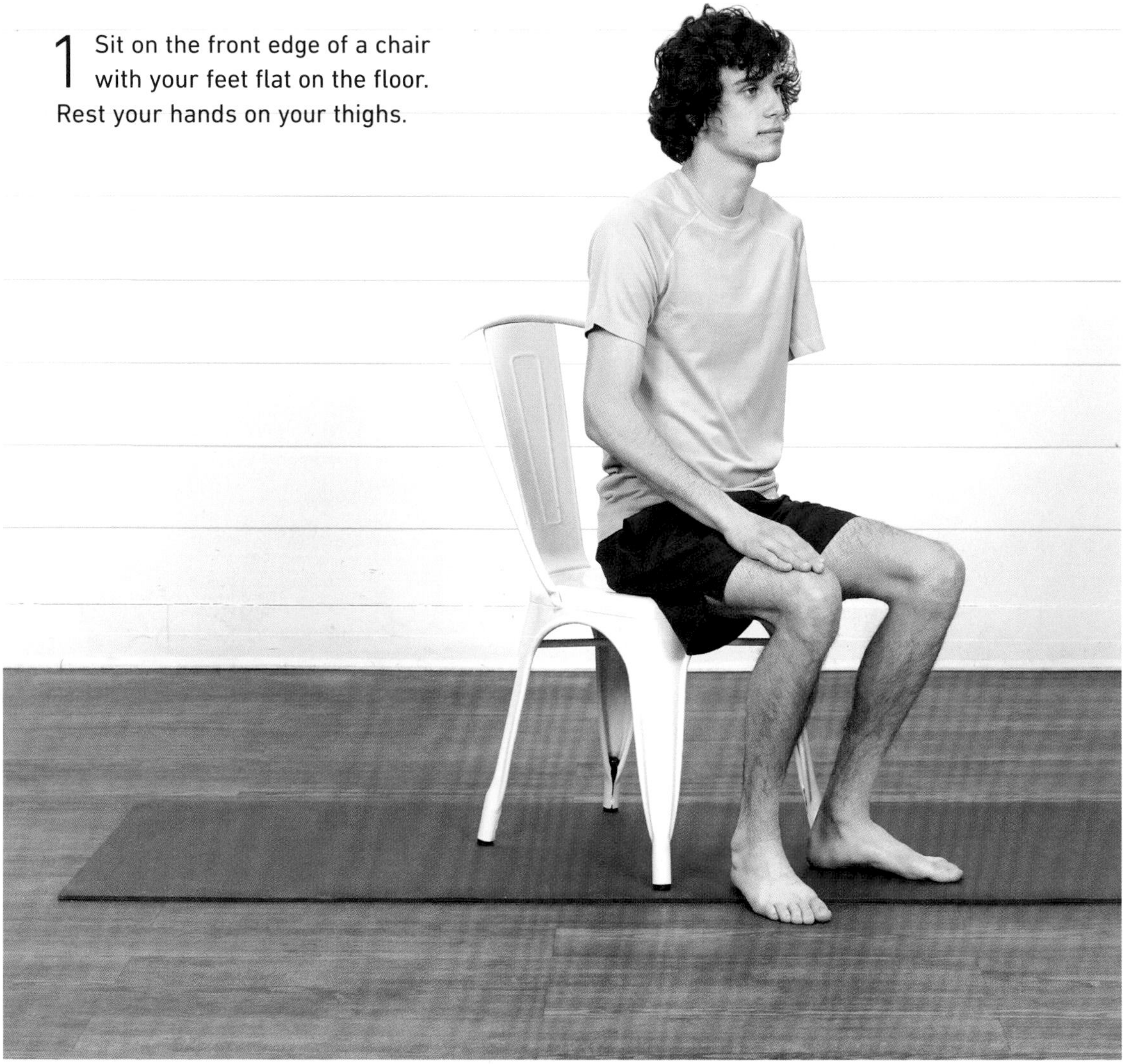

2 Bend your left knee and place your left ankle on top of your right knee. Place your right hand on top of your left ankle.

3 Bend forward at your waist and lower your chest toward your thighs. Hold this position for 10 to 20 seconds. Reverse your movements to return to your starting position in step 2. Perform the last two steps 3 times. Repeat these steps with your right ankle on top of your left knee.

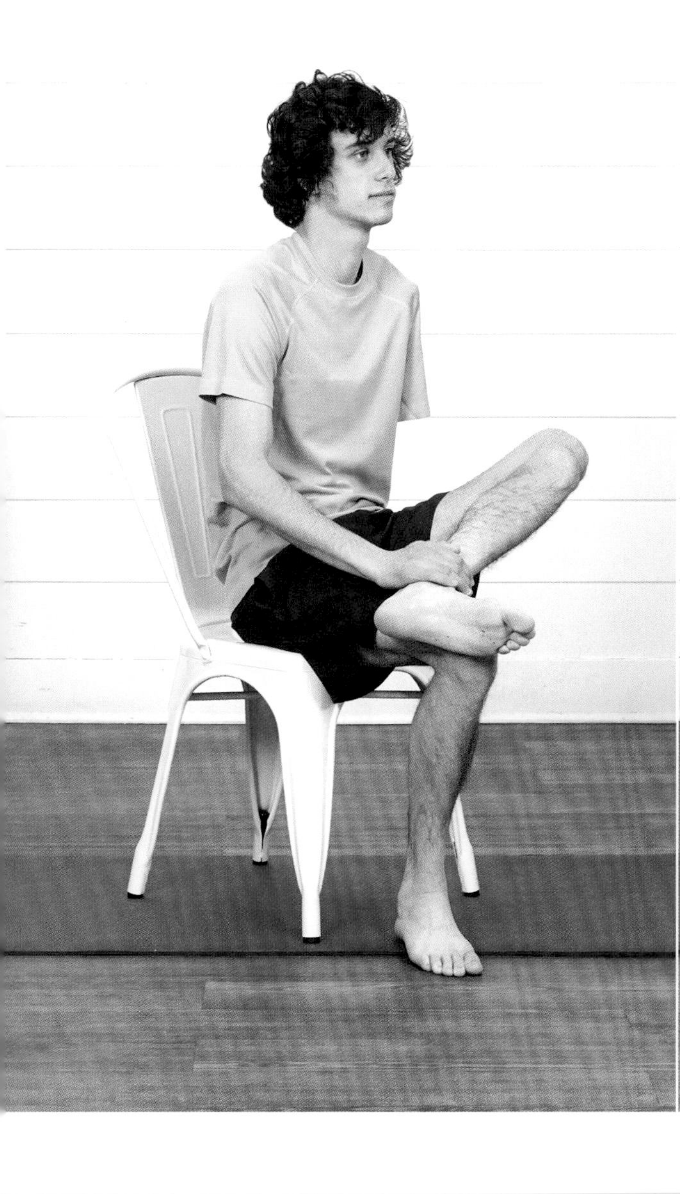

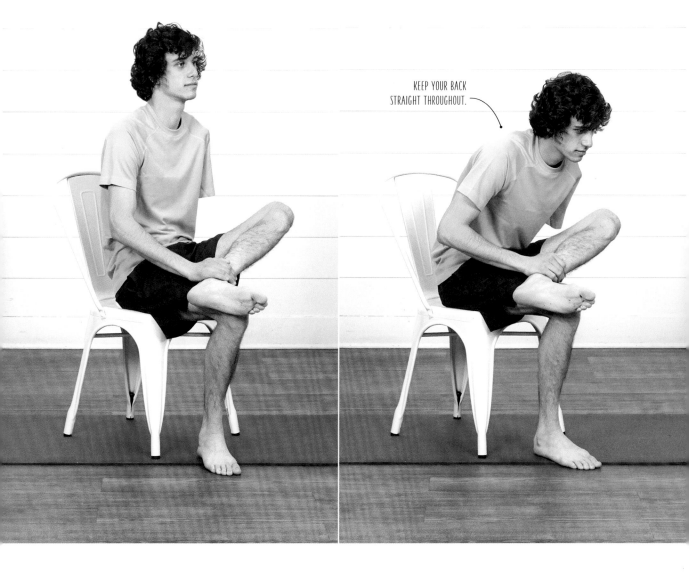

SEATED FIGURE FOUR STRETCHES

VARIATIONS

Incorporating a resistance band can help stretch the muscle groups involved with this exercise as well as aid in gradually helping you gaining more flexibility. Using a wall can also provide added lower back support.

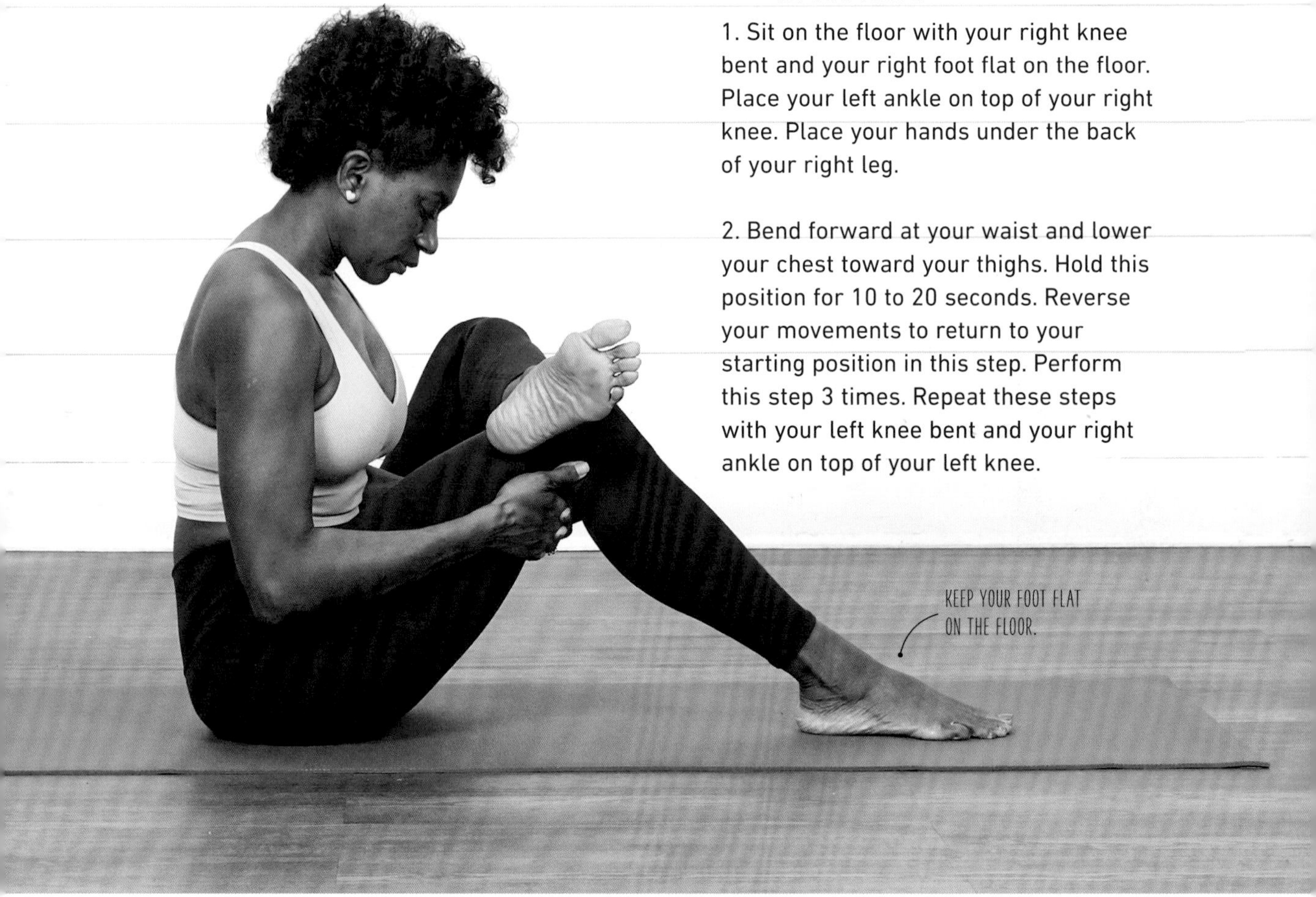
KEEP YOUR FOOT FLAT ON THE FLOOR.

ON THE FLOOR

1. Sit on the floor with your right knee bent and your right foot flat on the floor. Place your left ankle on top of your right knee. Place your hands under the back of your right leg.

2. Bend forward at your waist and lower your chest toward your thighs. Hold this position for 10 to 20 seconds. Reverse your movements to return to your starting position in this step. Perform this step 3 times. Repeat these steps with your left knee bent and your right ankle on top of your left knee.

<<< AGAINST THE WALL

1. Sit on the floor with your back against a wall. Bend your left knee and place your left foot flat on the floor. Place your right ankle on top of your left knee.

2. Bend forward at your waist and lower your chest toward your thighs. Hold this position for 10 to 20 seconds. Reverse your movements to return to your starting position in this step. Perform this step 3 times. Repeat these steps with your right knee bent and your left ankle on top of your right knee.

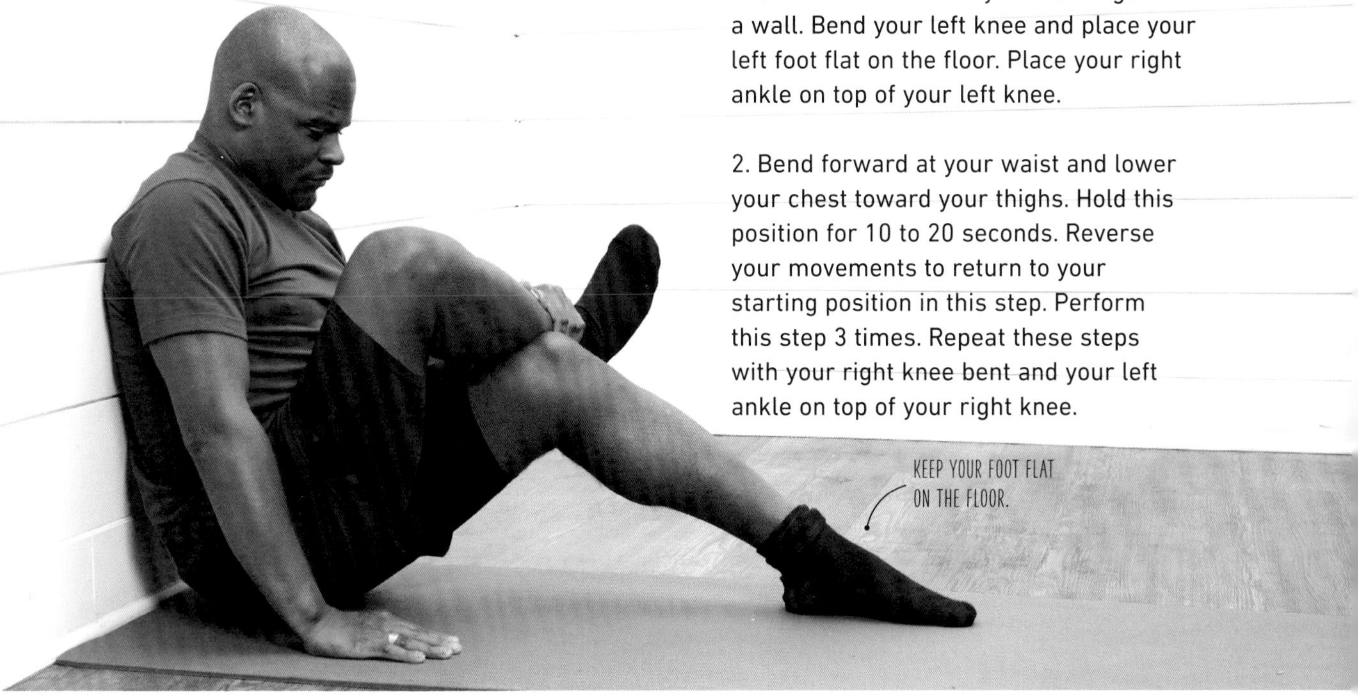
KEEP YOUR FOOT FLAT ON THE FLOOR.

<<< WITH A RESISTANCE BAND

1. Sit on the floor with your right leg extended flat on the floor. Place your left ankle on top of your right knee. Loop a resistance band around your right foot and hold the ends of the band with both hands.

2. Bend forward at your waist and lower your chest toward your thighs as you pull the resistance band toward your body. Hold this position for 10 to 20 seconds. Reverse your movements to return to your starting position in this step. Perform this step 3 times. Repeat these steps with your right ankle on top of your left knee and the resistance band around your left foot.

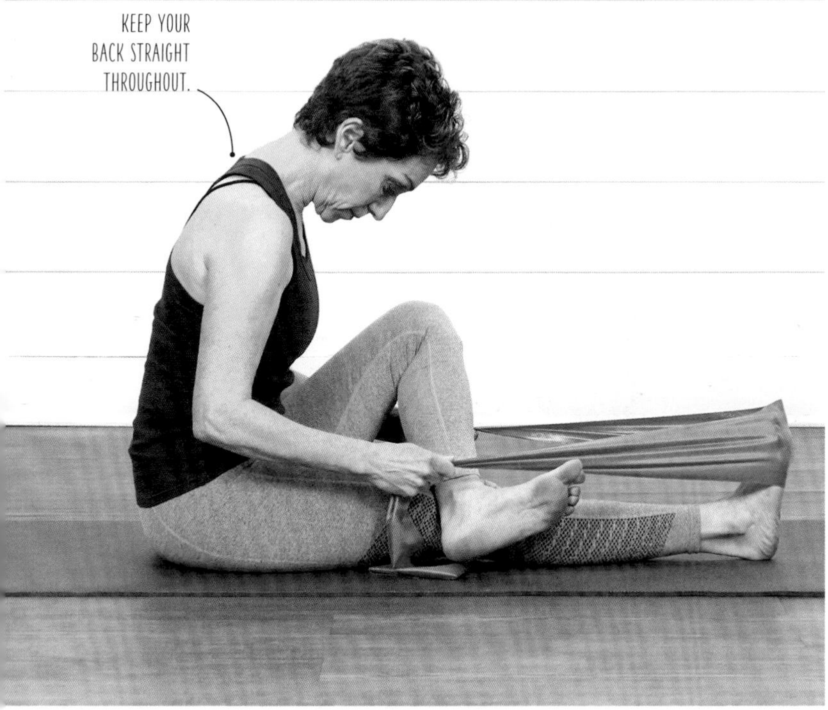
KEEP YOUR BACK STRAIGHT THROUGHOUT.

SUSAN HOLEWINSKI

In his book *Return to Life Through Contrology*, Joseph Pilates said: "The art of Contrology [Pilates] proves that the only real guide to your true age lies not in years or how you THINK you feel but as you ACTUALLY are as infallibly indicated by the degree of natural and normal flexibility enjoyed by your spine throughout life. If your spine is inflexibly stiff at 30, you are old; if it is completely flexible at 60, you are young." At age 59, Susan believes this is true. She practices Pilates daily and shares her knowledge with her Pilates clients, who range from middle school students and elite athletes to those recovering from injuries and surgeries. Pilates can be done by anyone of any ability at all stages of life.

According to Joseph: "Physical fitness is the first requisite of happiness." Susan embodies this philosophy. She's been physically active her whole life. She ran track and cross-country in high school and college, taught swimming, and competed in marathons. Her passion for movement led her to teaching everything from preschool fitness and step and spinning classes to coaching cross-country and track. A devastating foot injury from running led Susan to the healing world of Pilates—and a new career. As the years have gone by, she's adjusted her exercise regime and now she walks, swims, bikes, and practices Pilates and yoga. Her husband, two daughters, and their families often join her for a hike or bike ride. Her goal is to keep up with her three grandchildren and enjoy them as much as she can. Susan loves to travel and read about everything.

"Contrology develops the body uniformly, corrects wrong postures, restores physical vitality, invigorates the mind and elevates the spirit." Susan's passion is helping students of all ages and abilities discover and achieve their potential not only in movement but also in life. She knows by strengthening and lengthening the muscles and breathing deeply and fully, people develop self-confidence and poise that are reflected in their posture. They stand taller and radiate goodness. This complete sense of calm and well-being leads them to accomplish whatever physical task they set out to do and live life to its fullest with the stamina and endurance to accomplish "daily tasks with spontaneous zeal and pleasure"—from climbing Mount Everest to walking a block without pain after a knee replacement. Pilates offers these life skills to anyone willing to put in the time and energy to discover the joys of the method. Susan's life philosophy is "Keep the mind sharp, the body flexible, and the spirit renewed."

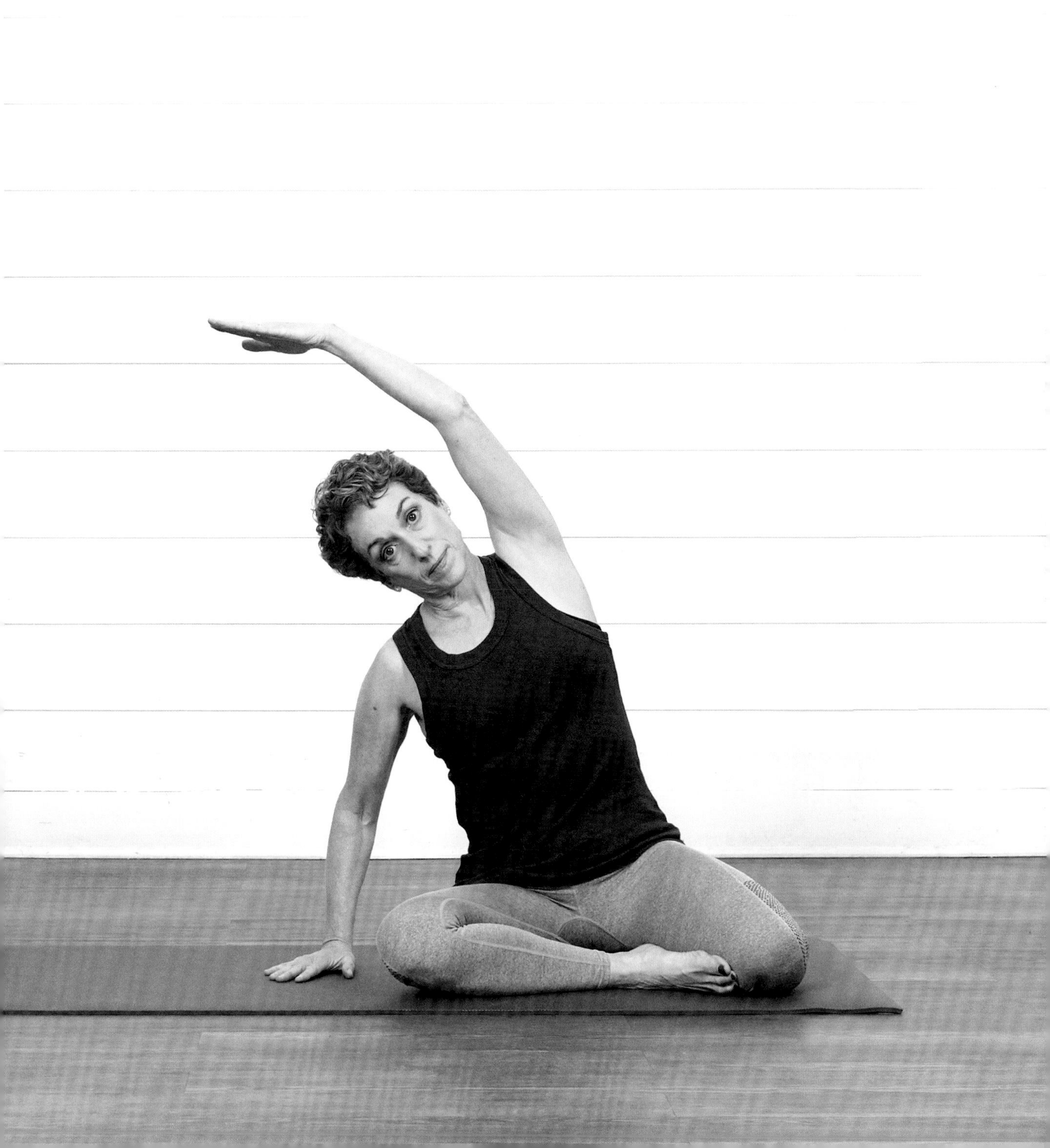

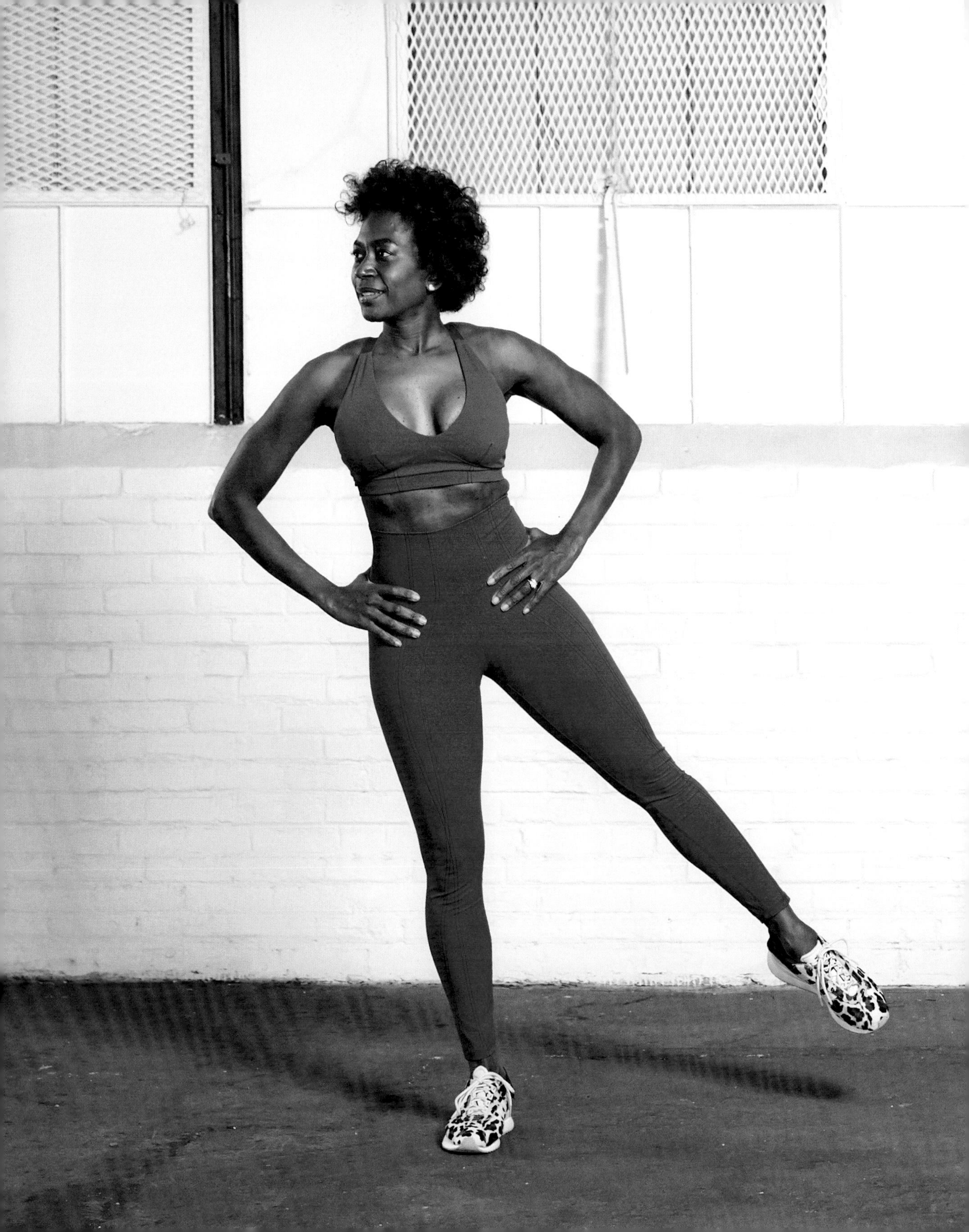

CHAPTER 7
Sequences

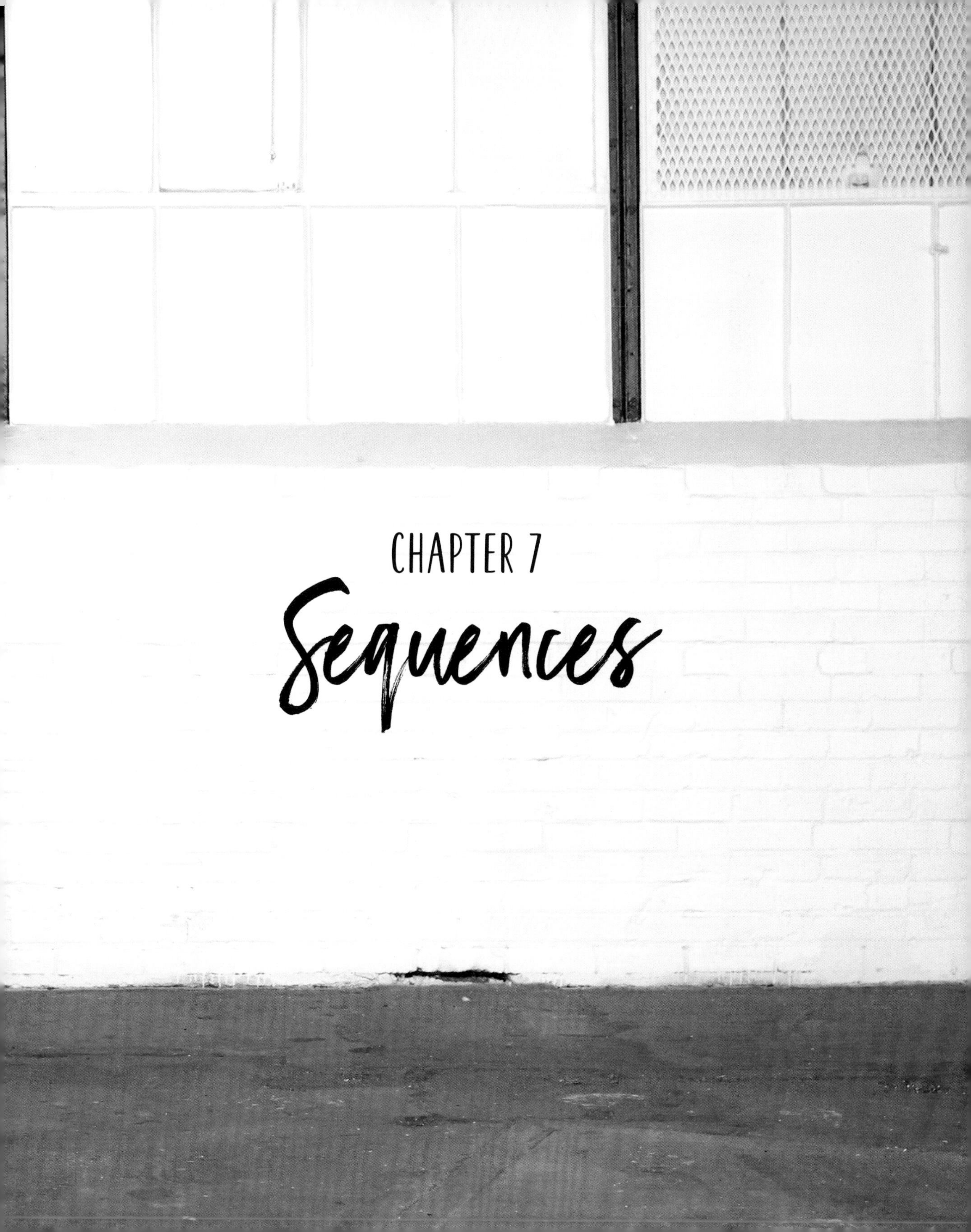

Office Workout

Perform each exercise 6 to 10 times. Perform this entire sequence for 1 to 3 sets.

SEATED HUNDRED (p. 216)
SEATED CRISS-CROSS (p. 220)
SEATED PUSH-UPS (p. 208)
SEATED BICEPS CURLS (p. 204)
SEATED SWIMMING (p. 212)
SEATED LEG LIFTS (p. 228)
SEATED TEASER (p. 224)
SEATED SPINE TWISTS (p. 232)
SEATED FIGURE FOUR STRETCHES (p. 236)

Strength & Stretch

Perform each exercise 6 to 10 times. Perform this entire sequence for 2 to 3 sets.

ROLL-UPS (p. 26)
FORWARD SPINE STRETCHES (p. 60)
PUSH-UPS (p. 44)
SCISSORS (p. 52)
SHOULDER BRIDGE (p. 70)
SIDE BENDS (p. 144)
SINGLE-LEG KICKS (p. 86)
SWIMMING (p. 126)
HEEL BEATS (p. 92)
SPINAL ROTATIONS (p. 64)

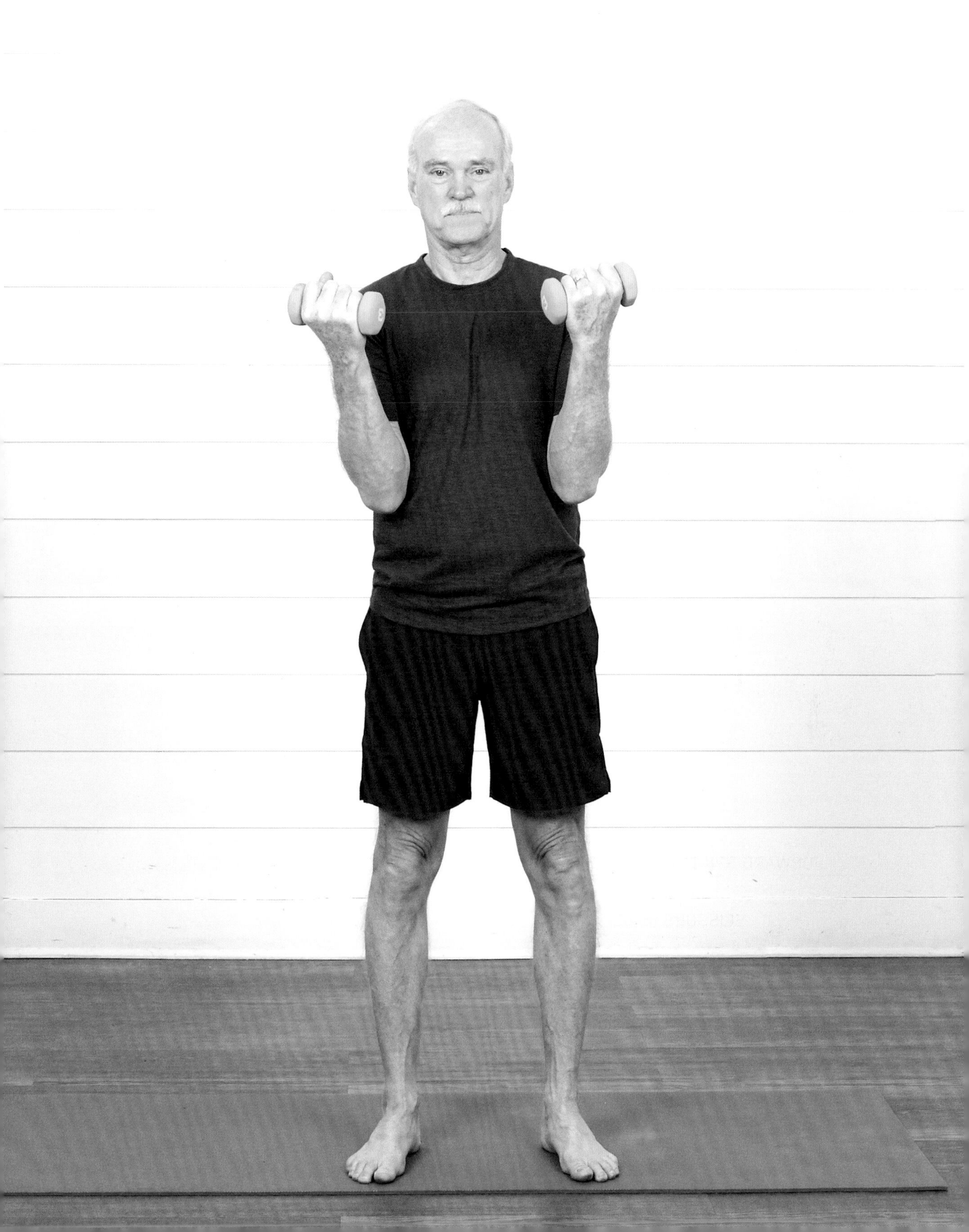

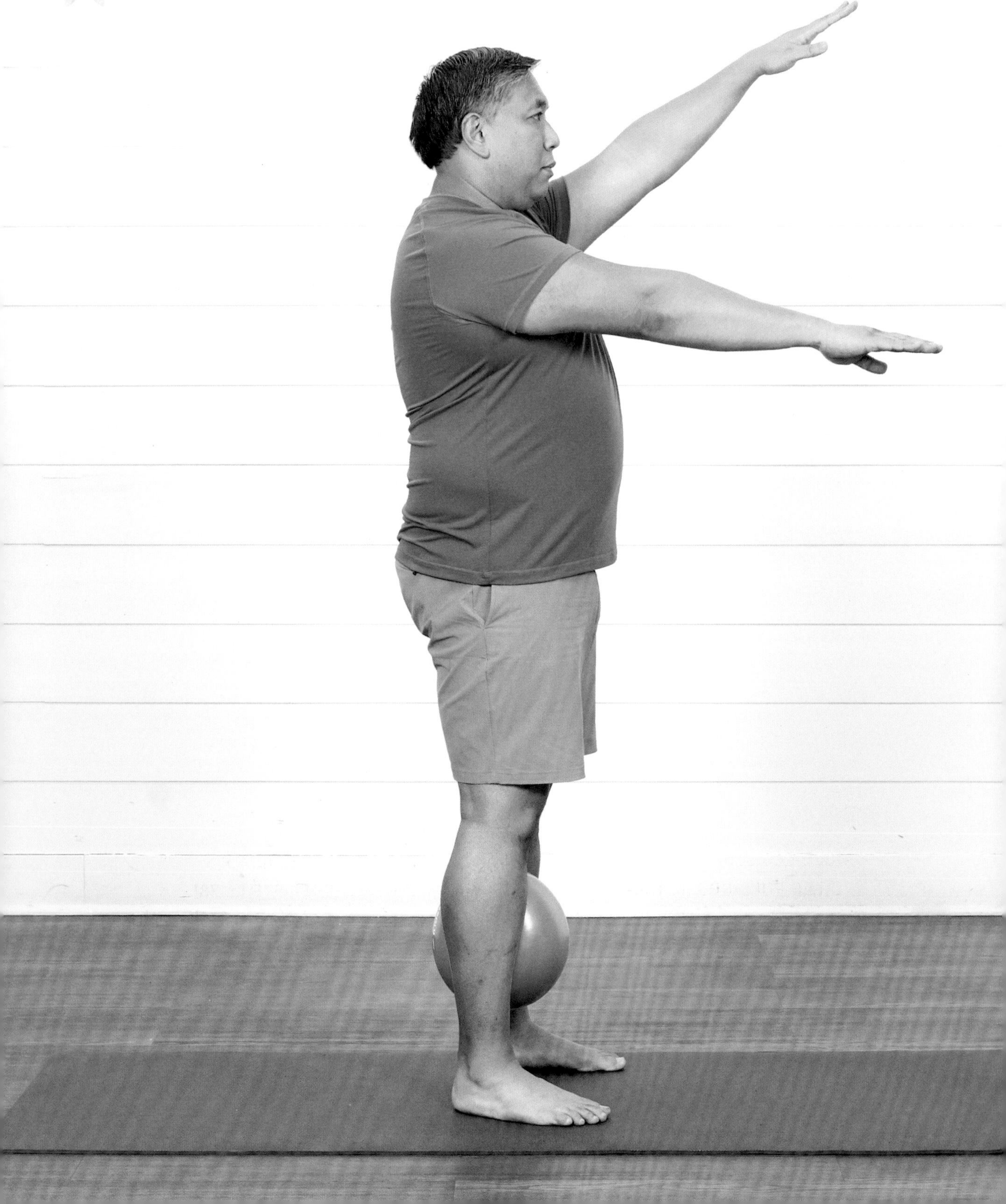

Core & More

Perform each exercise 5 to 8 times, except Cat-Cow, which you should perform 4 to 6 times. Perform this entire sequence for 2 to 3 sets.

THE HUNDRED (p. 22)
LEG CIRCLES (p. 96)
ROLL-UPS (p. 26)
TEASER PREP (p. 118)
TEASER (p. 122)
STANDING OBLIQUE CRUNCHES (p. 192)
STANDING SWIMMING (p. 176)
SINGLE STRAIGHT-LEG STRETCHES (p. 156)
SIDE BENDS (p. 144)
FORWARD SPINE STRETCHES (p. 60)
DOUBLE STRAIGHT-LEG STRETCHES (p. 100)
CAT-COW (p. 164)

Legs, Legs, Legs

Perform each exercise 6 to 8 times, except for Hamstring Lunge Stretches, Forward Spine Stretches, and Cat-Cow, which you should perform 6 times each. Perform this entire sequence for 2 to 3 sets.

SINGLE-LEG STRETCHES (p. 152)
LEG PULL-UPS (p. 134)
SINGLE STRAIGHT-LEG STRETCH (p. 156)
KNEELING SIDE KICKS (p. 138)
HIP CIRCLES (p. 148)
DOUBLE STRAIGHT-LEG STRETCHES (p. 100)
FOREARM V-LIFTS (p. 108)
SINGLE-LEG KICKS (p. 86)
SIDE KICKS (p. 82)
LEG CIRCLES (p. 96)
INNER THIGH LIFTS (p. 78)
BICYCLE (p. 56)
ONE-LEG CIRCLES (p. 30)
CLAM (p. 74)
FOREARM KICKS (p. 38)
HAMSTRING LUNGE STRETCHES (p. 112)
FORWARD SPINE STRETCHES (p. 60)
CAT-COW (p. 164)

Total Body

Perform each exercise 6 to 8 times.
Perform this entire sequence for 1 set.

STANDING HUNDRED (p. 172)

STANDING ARM CIRCLES (p. 184)

STANDING TRICEPS EXTENSIONS (p. 196)

STANDING SWIMMING (p. 176)

STANDING BOXING (p. 180)

STANDING BICEPS CURLS (p. 188)

STANDING OBLIQUE CRUNCHES (p. 192)

PUSH-UPS (p. 44)

CRISS-CROSS (p. 48)

SPINAL ROTATIONS (p. 64)

ROLL-UPS (p. 26)

SHOULDER BRIDGE (p. 70)

HEEL BEATS (p. 92)

SWIMMING (p. 126)

TEASER PREP (p. 118)

TEASER (p. 122)

LEG PULL-UPS (p. 134)

SIDE BENDS (p. 144)

FORWARD SPINE STRETCHES (p. 60)

DOUBLE STRAIGHT-LEG STRETCHES (p. 100)

FOUR-POINT BALANCE (p. 130)

SEATED LEG LIFTS (p. 228)

SEATED TEASER (p. 224)

SEATED FIGURE FOUR STRETCHES (p. 236)

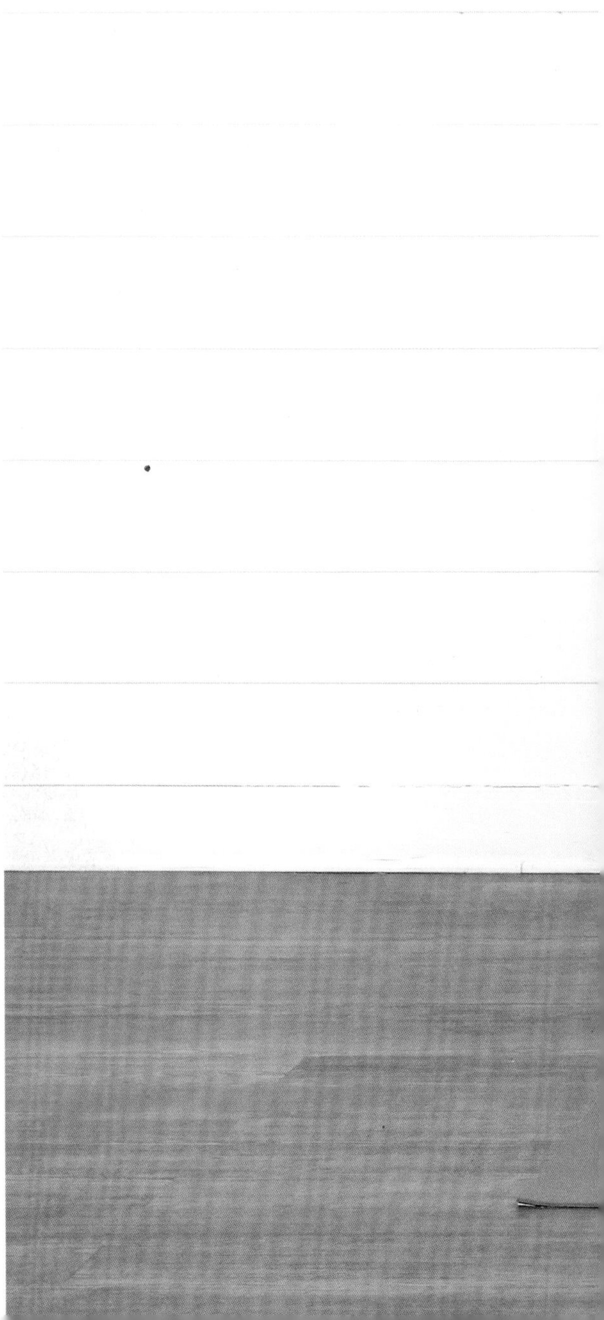

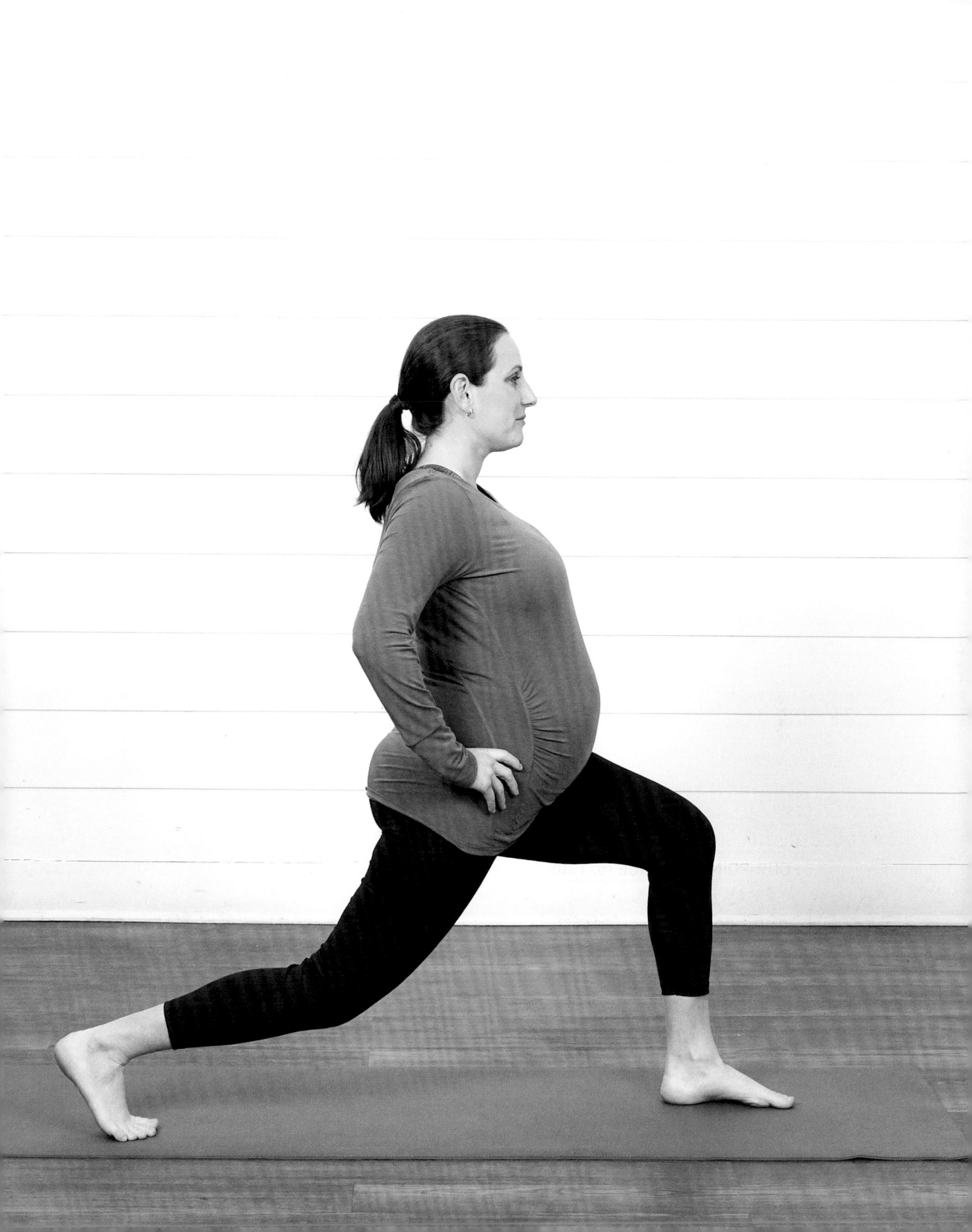

Index

F–G

H

I

K

L

S

T

U

W–X–Y–Z

ABOUT THE AUTHOR

Micki Havard is a Pilates instructor with more than 20 years of experience. She started practicing Pilates in preparation for her wedding and fell in love with the principles, movements, and results of Pilates. After practicing for a year, she became certified through Power Pilates as a Mat I and Mat II Pilates instructor. Micki is also certified through the American Council on Exercise (ACE) and the Athletics and Fitness Association of America (AFAA) as a wellness coach, strength coach, and group fitness instructor.

In 2011, Micki started a wellness coaching company called MickiPhit, through which she combines her knowledge of Pilates, group fitness, and nutrition to help her clients achieve their wellness goals. In 2018, MickiPhit launched a membership-based online Pilates studio that offers 24/7 access to step-by-step instructional Pilates videos. Micki provides simplified Pilates instructions for the home or on-the-go Pilates practice. In 2019, she created the PilatesPHIT and ChairPHIT fitness programs and their online certifications. She has an international following and has taught in Greece, Panama, Jamaica, and Aruba.

Micki currently lives in Atlanta, Georgia. When she's not teaching clients or filming videos, she loves spending time with her husband, Imari, and her two children, Autumn and Miles.

ACKNOWLEDGMENTS

First and foremost, I want to thank my amazing husband, Imari Havard. From setting up my office in our son's old room to rubbing my shoulders after a long day hunched over my laptop to pouring me a large glass of wine to celebrate each book milestone—thank you, babe, for always being there and supporting me in all my endeavors.

Thanks to my beautiful children, Autumn Lyles and Miles Havard, for putting up with my goofy jokes, weird quirks, and anxiety (before, during, and after writing this book)—and for loving me in spite of it all. You're the reasons I do what I do—my heartbeats and my biggest accomplishments.

Thanks to my sister, Jennifer Price, for proofreading my early drafts, assisting during the photo shoot, encouraging me from the very beginning of the process, and believing I could actually write a book.

Thank you to my mother and father, Donald and Mary Price, for instilling in us a work ethic, a confidence, and a desire to continue to learn new things.

Faith Butts, my legal counsel and friend, I literally couldn't have completed the contract without you. Thank you so much.

Big thank-you to my editor, Christopher Stolle, for guiding me through the entire process with patience, kindness, and knowledge.

PUBLISHER'S ACKNOWLEDGMENTS

The publisher wishes to thank Andrew Blum, Andrew Peterson, Jerry Denys, Jerome Pascua, Jillian Peterson, Susan Holewinski, and especially Micki Havard for being models for this book. We couldn't have created this book without you. You're aspirational and inspirational!